MW01414007

Textbook of
Cardiovascular Technology

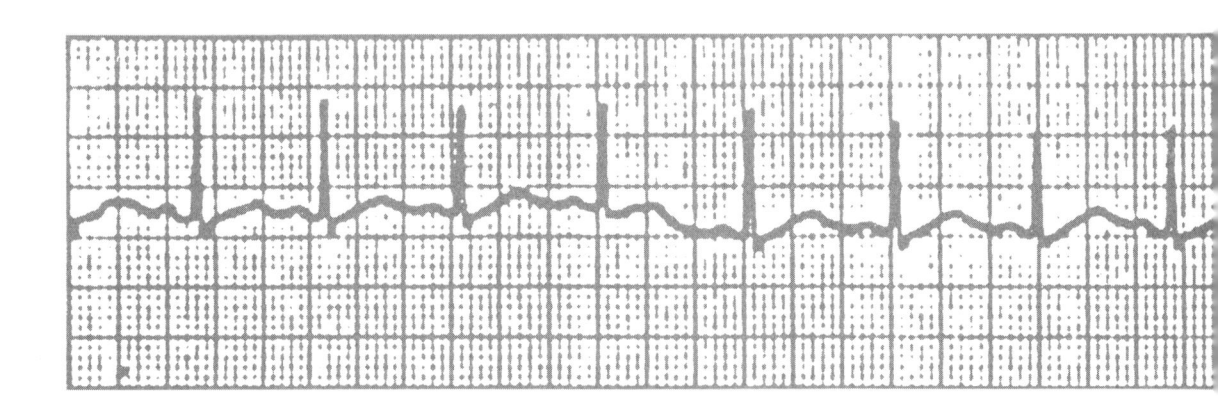

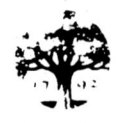

J. B. Lippincott Company
Philadelphia

London   Mexico City   New York   St. Louis   São Paulo   Sydney

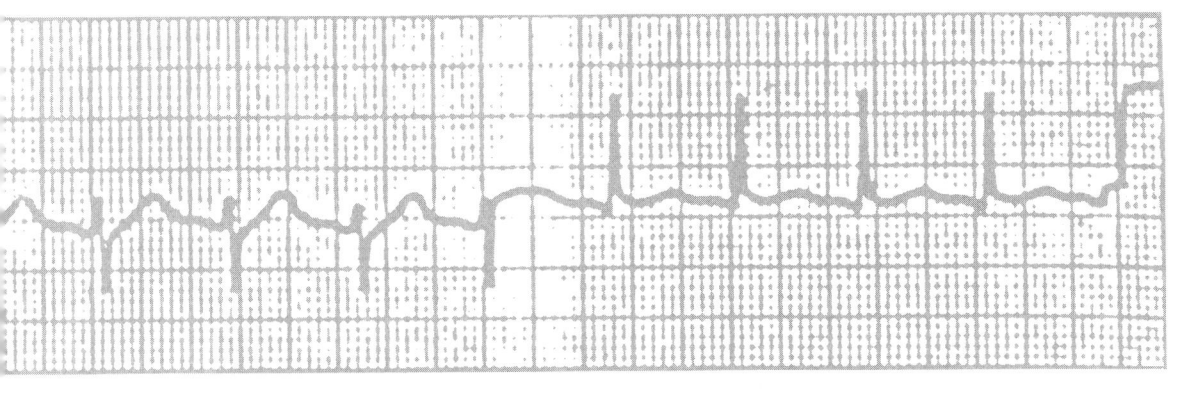

Textbook of Cardiovascular Technology

Lynn Bronson, R.C.T.
Past Director, Founder, and Instructor
School of Cardiovascular Technology
Morristown Memorial Hospital
Morristown, New Jersey

with 7 contributors

Acquisitions Editor: Lisa Biello
Manuscript Editor: Lorraine D. Smith
Indexer: Norman Duren, Jr.
Design Director: Tracy Baldwin
Design Coordinator: Anne O'Donnell
Designer: Katharine Nichols
Production Manager: Kathleen P. Dunn
Production Coordinator: Kenneth Neimeister
Compositor: Circle Graphics
Printer/Binder: R. R. Donnelley & Sons Company

Copyright © 1987, by J. B. Lippincott Company.
All rights reserved. No part of this book may be
used or reproduced in any manner whatsoever without written permission
except for brief quotations embodied in critical articles and reviews.
Printed in the United States of America. For information write J. B.
Lippincott Company, East Washington Square, Philadelphia, Pennsylvania
19105.

6 5 4

Library of Congress Cataloging in Publication Data

Bronson, Lynn.
　Textbook of cardiovascular technology.

　Bibliography: p.
　Includes index.
　1. Cardiovascular system—Diseases—Diagnosis.
2. Medical technology.　I. Title
RC670.B76　1987　　616.1′07′5　　87-3971
ISBN 0-397-50726-7

The authors and publisher have exerted every effort to ensure that drug
selection and dosage set forth in this text are in accordance with current
recommendations and practice at the time of publication. However, in
view of ongoing research, changes in government regulations, and the
constant flow of information relating to drug therapy and drug reactions,
the reader is urged to check the package insert for each drug for any
change in indications and dosage and for added warnings and precautions.
This is particularly important when the recommended agent is a new or
infrequently employed drug.

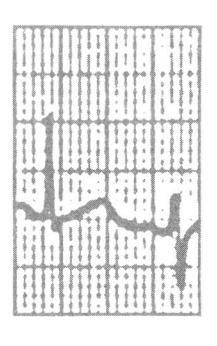

Contributors

Lynn Bronson, R.C.T.
Past Director, Founder,
and Instructor
School of Cardiovascular
Technology
Morristown Memorial Hospital
Morristown, New Jersey

Dale Davis, R.C.T.
Instructor, School of
Cardiovascular Technology
Morristown Memorial Hospital
Morristown, New Jersey

Gregg Harris, B.S., R.C.T.
ECG Systems Manager
Pitt County Memorial Hospital
Greenville, North Carolina

Linda Humston, R.C.T.
Manager, Pediatric Cardiology
Services
University of Michigan Hospital
Ann Arbor, Michigan

Stephen D. Kaniecki, R.C.T., C.C.P.T.
Supervisor of Cardiology Services
St. Luke's Hospital
Bethlehem, Pennsylvania

Linda Martin, R.C.T.
Chief, Cardiovascular Technologists
Instructor, School of
Cardiovascular Technology
Corvas Medical Center
Morristown, New Jersey

Mark A. Oliver, M.D.
Co-Director of Noninvasive
Peripheral Vascular Laboratory
Attending Physician, Department
of Internal Medicine
Morristown Memorial Hospital
Morristown, New Jersey

Doris Ottoson, R.C.T.
Supervisor, Cardiovascular
Technologists
Instructor, School of
Cardiovascular Technology
Morristown Memorial Hospital
Morristown, New Jersey

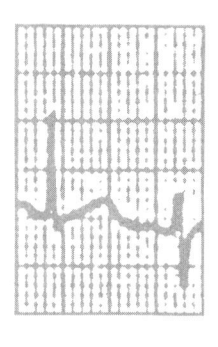

Preface

The aim of this "Textbook of Cardiovascular Technology" is to present to students and technologists the core material required in order to understand and to perform cardiovascular diagnostic testing.

A knowledge of the complete cardiovascular system in normal situations, and just how the heart functions, is later applied to an understanding of precisely what happens to the heart in diseased states and to a knowledge of the kinds of procedures, tests, and/or protocols that can be used in diagnosing a particular cardiovascular condition.

This text is designed to provide a foundation for future learning, and care was taken to instill simple, basic concepts without leading the student to any misconceptions or erroneous impressions. Some information may have been presented in a fashion that might be considered cursory, but that was done intentionally, because such information was considered more advanced than necessary for the student. Every attempt has been made to emphasize learning material that the student or technologist will use in his professional career.

"Textbook of Cardiovascular Technology" consists of two sections. Together, they comprise an integrated whole, although each can be used separately. In Section One, normal development, anatomy, and physiology of the heart are integrated with resultant diseases, thus setting the background for a proper understanding of the most commonly used modes of cardiovascular diagnostic testing, which are discussed in depth in Section Two.

Lynn Bronson, R.C.T.

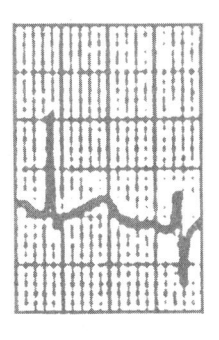

Acknowledgments

I particularly wish to express sincere appreciation to Robert Feinberg of Bio-Medical Imaging for his valuable assistance with the specialized graphics and artwork used in this text, to Joan Dennis, R.C.T., P.V.T., of Morristown Memorial Hospital, who shared her knowledge of peripheral vascular testing, and to Charles A. Shioleno, M.D., for his time and patience in teaching the mechanics of filming two-dimensional and m-mode echocardiography. Dr. Shioleno's precise critiques were of great help in clarifying content for the chapter on echocardiography.

Special thanks are due all the contributors who helped put this book together. Without them, none of this would have been possible.

Finally, thanks are extended to all the people who worked with me—my husband, family, friends, students, and my editors at J. B. Lippincott. Their encouragement helped me bring this project to fruition.

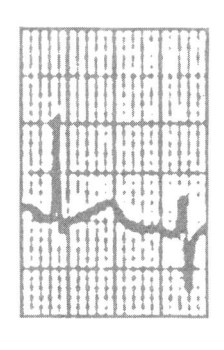

Contents

Section One
Basic Understanding of Normal and Abnormal Heart Function and Circulation

1 Normal Cardiovascular Anatomy Gregg Harris 3

The Circulatory System 3

2 Disease States Gregg Harris 18

Developmental Diseases 18

3 Cardiovascular Pharmacology Lynn Bronson 31

Vasodilators 31

Sodium Nitroprusside 31

Hydralazine 32

Prazosin 32

Antiarrhythmic Agents 32

Slow Channel Blockers 33

Thrombolytic Agents 33

Anticoagulants 33

Adrenergic Pharmacology   34
Beta-Adrenergic Blocking Agents   34
Alpha-Adrenergic Blocking Agents   34
Alpha-Adrenergic Receptor-Stimulating Drugs   35
Beta-Adrenergic Receptor-Stimulating Drugs   35
Alpha- and Beta-Adrenergic Receptor-Stimulating Drugs   35

4 Cardiovascular Terminology   Lynn Bronson   **38**
Roots   39
Prefixes   39
Suffixes   40
Systems Associated With the Body   40
Cardiovascular Terms and Definitions   41

5 The Heart and Electrical Hazards   Lynn Bronson   **54**
Basic Electricity   54
Electric Shock   56
Electric Shock in the Hospital   57
Precautions in Patient Care Areas   61
Special Precautions   63

Section Two
Diagnostic Techniques or Directions in Cardiovascular Technology

6 Electrophysiology   Stephen D. Kaniecki   **67**
Conduction System of the Heart   67
Cellular Anatomy and Electrophysiology   69
Excitation-Contraction Coupling   84

7 Electrocardiography and Arrhythmias   Dale Davis   **86**
Standard Leads   86
Augmented Leads   86
Precordial Leads   87

Depolarization and Repolarization 89
Electrical Conduction System 89
ECG Graph Paper and Measurements 92
Ischemia, Injury, Infarction 114
Miscellaneous ECG Patterns 121
Sinus Rhythms 127

8 Graded Exercise Testing (Stress Testing) Doris Ottoson 144
Basic Exercise Physiology and Normal Responses 145
Interview 147
Indications for Stress Testing 148
Maximal and Submaximal Testing 151
Interpretation of the Exercise ECG 156
Thallium Stress Testing 169

9 Basic Echocardiography Linda Martin 171
Types of Echocardiography 171
Machine and Instrument Control 172
Types of Real-Time Echocardiography 174
The Examination 175
Disease States 209

10 Basic Doppler Echocardiography Linda Martin 239
The Examination 244

11 Cardiac Catheterization Linda Humston 280
Catheterization: A Diagnostic Tool 281
Catheterization: A Therapeutic Tool 281
Catheterization: An Invasive Technique 282
Technical Aspects of Catheterization 287
Disease Processes Confirmed 305
Therapeutic Catheterization Procedures 319

12 Peripheral Vascular Testing Mark A. Oliver **325**

Noninvasive Techniques 325

Arterial Evaluation 334

Cerebrovascular Evaluation 349

Venous Evaluation 362

Index **379**

Section 1

Basic Understanding of Normal and Abnormal Heart Functions and Circulation

Chapter 1

Normal Cardiovascular Anatomy

Gregg Harris

Anatomy is often presented as a collection of Latin and Greek words and phrases assigned to specific locations on illustrations of biological structures. As a result, the science is reduced to a memory exercise. This chapter presents the anatomy of the cardiovascular system from a functional point of view that, hopefully, will add a component of understanding to the tedium of memorization.

The Circulatory System

The circulatory system represents the evolutionary development that makes possible multicellular vertebrate existence. It has three major functions. First, it allows for intercellular communication via the endocrine and the nervous systems. Second, it provides a means of waste removal, with the aid of the kidneys, liver, and gallbladder. Third, it efficiently distributes and delivers nutrients to the cells. It is the latter process with which Chapters 1 and 2 are most concerned.

All nutrients that sustain tissue life are transported throughout the body by the circulation of blood. Organic fuels enter the blood from ingested food via the digestive and hepatobiliary systems, while oxygen enters the blood by way of the lungs. Both the fuel and the oxygen are carried to every living cell by the cardiovascular system. The remainder of this discussion will concentrate on oxygen delivery to the tissues.

Fluid Transport/Delivery

In order to deliver something, a vehicle is required, to carry the goods, as is a route for transporting these goods to the consumer. In the case of oxygen delivery, the vehicle is the red blood cell, and the transport mechanism is the cardiovascular system. This system is designed to overcome several problems, the most significant of which are the high volume/high velocity demands contrasted with the slower velocities needed in order that diffusion may take place.

Diffusion is a process by which dissolved substances flow from a state of high concentration to a state of low concentration. In a moving liquid, the effectiveness of diffusion is limited by three factors: the size of the concentration gradient, the distance over which diffusion must take place, and the velocity of the moving fluid. Diffusion is most effective with large concentration gradients, small distances, and slow velocities.

This presents a problem of fluid dynamics. The optimum design for an oxygen delivery system is one that features high oxygen concentration, small vessels, and slow blood flow. However, the most efficient means by which fluids can be transported is in large, high-flow vessels. How can one system satisfy both of these requirements? The answer to this question could be found in an in-depth discussion of physics and mathematics, but it can be illustrated quite simply by the following analogy.

Imagine that you are the circulation manager of a major newspaper and you depend solely on trucks for delivery of your papers to your readers in every neighborhood throughout the state. In order to serve customers hundreds of miles away, your delivery trucks must travel at 55 miles per hour on the state turnpike. Obviously they can't drop newspapers on people's driveways at that speed. However, if the trucks were to travel at speeds slow enough to permit them to deliver everyone's newspaper along the way, they would never get to those far-distant customers before the news would be outdated. In addition, the fuel economy of trucks (as with all motor vehicles) is significantly greater on the open highway. Thus a large number of trucks must travel quickly along the turnpike, then some must exit onto slower county and municipal roads near each population center. Even though each vehicle is moving more slowly after leaving the turnpike, the truckers are now traveling in different directions and their *total* mileage is greater. For example, two vehicles traveling along the same highway at 55 miles per hour cover 55 miles of countryside every hour; however, if the two trucks now travel at 40 miles per hour on two separate roads, they each cover 40 miles of the delivery area or a total of 80 miles. To put this in perspective, 1000 trucks on the turnpike can still only cover the same 55 miles per hour, but when the trucks exit and each travels its own delivery route at 5 miles per hour, the fleet covers 5000 miles of local roadway per hour. Thus mass transport of newspapers is best accomplished over larger high-speed highways, but individual deliveries are made on many small, dispersed roads at lower speeds.

The circulatory system is designed in a similar fashion. The large major artery corresponding to the state turnpike is called the *aorta*. There are ten major "exits" along this system, each leading towards high-consumption areas (major organs and muscle masses), which would compare to population densities in the preceding analogy. Exits 1, 2, and 3 are known as the *brachiocephalic* branches because they supply the head and upper extremities. The fourth exit, called the *celiac axis*, divides into arteries supplying the stomach, spleen, and liver. The *superior mesenteric artery* is exit 5, which supplies the small intestine and most of the colon. The descending colon and rectum are supplied by the *inferior mesenteric artery* at exit 8. Exits 6 and 7 are the right and left *renal arteries* leading to the kidneys. Finally, this "circulatory turnpike" ends in the pelvic region where it divides into exits 9 and 10, called the *common iliac arteries*, which provide access to the pelvis and lower extremities. Our circulatory turnpike is graphically illustrated in Figure 1-1.

Each major branch of the arterial structure, in turn, divides into smaller vessels supplying more specific tissue groups. Eventually every "road" narrows into the smallest vessels used to reach the target cells; these vessels are called *arterioles*. The *capillaries* are the minute vessels that connect the arteries and the veins.

The structure of the venous system (Figure 1-2) is reciprocal to that of the arteries. As the capillaries complete their deliveries they merge into larger and larger vessels, the final two being the *inferior vena cava* from the lower body, and the *superior vena cava* from the head and upper extremities. Using the reverse principle to describe the velocities of the "trucks" returning to the heart, one realizes that, as hundreds of trucks from smaller side roads merge into a major highway, they must accelerate in order to make room for those behind them.

In short, whether you are a publisher delivering newspapers, or the circulatory system delivering oxygen, it is most efficient to travel long distances at high speeds in a few large arteries. This conserves fuel and provides for remote deliveries in a timely fashion. It is also necessary to move very slowly during the actual deliveries to the millions of "consumers" located along the small local routes. It is during this time that the majority of the energy is expended.

The Heart

Now that the overall design of the circulatory system has been considered, it is necessary to examine the principal organ in that system, the heart.

The heart is a muscular pump that supplies the driving force to circulate blood throughout the body. It is a link between two circulatory systems that together make up the cardiovascular system. These two networks are known as the systemic circulation system (discussed in preceding paragraphs) and the pulmonic circulation system, which follows the same conceptual design

(Text continues on page 8)

6 Normal Cardiovascular Anatomy

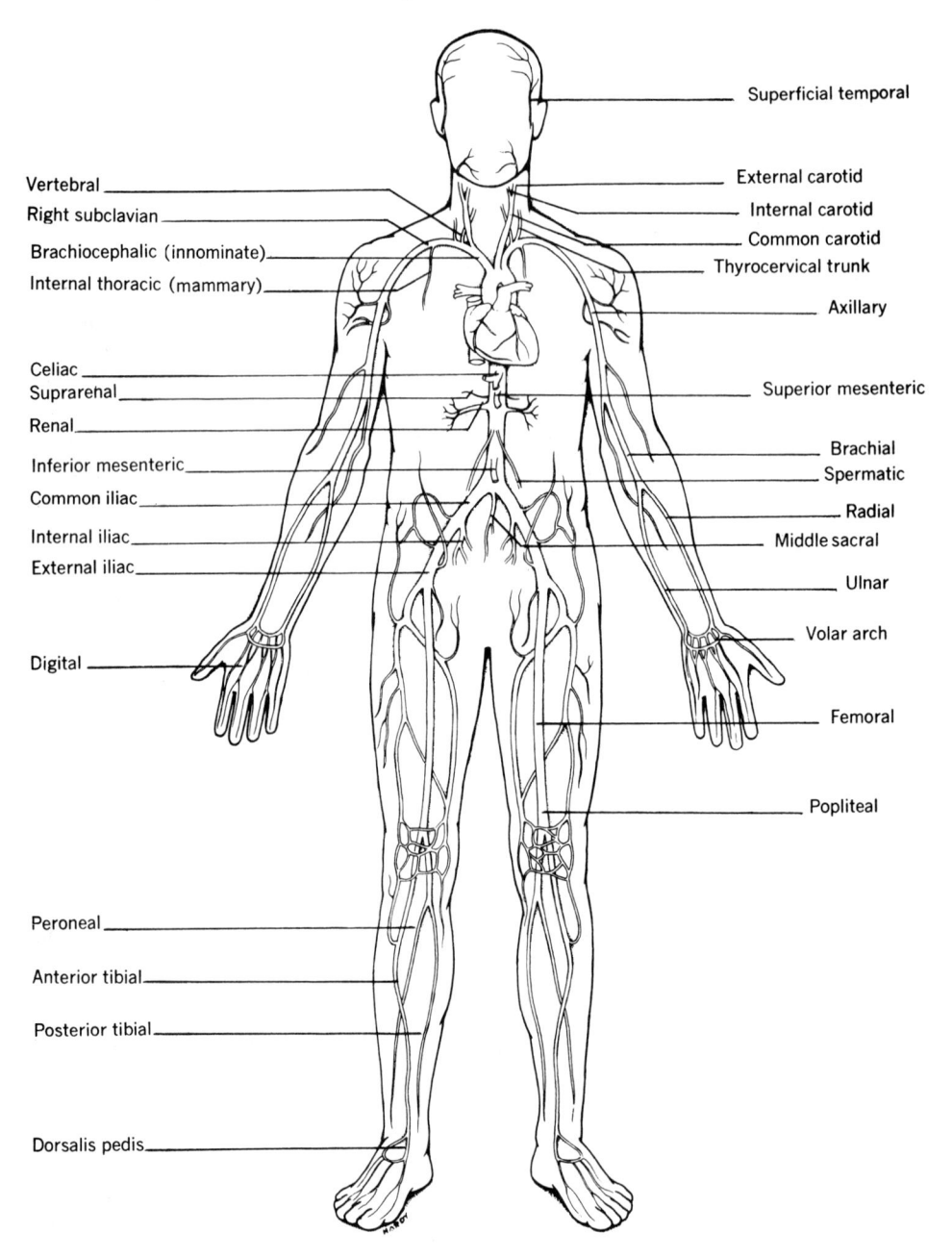

Figure 1-1 Arterial vascular system. (Chaffee EE, Lytle IM: Basic Physiology and Anatomy, 4th ed. Philadelphia, JB Lippincott, 1980)

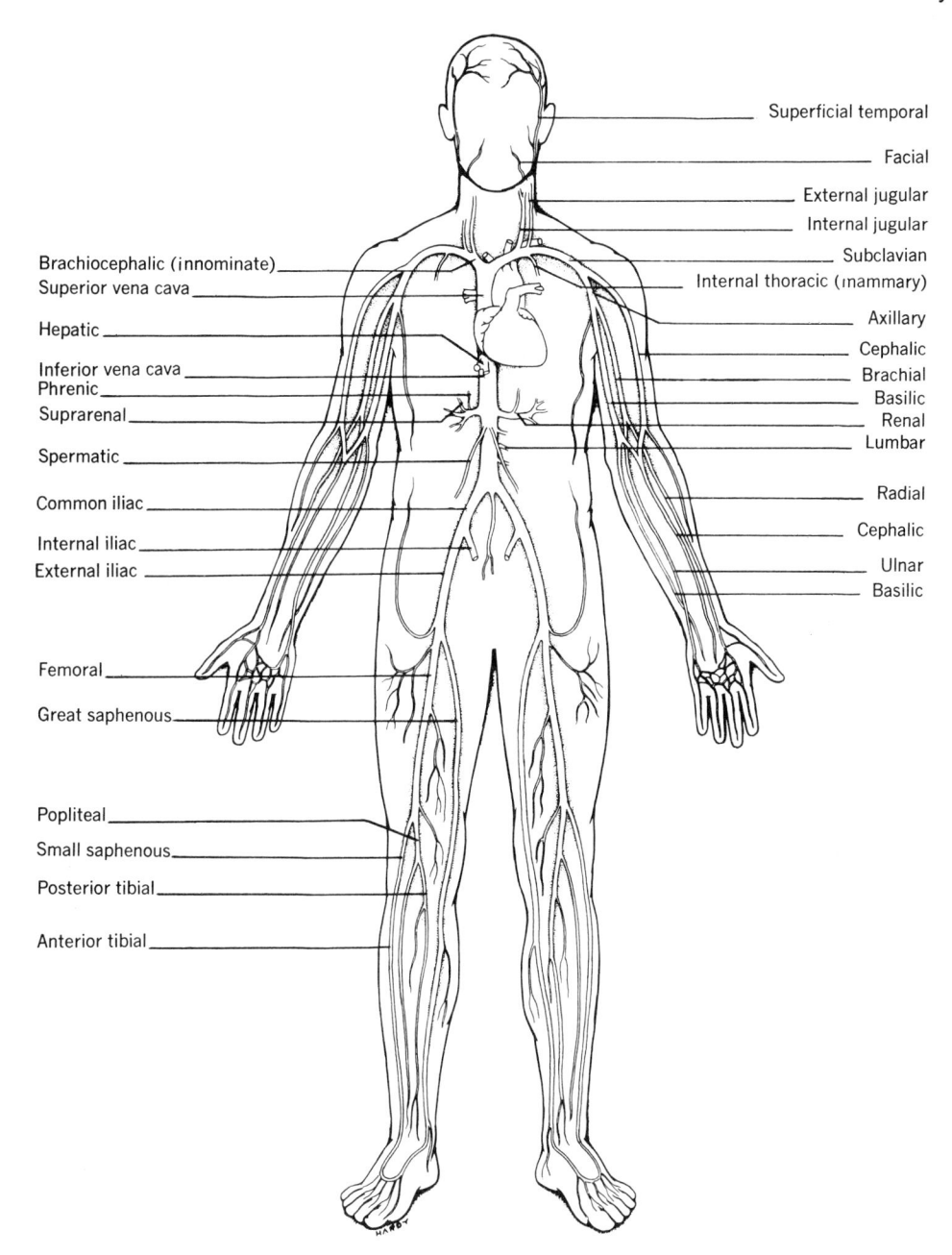

Figure 1-2 Venous vascular system. (Chaffee EE, Lytle IM: Basic Physiology and Anatomy, 4th ed. Philadelphia, JB Lippincott, 1980)

of large arteries for mass transportation with millions of tiny vessels along which the exchange of goods takes place. The primary difference between the two is that the systemic circulation system carries oxygenated blood from the left ventricle to various tissues of body, then returns venous blood to the right atrium. The pulmonic circulatory system, in contrast, carries venous blood from the right ventricle to the lungs and returns oxygenated blood to the left atrium (Figure 1-3).

Because the heart acts as the pump for both of these systems, its structure is extremely important. In an attempt to simplify this discussion, the structure of the heart will be divided into two sections. First, *functional anatomy* will be described, and then, *geographic anatomy*.

Functional Internal Cardiac Anatomy

The heart consists of four chambers. Two of these, the atria, are receiving compartments for blood. The other two, the ventricles, are the pumps associated with systemic (left) and pulmonic (right) circulation. The atria are composed of two parts: the atria proper and the atrial appendages, or auricles. The atria proper are smooth-walled cavities into which the blood is returned to the heart. On the other hand, the auricles are lined with a muscular lattice called *trabeculae*; these are the vestigial remnants of the embryonic atria. The two atria are separated by the interatrial septum, which is a muscular wall with an oval fibrous area in its central region. This "window" is known as the *foramen ovale*, which will be discussed later in this chapter.

The atria are divided from the ventricles by the atrioventricular valves—the tricuspid valve on the right and the mitral valve on the left.

The ventricles are much larger than the atria from the perspectives of both cavity volume and wall thickness. (The wall thickness of the left ventricle is three times that of the right ventricle.) They are also separated by a muscular septum; however, the membranous area of the ventricular septum is its most superior portion. This area also bends to the right to form the left ventricular outflow tract. In addition to many trabeculae, as in the atrial appendages, the ventricles also have specialized muscular projections arising from the apices called *papillary muscles*, which are responsible for controlling the atrioventricular valves.

Each chamber of the heart has major blood vessels associated with it. On the right side of the heart there are the superior and inferior venae cavae, which lead into the right atrium through a common orifice from the systemic circulation system. In addition, the coronary sinus returns venous blood from the coronary circulation system through the posterior wall of the right atrium. The right ventricle is served by the pulmonary artery, which carries blood from the right side of the heart to the lungs for oxygenation. On the left side of the heart, the four pulmonary veins return oxygen-rich blood from the lungs and each individually empties into the left atrium. Finally, the major artery leaving the left ventricle is called the *aorta*. All of these together are known as the *great vessels*.

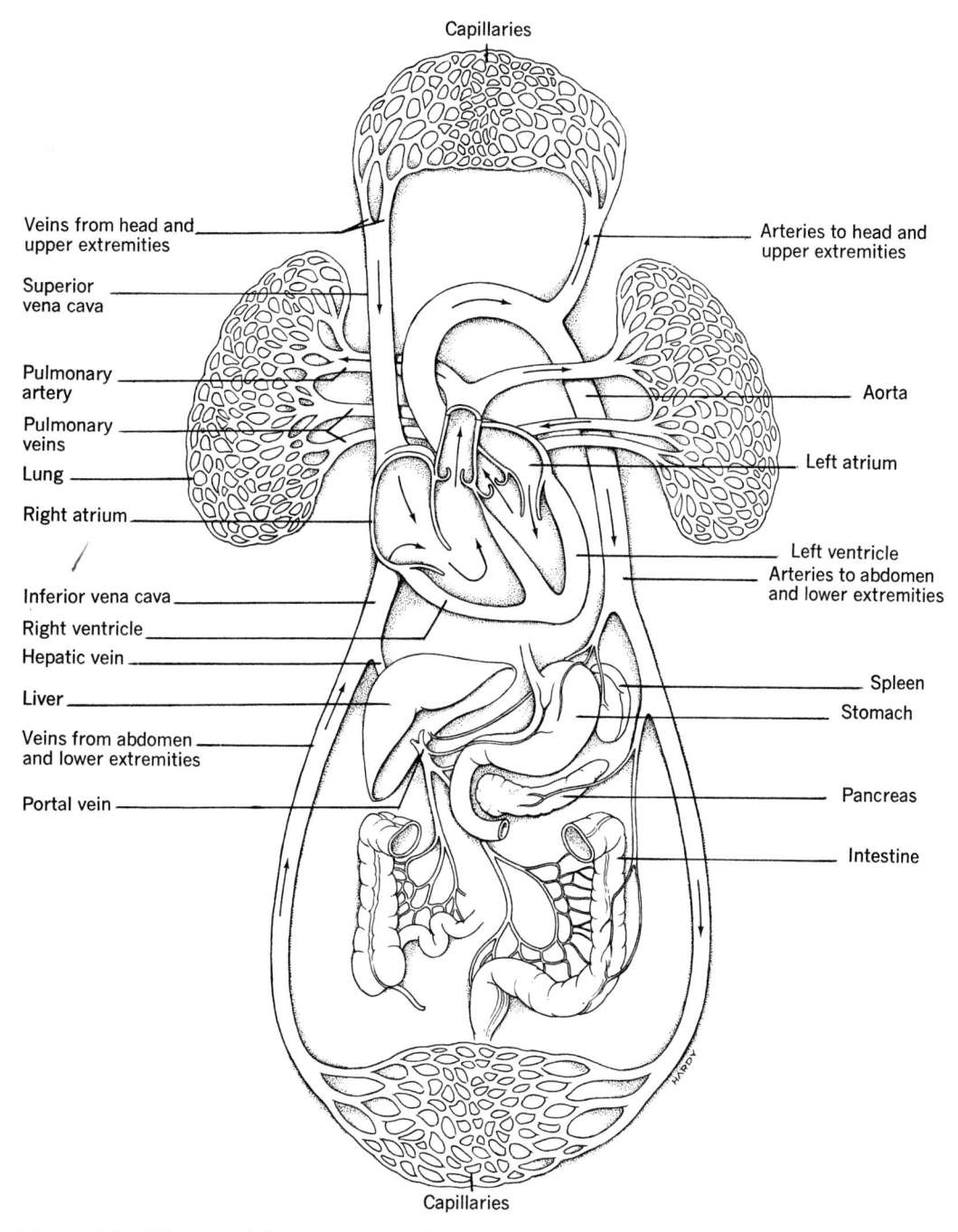

Figure 1-3 Diagram of the pulmonary and systemic circulations. The pulmonary circulation includes the pulmonary arteries, capillaries, and veins. The systemic circulation includes all the other arteries, capillaries, and veins of the body. (Chaffee EE, Lytle IM: Basic Physiology and Anatomy, 4th ed. Philadelphia, JB Lippincott, 1980)

All of the great vessels, with the exception of the pulmonary veins and superior vena cava, are separated from their respective cardiac chambers by one of two types of valves. The *venous valves*, which are at the ostia (or openings) of the inferior vena cava (the eustachian valve), and the coronary sinus (the thebesian valve) in the right atrium, are no more than an extra fold of the lining tissue that hinders reverse blood flow. The second type of valve is one with three tissue folds known as *cusps*. The folds arise from the arterial walls of the pulmonary artery and the aorta and curve inward and upward into the lumens, forming three pockets on the arterial side of the valve, known as the *sinuses of Valsalva*. As blood begins to flow backward, these pockets fill up and force the valve cusps together, thus preventing reverse blood flow. These valves are also known as *semilunar valves* because of the half-moon shape of each cusp. There is one other kind of valve that needs to be discussed. Mentioned earlier, these valves are known as atrioventricular valves, and are the most intricate of the cardiac valves. The primary difference between the valve on the right side of the heart, the tricuspid valve, and the valve on the left side, the mitral valve, is the number of leaflets that make up the closure apparatus. From its name, one could guess the tricuspid valve has three leaflets; however, the mitral valve has only two. With this difference in mind, we may now discuss the structure of the atrioventricular (AV) valve in general.

The AV orifice is encircled by a structure called the *anulus fibrosis* or the fibrotic ring. The valvular cusps arise from this ring and meet in the center of the orifice. On the ventricular surface a number of tendonlike structures (*chordae tendineae*) are attached to each leaflet, and anchor the leaflets into the papillary muscles near the ventricular apex. During ventricular contraction, this provides an active means of maintaining a fluid-tight seal. As the systolic pressures increase the valve leaflets tend to be forced upward into the atria. However, these papillary muscles are also contracting, pulling the leaflets *down* into the ventricles. Thus, the hydrostatic pressure of the blood forces the valve to close, and the tensile strength of the papillary muscle complex prevents the leaflets from prolapsing into the atria and allowing retrograde blood flow.

The final aspect of functional or internal anatomy of the heart involves a discussion of various types of tissue. The most important, of course, is the *cardiac muscle*, or the *myocardium*. This muscle makes up the walls of the cardiac chambers and the bulk of the atrial and ventricular septa. It is composed of three layers: the endocardium, the myocardium, and the epicardium. The endocardium is the lining of the interior chambers. The epicardium is an external membrane covering the surface of all four chambers, and the myocardium is the actual contractile muscle that provides the pumping action of the heart. Another type of tissue important to the function of the heart is the *fibrous tissue*. This tissue has been referred to earlier as comprising portions of the septa and the support of the AV orifices. In addition to its supportive nature, this tissue also allows the heart to mature from its fetal stages into adulthood. The last type of tissue that is crucial for the normal functioning of the heart is a *specialized conductive tissue*. This tissue coordinates the cardiac cycle much as the distributor of a car coordinates the internal combustion engine.

The conductive tissue composes several structures of the heart. First, the sinoatrial (SA) node, lies in the wall of the right atrium near the junction of the superior vena cava. It is responsible for initiating the electrical impulses that cause the myocardium to contract. In the heart there are several "wires" that connect the SA node and the atrioventricular (AV) node. These cardiac wires are called internodal pathways, and in the process of conducting the impulses between the two nodes they cause the atria to contract, with a resulting surge of blood into the ventricles. The AV node is situated in the lower left wall of the right atrium. The density of the specialized conductive tissue accepts the stimuli from the internodal pathways, reconcentrates them, and distributes them to the ventricles. At this point the conduction system of the heart becomes even more complicated than that of an automobile engine. The heart has one primary conduit that is called the *bundle of His*. This initial conduit divides into two bundle branches, one to the right ventricle and the other to the left ventricle. Due to the larger size of the left ventricle, the left bundle branch also divides into two tracts called *fascicles*. One leads posteriorly and the other anteriorly. These two fascicles and the right bundle branch divide into a network of tiny strands that disperse from the apices of the ventricles. Called Purkinje's fibers, these strands transfer the impulses into the myocardium, resulting in ventricular contraction (Figure 1-4).

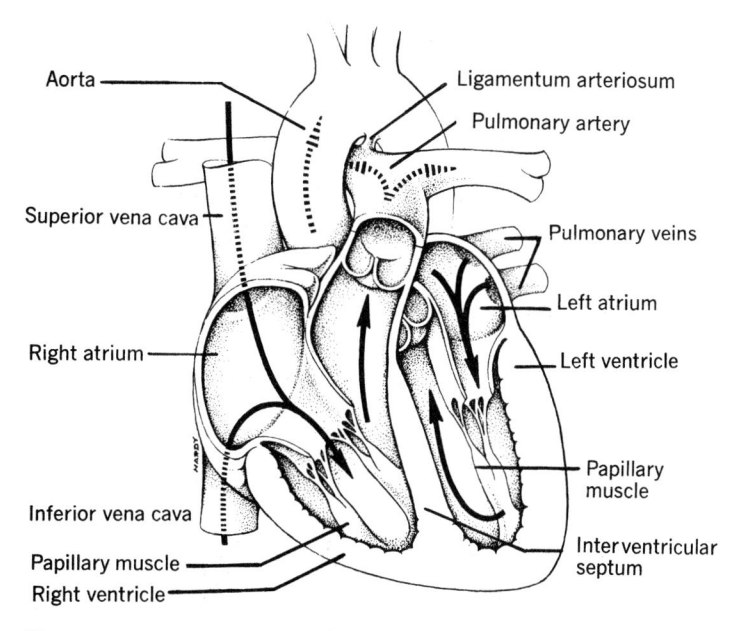

Figure 1-4 Interior of the heart. Arrows indicate the direction of blood flow. (Chaffee EE, Lytle IM: Basic Physiology and Anatomy, 4th ed. Philadelphia, JB Lippincott, 1980)

Geographic Anatomy

The remainder of the cardiac structures to be discussed here are not enclosed within the walls of the heart. They are also generally of a less dynamic nature than those described thus far. For these reasons, they have been labelled "geographic structures."

Before a dicussion of the cardiovascular system continues, it is necessary to become familiar with some descriptive terms from the field of medicine. Tables 1-1 and 1-2 are a collection of the most common of these terms and it is highly recommended that these lists be committed to memory before proceeding beyond Chapter 1.

The geography of the heart, just as that of the earth, begins with a description of its position in space. The heart lies within the thoracic cavity just to the left of the midline. The north-south axis of the globe is not vertical and, similarly, the long axis of the heart is angled within the chest in such a manner that the ventricular apex is pointed toward the left and slightly forward.

Table 1-1 **Terminology of Position**

Term	Meaning
1. Anterior (ventral)	Front, or chest, side of body
2. Posterior (dorsal)	Back
3. Inferior (diaphragmatic)	Below, lower, or toward the feet
4. Lateral	Away from the midline
5. Apical	Area around the apex
6. Septal	Area of the septum
7. Medial	Towards the midline
8. Anterolateral	Anterior and lateral
9. Posterolateral	Posterior and lateral
10. Inferolateral	Inferior and lateral
11. Inferoposterior	Inferior and posterior
12. Anteroseptal	Medial portion of anterior wall
13. Superior (basal)	Above, higher, or toward the head
14. Distal	Away from the origin
15. Proximal	Near the origin
16. Antegrade	Forward
17. Retrograde	Backward, reverse

Table 1-2 **Terminology of Dissection**

Term	Meaning
Sagittal	A cut parallel to spinal column, dividing left and right
Midsagittal	A sagittal cut through the midline
Transverse	A cut perpendicular to the long axis
Coronal	A vertical cut dividing anterior and posterior

While the earth is blanketed by its atmosphere, the heart is contained within a saclike structure called the *pericardium*. In order to examine the topographical appearance of the heart, one must first pass through this structure. In a very schematic way the epicardial surface of the heart can be compared to that of our planet. There are exposed regions of cardiac tissue separated by trenches, most of which are filled predominantly with fat. With the exception of color, it is quite similar to the land masses of the earth separated by the water-filled canyons we call oceans.

In the frontal view of the heart there are three major areas of exposed epicardium. On the left is the right atrium and the right atrial appendage. The central region is the anterior surface of the right ventricle, and on the right is the anteroseptal and apical walls of the left ventricle. The depression separating the right atrium and the right ventricle is known as the *coronary sulcus* or the right atrioventricular (AV) groove. The right ventricle and the left ventricle are separated by the *anterior interventricular sulcus* (groove), which is an external ramification of the ventricular septum. Three of the great vessels arise from the top of the heart. They are the superior vena cava, the aorta, and the pulmonary artery. Immediately after the main pulmonary artery exits the pericardial sac, it bifurcates or divides into the left and right pulmonary arteries (Figure 1-5).

If one now turns over the heart and examines its inferoposterior aspect, the left atrium and all the great vessels form a crownlike structure atop the left ventricle and the right atrium and right ventricle. As in the frontal view, the atria are partitioned from the ventricles by the AV groove, and the ventricles are separated from each other by the interventricular sulcus.

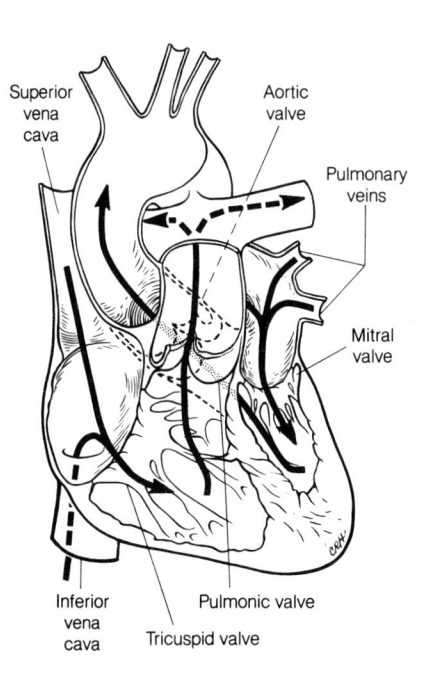

Figure 1-5 The valvular structures of the heart. The atrioventricular valves are in an open position and the semilunar valves are closed. There are no valves to control the flow of blood at the inflow channels (vena cava and pulmonary veins) to the heart. (Porth CM: Pathophysiology, Philadelphia, JB Lippincott, 1986)

The atria are divided by the union of the superior and inferior venae cavae. The last structure of geographic anatomy that bears mentioning is the groove at the junction of the superior vena cava and the anterior portion of the right atrium. This groove is called the *sulcus terminalis* and is a ramification of the *crista terminalis*, which is the ridge marking the superior vena caval orifice. This is used to approximate the location of the SA node within the myocardium (Figure 1-6).

Regional Vascularization

The final aspect of anatomy that will be necessary to the total understanding of the subsequent chapters is that of regional vascularization.

Before discussing the vascularization of any specific regions, it is necessary to review the structure and function of the vascular system as a whole. All blood vessels in the body can be divided into three categories: arteries, veins, and capillaries. Arteries are vessels that carry blood away from the heart. They are surrounded by a relatively thick layer of muscle tissue (vascular smooth muscle) that maintains the pressure in the system and

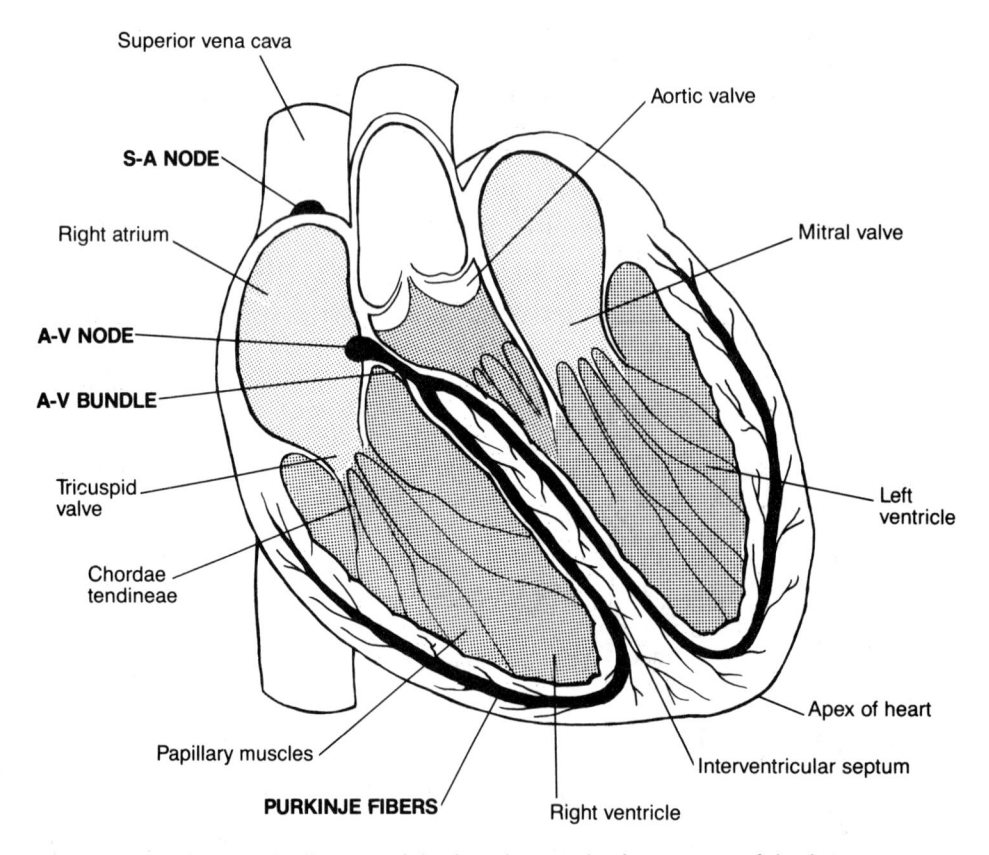

Figure 1-6 Schematic diagram of the impulse-conducting system of the heart. (Cormack DH: Introduction to Histology. Philadelphia, JB Lippincott, 1984)

forces blood flow forward. The structure of the veins is similar to that of the arteries, with several exceptions. A significant muscle layer is absent, and veins have involutions of the vessel lining that act as valves to hinder reverse blood flow. This will be discussed further in Chapter 2. The venous system is responsible for returning the blood to the heart.

Finally, the capillaries are very tiny, thin-walled vessels that allow for the exchange of nutrients and waste. They also serve to connect the arterial system (via arterioles) and the venous system (via venules).

The easiest way to think of the vascular system is to compare it to the plumbing in a house. The arterial side is the pressurized pipe that supplies all the faucets with water from the water company. The sinks, showers, and so forth, where the water is actually put to work, correspond to the capillary beds, which are the functional areas of nutrient delivery. Finally, the drains lead the used water back to the point at which it can be processed and used again, much as the veins do with blood. Additionally, the driving force in the veins is primarily due to the momentum of the blood entering the system from the capillaries, as the force that keeps water moving through your drains is attributable to gravity.

Before concluding the discussion of the anatomy of the heart, it is important to consider the blood supply that provides the essential nutrients to the myocardium. Oxygen is delivered to the muscle tissue of the heart through the coronary arteries. These arteries, that arise from the Valsalva's sinus, are divided into two systems: the right and left coronary arterial systems.

The right coronary arterial system is the simpler of the two. The main right coronary artery (RCA) originates immediately above the base of the right aortic cusp. In about 90% of persons a small branch, known as the *conus branch*, arises shortly after the origin of the right coronary artery. This branch supplies the SA node with blood. As the right coronary artery travels beneath the fatty tissue that occupies the AV groove, it produces one other major branch on the anterior surface of the right ventricle. This right margin branch and its sub-branches feed the anterior wall of the right ventricle, the inferior wall of the left ventricle and, in about 60% of individuals, the AV node. Distal to the right marginal branch, the RCA continues in the AV groove around the right lateral wall of the heart and across the posterior aspect until it reaches the posterior intraventricular groove. At this point it either divides into the posterior descending branch and a transverse branch in persons who have right dominant systems (approximately 70% of the population), or it joins with the left coronary artery (LCA).

In about 10% of human hearts, the LCA gives rise to the posterior descending artery and the left transverse branch. This is considered a left dominant system. The remaining 20% of cases are considered codominant systems, since the responsibility for supplying the posterior aspect of the heart is fairly equally shared between the RCA and LCA.

The LCA originates in the posterior sinus of Valsalva and travels in the left AV groove. The LCA bifurcates into the left anterior descending artery

(LAD) and the left circumflex artery (CIRC) soon after its origin. The CIRC is found in the AV groove until it intersects with the RCA along the posterior wall. By means of its marginal branches the CIRC is the primary blood supply for the left atrium, the lateral wall of the left ventricle and, in some cases, the posterior wall and the AV and SA nodes.

The other major artery of the left coronary system, the LAD, is the most important of the three major coronary arteries (RCA, CIRC, LAD). It supplies the largest portion of the left ventricle through a network of diagonal branches. The LAD travels in the left anterior AV groove until it turns toward the apex along the anterior interventricular sulcus. In most cases the LAD wraps around the apex, and anastomoses or forms a link with the posterior descending artery.

As discussed earlier, a circulatory sytem has delivery and return components. The venous portion of the coronary circulation is dominated by one major vessel, the coronary sinus. The coronary sinus runs along the posterior AV groove and empties into the inferoposterior portion of the right atrium.

The next regions to be discussed are the upper extremities. The primary difference between the left and right sides of the body occurs at the arch of the aorta. The left side has separate branches of the aorta for cerebral vessels and for those of the arm and chest. On the right side, the innominate (or nameless) artery branches off the aorta and subsequently divides into the subclavian and carotid arteries. As the subclavian artery travels toward the upper extremity, the first major "intersections" encountered are the vertebral and the internal mammary arteries. The subclavian artery soon narrows within the shoulder joint and becomes the axillary artery. This in turn narrows a bit more and is renamed the brachial artery in the upper arm. At the elbow the brachial artery divides into the radial and ulnar arteries that traverse down either side of the forearm only to divide further within the hand. Venous return from the upper extremity uses the same nomenclature, with the exception of the area between the shoulder and the elbow. The major veins in this area are called the *cephalic* and the *basilic veins*. The journey is complete when the subclavian vein merges with the superior vena cava, and return to the right atrium is complete.

The arterial tree of the lower extremity is slightly more complicated. The common iliac artery splits off the abdominal aorta and almost immediately divides into internal and external branches. The internal iliac artery supplies the pelvic girdle, and the external iliac artery continues down the leg. Between the hip and the knee, the major artery is called the *femoral artery*, which becomes the *popliteal artery* just above the knee. Within the knee joint the popliteal trifurcates into the anterior and posterior tibial arteries and the peroneal artery. The anterior tibial artery is renamed the *dorsal pedal artery* as it crosses the top of the foot.

Again the venous system has similar nomenclature with one exception. Within the area between the foot and the knee, the two major veins are known as the *internal* and *external saphenous veins*.

The last region of the adult circulation to be explored is the cerebral vasculature. This subsystem follows the same pattern as the others discussed; the arteries and veins share common names. The one notable exception is in the cervical (neck) region. The arterial vessels that supply the head are called the *carotid arteries*, and the jugular veins are the *cerebral "drains."* Both systems have internal and external branches of the cervical vessels. The external branches serve the sense organs and the cerebral cortex via the facial, occipital, and temporal divisions. The internal branches are responsible for oxygen delivery to the base of the brain. In order to preserve oxygen supply to the base of the brain, an interesting circuit has developed between the right and left internal carotid arteries and the vertebral artery, so that, should an obstruction occur in any of them, the others would compensate for this malfunction. This protective development is known as the *circle of Willis*.

There is one final aspect of the cardiac system that needs to be described—the transition from the fetal to the adult heart.

In utero, a fetus depends on the mother's circulatory system to supply all necessary nutrients. The two circulatory systems are not united; however they both innervate a specialized organ, the placenta, which permits an exchange of materials. As a result, oxygen is transferred to the fetal blood and transported through the umbilical vein into the fetal circulatory system. This oxygenated blood enters the iliac vein, is detoured around the liver via the *ductus venosus* and into the inferior vena cava. The septal wall in the right atrium has a passage into the left atrium called the *foramen ovale*. Because of the direction of blood flow from the inferior vena cava, the oxygen-rich blood is shunted through the foramen ovale and enters the fetal systemic circulation. The majority of the blood leaving the left ventricle flows through the brachiocephalic branches toward the brain and returns through the superior vena cava. The blood flow from the superior vena cava is directed downward through the tricuspid valve. The outflow of the right ventricle leaves through the pulmonary artery and is shunted into the aorta via the ductus arteriosus, and the deoxygenated blood is transported to the umbilical artery and back to the placenta. Shortly after birth, the ductus venosus, the foramen ovale, and the ductus arteriosus are closed by fibrotic tissue. If this process does not take place a congenital shunt will result.

The purpose of this chapter was to present normal cardiovascular anatomy from a functional point of view. It is hoped that the analogies have been helpful in adding a conceptual element to the structural analysis of biological systems.

Chapter 2

Disease States

Gregg Harris

According to Webster's Dictionary, a disease is any abnormal condition in living systems that impairs normal vital functions. The abnormal condition can be caused by biochemical, bacterial, viral, or mechanical forces, and can affect any aspect of the physiology of the biological system. This chapter will explore cardiac diseases that result from anatomical abnormalities, such as abnormal development, toxic effects, and atherosclerosis.

Here, as in Chapter 1, an effort has been made to simplify the complexities of this subject wherever possible by the use of analogies.

Developmental Diseases

The first category of diseases to be discussed arises from improper formation of the cardiac structures during fetal development. Because of the complexity of embryology, there are countless numbers of potential defects that could occur. This section will deal only with the most common of these, which result in abnormal junctions between the systemic and pulmonic circulations.

Five Common Defects

The most common defects arise from the malformation of the chambers of the heart. The malformations appear as incomplete or improper "construction" of the atrial or ventricular septa.

The ventricular septum forms as the anterior and posterior walls pinch into the cavity of the primitive heart, beginning at the apex and progressing toward the atria. As this process proceeds, the trabeculae form across the septum as the teeth of a zipper interact. At any point in this seam, where the two surfaces join, an imperfection can occur. This would create an area of discontinuity similar to a zipper with a missing tooth.

A ventricular septal defect (VSD) can occur in the membranous region of the septum as well as in the muscular septum. The mechanisms by which defects in this area arise are quite different. The fibrous region of the ventricular septum is formed by the fusion of the muscular septum and the aortic and pulmonary arterial walls. If any of these structures is out of position, they cannot fuse and a duct is formed between the two ventricles. This is the most common etiology of a discontinuity of the ventricular septum.

In either case of VSD, a shunt exists. This means that instead of all the blood in the high-pressured left ventricle being ejected through the aortic valve, the cardiac output is divided between the sytemic circulation and right ventricle, which exerts far less pressure in systole. In addition to decreasing effectively the blood flow to the body tissues, a left-to-right shunt decreases the efficiency of the cardiovascular system by sending oxygenated blood back to the lungs, and increasing the pulmonary pressures. Elevated pulmonary pressures will be discussed in a subsequent section of this chapter.

There are also two conditions in the atria that could result in shunts within the heart. The first is true atrial septal defect (ASD), similar to a VSD in the muscular septum. These defects usually occur near the opening of the superior vena cava or in the region of the AV valves. A major difference is the potential for a right-to-left shunt in the atria. Due to the lack of a large pressure difference between the atria, it does not require an extreme right atrial hypertrophy to force oxygen-poor blood from the right atrium into the systemic circulation. Although this would effectively increase the amount of blood being circulated systemically, the oxygen concentration is reduced. Since diffusion depends on the concentration gradient a right-to-left shunt would significantly affect oxygen delivery.

The second type of ASD is created by incomplete fusion of the foramen ovale with the atrial septum. This condition exists in about one in five persons; however, most of those cases are known as *"probe patent" foramen ovale*. That is, although it is possible to cross through this window with a probe (or sometimes a catheter) from the right atrium to the left, a shunting of blood flow does not occur. In contrast to the true ASD in which shunting in either direction is possible, a patent foramen ovale can only allow for right-to-left shunting because of the valvelike nature of the fibrous patch.

There is one other common detrimental connection of the pulmonary and systemic circulations. Similar to the patent foramen ovale, this condition also stems from the failure of a structure, critical for fetal circulation, to close after birth. The specific structure in question is known as the *ductus arteriosus*.

As discussed in the preceding chapter, the ductus arteriosus joins the pulmonary artery and the aorta *in utero* in order to bypass the inactive fetal lungs. The condition known as *patent ductus arteriosus* (PDA) exists when this fetal vascular detour fails to close and transform into the *fibrous ligamentus arteriosus* which is a supportive structure in the adult anatomy.

Although a PDA results in a left-to-right shunt similar to a VSD, it is often not discovered for several years after birth. This is because the vessel is small and the majority of the blood flow in the systemic system continues normally through the aorta. Only a small fraction of oxygenated blood is shunted back to the pulmonary artery; however the pressure in the systemic circulation system does tend to be reflected in increased pulmonary pressures, and gas exchange in the lungs is hampered. This results in decreased stamina and endurance in the more active years of childhood.

The preceding section has attempted to reveal to the reader five of the most common forms of congenital heart disease in basic terms. As mentioned earlier, the miracle of embryology is so complex that defects can arise at any stage of development. This section has concentrated solely on abnormalities that misdirect blood flow. Other areas of congenital disease that may be of interest to the reader are malformation of the conductive tissues or abnormal structure of the myocardium itself.

The Myocardial Infarction

The myocardial infarction (MI) or "heart attack" is the most common and most widely publicized result of cardiac disease. It is just that: the result of an underlying disease. Such diseases limit and eventually stop blood flow to an area of myocardium. This obviously stops the delivery of oxygen and nutrients to those cells in the area, and the cells soon die. An MI is simply an area of myocardial tissue that has died due to the lack of oxygen.

Think of the cardiac cells as soldiers in a well-disciplined, highly organized army in a war to keep the individual alive. The enemy is heart disease. Its strategy is to cut off fuel lines and the supply lines, to make the troops' position untenable, then to starve them. This may be accomplished in two ways: first, the enemy can barricade the routes and stop all deliveries, or he can sabotage the pipelines so that the fuel is spilled all over the countryside. In either case the result is similar; the battalions served by the affected fuel lines and supply lines will die. Detours and alternate routes could be built, but only if there were enough time between the initiation of the road block and its completion. If the pipelines have been weakened or ruptured the only chance is to patch or to replace them, which is very difficult under hostile conditions. Another factor that comes into play is that the closer to the supply depot the barricade is erected, the greater is the number of troops jeopardized.

The two tactics discussed above illustrate the forms that coronary artery disease (CAD) can take. First, the effects of atherosclerotic lesions can inhibit coronary blood flow, which will be discussed shortly in greater detail. Second, the effects of coronary aneurysms (weaknesses of the arterial walls) can be simulated. One other scenario should also be mentioned. A condition known as *coronary artery spasm* may result in a MI due to temporary restriction of blood flow, caused by the spasm of the vascular smooth muscle in the coronary arteries.

In short, regardless of the method the enemy uses to cut off supply lines, the result is the same: a portion of the friendly forces dies. Similarly, whether there are lesions, aneurysms, or spasms in the coronary arteries, an MI will occur.

As a result of cellular death in an area of the myocardium, a process begins that removes the necrotic tissue and replaces it with a scar. This process decreases the risk of infection by removing the decaying matter that would be a prime culture medium for bacteria; however, at the same time, it temporarily increases the risk of a ventricular aneurysm (the most common complication of an MI).

This healing process begins with white blood cells, known as *polymorphonuclear leukocytes*, engulfing the necrotic tissue, which thins and weakens that region of the ventricular wall. Over the course of about 2 to 8 weeks this necrotic tissue is replaced by a fibrous material composed mainly of a substance called *collagen*. Once the "collagen patch" has been completed, the area of the MI is well protected from rupture. However, in those crucial weeks immediately after the infarct, the weakened area can bulge like the lining of a football protruding through broken laces. This condition decreases the effectiveness of the patch formation and may lead to ventricular rupture or necessitate surgery to remove the aneurysm and suture together the edges of myocardium.

In the cases in which a scar successfully forms over an old infarction, there are two other clinical ramifications of the MI. The first is the obvious loss of functional muscle tissue. The scar does not contract, as does healthy myocardium, and it also does not stretch during diastole. Thus the amount of blood that can be pumped per contraction (stroke volume) is decreased, and must be compensated for if the deficit is significant.

The second common by-product of an MI is the development of cardiac arrhythmias. If a portion of the electrical conduction system is involved in the infarction, one of a number of "blocks" may occur. Usually these conditions can be managed easily through medication and/or artificial cardiac pacing. The more dangerous conditions of tachyarrhythmias (fast rates) arise due to an increased irritability of the tissue immediately surrounding the infarcted area. Such patients require extensive monitoring and aggressive therapy (including medication, electrophysiological treatments, or surgery) to prevent sudden death. The chapters concerned with electrocardiograms (ECG) and electrophysiology will demonstrate and explain these conditions in greater detail.

Because of an unsettled controversy over the origins of spasm, this condition will not be discussed in detail in this chapter. However, aneurysmal disease and atherosclerotic disease will be discussed further in the following section.

Coronary Artery Disease

As mentioned previously CAD primarily takes two forms that are aneurysmal and atherosclerotic in nature. Aneurysmal disease is generally thought to have viral or toxicological etiology. One identified disease, known as *Kawasaki's syndrome*, affects children primarily and is documented to cause aneurysms of the coronary arteries as well as the other aortic branches.

There are two major complications involved with coronary aneurysms. The first is the risk of the artery rupturing, because of weakness in the wall. The resulting hemorrhage probably would be catastrophic. The second risk is just as dangerous but somewhat harder to visualize.

Try to imagine the aneurysm as a tidal pool at the beach. During high tide (systole) the ocean fills the pool with currents and allows particulate matter (red blood, platelets, etc.) to be circulated. However, at low tide (diastole), whatever particles are trapped in the pool can settle and accumulate on the bottom. Eventually these sediments adhere to each other and form large aggregates that remain in the tidal pool until an unusually strong current arises and carries them out to sea. In the above analogy, there is no detrimental result when the aggregate is swept away. However, in the coronary aneurysm, the aggregate would be in the form of a thrombus that would become lodged in the narrowing vessel, occlude blood flow, and produce an MI. These thrombi can remain in an aneurysm indefinitely, or they can be dislodged by any transient increase in blood pressure due to exercise or excitement. Thus, whether the weakened wall of an aneurysm ruptures, or the variable blood currents allow clots to form, this form of CAD can be devastating.

Although the prognosis of diffuse aneurysmal coronary disease is poor, the usual treatment is aimed at minimizing the risk of clots through anticoagulant therapy. In cases of isolated coronary aneurysms (usually in conjunction with atherosclerotic lesions) surgeons have developed means of "patching"—removing and bypassing the diseased area of artery. Such patients have a much brighter outlook than those with widespread multiple aneurysms, as do those patients who suffer from atherosclerotic CAD. Atherosclerosis is now being treated successfully with medication, catheter dilatation, surgery, and soon will be managed with laser therapy. Following is a comprehensive discussion of this disease, which is the major cause of heart attacks.

Atherosclerosis has three stages: initiation, progression, and clot formation. The primary cause of atherosclerosis is damage to the endothelial or intimal layers of the arterial wall. This damage may be a result of biomechanical forces that can result in endothelial or intimal discontinuities. Some biochemical factors contribute to the pathogenesis of coronary artery disease.

The first unavoidable mechanism that can create endothelial damage is the presence of unbalanced external forces applied to the coronary arteries. As the heart expands and contracts with each beat, the blood vessels are stretched and compressed. Over many years this constant stress of the arterial walls in itself will cause damage to the material of which they are composed. The endothelium and intima of the arteries crack and separate after years of myocardial contraction. Any factor that decreases flexibility of vessels will tend to accelerate this process.

Another inherent force that can cause vessel damage over extended periods of time is called *shear force*. This is a force exerted by the blood that tends to make the layers of the vessel "slide over" each other. In the process the continuity between the layers is disrupted, allowing for the formation of a lesion. This is much like the heel of a shoe causing the outer layers of skin to slide over the inner ones, permitting fluid build-up and the formation of a blister.

A biomechanical force that can be minimized and treated and that most definitely can contribute to CAD is hypertension (high blood pressure). Hypertension magnifies the two conditions already mentioned and increases the muscle thickness and oxygen demand of the vascular smooth muscle layer (muscular hyperplasia). It also causes an increased permeability of macromolecules (such as fats and fatty acids) that are the building blocks of atherosclerotic lesions.

With the exception of hypertension, the biomechanical forces exerted on the coronary arteries are intrinsic to the design of the system. It could be argued that, since they can be the initiating step for CAD, the latter may be a normal part of the aging process. It is probably the biochemical forces that initiate this disease prematurely, so some of these forces should be examined.

The biochemical forces that have been shown to contribute to the initiation of CAD do not necessarily physically change the structure of the endothelium but alter the permeability characteristics for macromolecules. Some of the more common forces include immunological reactions to both viral and bacterial infections, radiation, and toxins such as certain fats, fatty acids, and nicotine. The most thoroughly investigated biochemical stimulus for CAD is the role of lipoproteins in lesion formation.

There are three categories of important lipoproteins; low-density lipoproteins (LDL), also known as beta-lipoproteins, are the major carriers of cholesterol. They can cross the endothelial boundary but tend to accumulate in the intima once they have done so. They sequester on the smooth medial cells. Their presence increases cell activity, cell division, and cell proliferation due to increased nutrient supply. The thickening of the intimal space decreases the effectiveness of oxygen delivery while the oxygen demand is increased. This leads to the establishment of an oxygen debt and eventually necrosis and a focal injury of the endothelium. (The importance of a focal injury will be discussed shortly). This whole process is dependent on the permeability of the endothelium to LDL, which is determined by diet and metabolism.

High-density lipoproteins (HDL) are much more compact molecules and easily cross the endothelial boundary in both directions. These molecules may be responsible for the removal of LDL from the intima. However, they are not effective enough to compensate for poor diet, bombardment of endothelial irritants, and all the natural factors that can initiate LDL accumulations within the vessel walls.

The last general category of lipoproteins is very low-density lipoproteins (VLDL). The importance of these molecules in regard to CAD has not been well documented. Their characteristics of intimal mobility seems to be intermediate to that of LDL and HDL, and further research is needed to disclose any significant relationship.

Now that the initiating factors of atherosclerosis have been discussed, the manner in which the disease progresses is next to be considered. The first concept that must be understood is that atherosclerosis is rarely confined to a single system. If a patient has coronary lesions, he most probably has lesions in peripheral, renal, and/or cerebral vessels as well. The question is which lesions are symptomatic and threatening to life or limb. In this example, let us consider the coronary arteries to have these lesions.

In most cases, as blood flow to the myocardium is diminished because fatty buildup encroaches on the lumen of the coronary arteries, the patient develops angina pectoris. Angina is chest pain (occasionally the discomfort is localized in the arm(s), jaw, back, or upper abdomen) associated with exercise or increased oxygen demand. The pain is caused by insufficient oxygen supply and is analagous to soldiers under siege who radio for more ammunition when they are ordered to attack. As the lesions become "tighter," less physical activity is required to produce the symptoms, and eventually the symptoms develop even at rest. This pain would be similar to the troops' frantic plea for supplies needed just to maintain their position. The final phase of the disease results from the total occlusion of an artery. When this occurs a MI ensues, as when military supply lines are cut off completely and troops die.

Artery occlusion occurs by three methods. First, the lesion itself may seal the entire lumen. Second, after a lesion creates a critical narrowing, a thrombus (a circulating blood clot) may block the tiny passage available. Finally, a clot may form at the site of a constriction, thus stopping blood flow. Since the latter two situations involve blood clots, and are probably responsible for more extensive infarctions, the remainder of this section will be devoted to an understanding of thrombogenesis.

Thrombogenesis, the formation of blood clots, is a complex biochemical reaction of the body to blood vessel injury. It is designed to decrease or stop a hemorrhage. The final step in the chemical reactions that take place is the conversion of fibrinogen, an inactive blood protein, to fibrin, which is the material used to manufacture the clot. This conversion is the end product of a series of approximately eight previous conversions which were initiated by a substance released from the intima when the endothelium was damaged. The damage may be caused by a laceration, a blunt injury (bruise), or a focal injury at the site of an atherosclerotic lesion (discussed earlier).

The initial response to an interruption of the endothelial continuity is the formation of a platelet plug and localized vasoconstriction. Next, the sequential reactions begin to catalyze the following step in the chain to the activation of fibrin. The reason for the long series of reactions required to form fibrin is one that demonstrates the great amount of fibrin created with very little initial catalyst. Think of a guru seeking to establish a new cult. The first day he converts two individuals into his religion. The next day each of these two converts recuits two more members. This goes on for eight days, until there are 256 followers. Had the guru needed to recruit the same number of persons by himself, it would have taken 128 days. Thus, one can see that although the cascading of chemical reactions may not be direct, it does produce large quantities of the desired end product in much less time than a direct approach. Ultimately the fibrin will form a tiny netlike structure, which catches material such as platelets and other proteins in the blood stream and forms the patch to cover the endothelial injury. It is not hard to imagine that if the endothelial damage is a focal injury at the site of a critical lesion, this defense mechanism could easily be detrimental to the myocardial tissue beyond the initial site. Likewise, if clots form in another area and break free, they can become obstructions in a narrow vessel.

Valvular Disorders
In addition to decreasing the amount of muscle available to pump blood to the body, an MI can seriously impair the ability of other cardiac structures to function properly. Primary examples of this are the AV valves. If an infarction occurs in the area of the papillary muscles, the valve leaflet attached to that muscle would be able to open into the atrium as well as the ventricles. This condition is known as *prolapse*. It is usually seen in the mitral valve, and can be a source of reverse blood flow or mitral regurgitation.

Although mitral prolapse can be caused by an MI, it is not always associated with regurgitation. Mitral regurgitation can be present; it can be induced by exercise, or it may be absent. In the case of severe regurgitation, the valve would have to be replaced. Thus mitral prolapse can be serious or benign depending on its effect on blood flow.

The other common diseases of the cardiac valves stem from the calcification or fibrosis of the valvular structures. These processes decrease the pliability of the cusps and limit the size of the aperture, hampering forward blood flow.

All four cardiac valves are subject to stenosis (narrowing); however, it is more common on the left side of the heart. This is probably due to greater pressure exerted on these valves. As well as hindering forward blood flow, valvular stenosis can also prevent proper closure and thus allow retrograde flow or valvular insufficiency. One disease that can result in valvular stenosis (usually mitral or aortic) is rheumatic fever. Rheumatic fever can affect the endocardial surfaces of the valve cusps. This usually causes erosion and irritation along the edges where the cusps meet. During the healing process "growths" form around the irritation and scar tissue can fuse portions of the cusps, creating a stenosis. These growths along the closure site are referred to as *vegetations*, and they, themselves, can prevent proper valve closure.

We have now looked at diseases that affect development, the valves, and the blood vessels. The final group of diseases discussed are those that hinder directly the function of the muscle. These diseases are known as *cardiomyopathies*.

Cardiomyopathies

Literally, "cardiomyopathy" means disease of the muscle of the heart. These conditions affect the muscle tissue directly. An MI obviously affects the muscle but, as stated earlier, it is an indirect result of CAD, a disease of the blood vessels. There are three general categories of cardiomyopathies: congestive, hypertrophied, and constrictive.

Congestive cardiomyopathies are more accurately known as dilated myopathies because that is their effect on the heart. They are characterized by enlarged hearts with relatively thin walls and large chamber sizes. This results in decreased strength of contraction, thus decreasing the heart's ability to force the blood around the body. In some ways this is similar to the elastic in clothing when it becomes "stretched-out."

If a myopathy causes the myocardium to become "stretched-out," several physiological complications arise. Although the chamber volumes are larger, the amount of blood pumped out of the heart during each contraction (stroke volume) decreases because of the decreased force of contraction. As a result, there is an increased amount of residual blood in the ventricles after systole, which causes increases in the diastolic filling pressures. The final outcome is congestive heart failure; thus the terminology, congestive cardiomyopathy.

The second kind of myopathy umder discussion is called a *hypertrophic cardiomyopathy*. In this case, the walls of the heart are thickened (hypertrophied), thus decreasing the chamber's volume and elasticity (compliance), and requiring an increased oxygen supply. This category of myopathies can be subdivided into two conditions: obstructive disease and nonobstructive disease.

Nonobstructive hypertrophic cardiomyopathies are characterized by concentric and uniform thickening of the global muscle mass. The greatest concern in these cases is decreased stroke volume due to decreased end diastolic volume and increased oxygen demand due to increased muscular activity.

The obstructive type of this disorder is more commonly known as idiopathic hypertrophic subaortic stenosis (IHSS). In this form of the disease, the septal hypertrophy is significantly greater than that of the lateral free wall. In addition, it is the superior portion of the septum that is most affected; thus, during ventricular contraction, the thickened septum encroaches on the outflow tract below the semilunar valves. This simulates valvular stenosis and, due to anterior papillary muscle involvement, it can be accompanied by mitral/tricuspid regurgitation. In contrast to the congestive myopathies that are caused by alcoholism or some other toxicological source, IHSS is genetically determined.

The last form of cardiomyopathy to be discussed is known as a *constrictive cardiomyopathy*. This is a condition that decreases the diastolic elasticity (compliance) of the myocardium. Although this does not affect the systolic function of the heart, it restricts diastolic filling and thus limits stroke volume. The most common causes of decreased compliance are fibrosis (the buildup of fibrotic tissue) or amyloidosis, which is an infiltration of a glycoprotein (a compound substance consisting of sugar amd protein) into the muscle tissue. In short, each of the three types of cardiomyopathies is unique etiologically, anatomically, and physiologically. However, the end result of all three is decreased stroke volume. The constrictive type impairs diastolic filling; the congestive type impairs systolic efficiency, and the hypertrophic type impairs both diastole and systole.

Heart Failure

Heart failure is a condition in which blood is no longer circulated in sufficient quantity to maintain a normally active life. In general it is referred to as congestive heart failure (CHF). However, there are actually two types of failure. First, there is true congestive failure in which resistance to flow inhibits adequate cardiac output. Factors that could cause such resistance are valvular stenoses, IHSS, or increased vascular resistance. The second type of heart failure is myocardial failure. This occurs when the cardiac muscle no longer supplies enough force to perfuse the body sufficiently, such as following an extensive MI, or in patients with congestive cardiomyopathies. The two are often combined because, although their mechanisms are different, the clinical pictures are the same. Before expanding upon this discussion of CHF, some cardiac physiology should by examined, which will relate to all of the diseases in this chapter.

The primary function of the circulatory system is to deliver nutrients (oxygen for our purposes). The flow chart in Figure 2-1 illustrates all of the factors affecting oxygen delivery. Take a moment and try to find each one of the diseases we have discussed. How does each affect the proper distribution of oxygen?

Oxygen delivery is directly determined by two processes: absorption (getting oxygen into the red blood cell) and perfusion (transporting the red blood cell to the cells). Both of these processes depend on diffusion as a driving force, thus their efficiency is limited by those factors described in Chapter 1. Absorption can be measured via the oxygen saturation on the left side of the heart and can be adversely affected by hematological (blood) abnormalities, pulmonary dysfunction, and right-to-left shunts. Perfusion depends on the amount of blood being pumped (cardiac output) and the condition of the blood vessels in a particular region. It is easy to determine the amount of oxygen that is delivered to all the tissues of the body by

28 Disease States

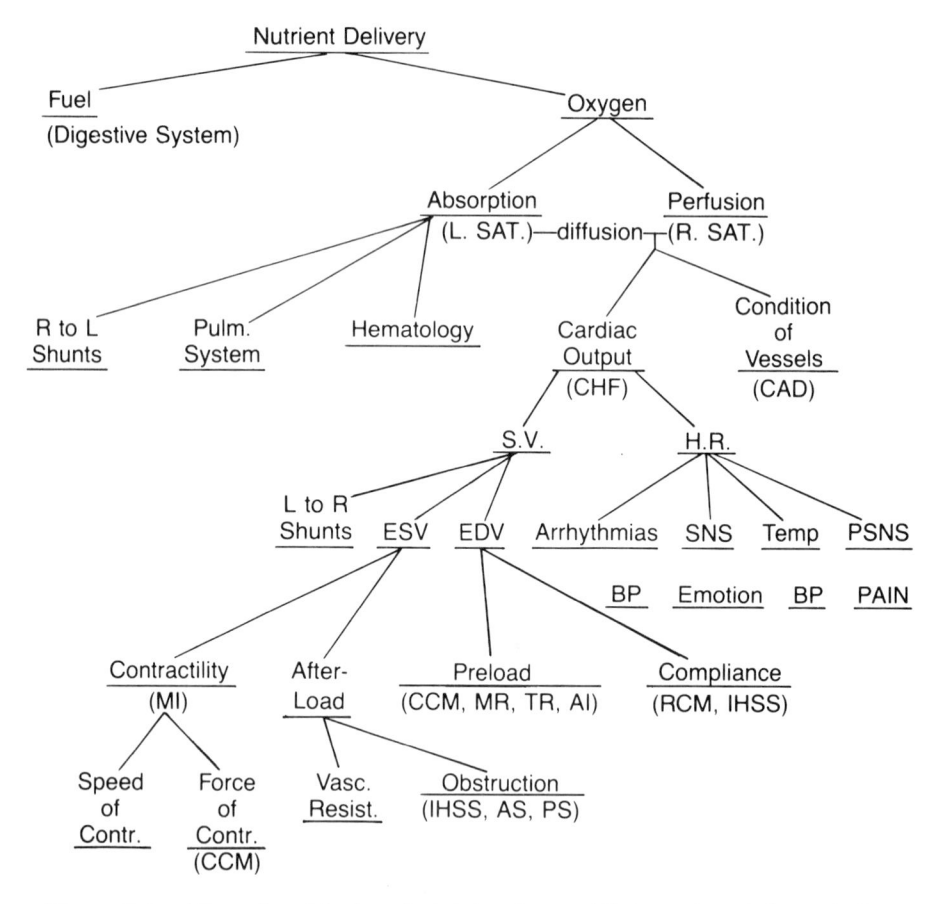

Figure 2-1 Hierarchy of factors that determine and limit nutrient delivery. Left heart O₂ saturation (L. SAT.); right heart O₂ saturation (R. SAT.); congestive heart failure (CHF); coronary artery disease (CAD); stroke volume (SV); heart rate (HR); end-systolic volume (ESV); end-diastolic volume (EDV); sympathetic nervous system (SNS); parasympathetic nervous system (PSNS); congestive cardiomyopathy (CCM); myocardial infarction (MI); restrictive cardiomyopathy (RCM); idiopathic hypertrophic subaortic stenosis (IHSS); aortic stenosis (AS); pulmonic stenosis (PS); mitral regurgitation (MR); tricuspid regurgitation (TR), and aortic insufficiency (AI).

measuring the oxygen concentrations of arterial and venous blood or even inspired and expired air. However, this method does not specify where the oxygen was delivered. A particular region may not have received enough or any oxygen, even though oxygen consumption for the body was normal. To determine whether or not there is adequate perfusion of a specific organ or extremity, one or more specialized tests must be performed, such as vascular Doppler studies, radioisotope scans, or angiography. Since CHF is basically a condition of decreased cardiac output (CO), the remainder of this discussion will concentrate on the factors that affect CO.

Cardiac output is defined as the amount of blood pumped out of the heart per minute, and it is usually measured in liters per minute. It can be determined by the amount of blood ejected during each ventricular contraction, stroke volume (SV), and the number of contractions per minute, heart rate (HR). Thus, $SV \times HR = CO$, and increases or decreases in either factor affect the CO proportionately. In certain circumstances, such as tachyarrhythmias, both SV and HR are involved as opposing determinants. In such a situation the HR tends to increase CO, but the decrease in SV outweighs the increased HR to create a net decreased CO.

With the exception of bradyarrhythmias the HR is usually not the impaired factor causing CHF. HR is primarily controlled by chemicals in the autonomic nervous system and, to some extent, by body temperature. The sympathetic nervous system (SNS) accelerates the HR by means of epinephrine (adrenaline) in response to decreased blood pressure or emotional stress (fear, anger, etc.). The parasympathetic nervous system (PSNS) tends to slow HR in response to several factors such as elevated blood pressure (BP), pain, and anxiety. Acetylcholine is responsible for this mechanism, often referred to as the vagal reaction after principal parasympathetic nerve, the vagus nerve.

On the other hand all of the diseases that have been discussed in this chapter decrease stroke volume either directly or indirectly. As defined earlier, SV is the amount of blood ejected from the ventricle during each contraction. Another way to describe SV would be to subtract the chamber volume at the completion of contraction (end systolic volume) from the maximum volume obtained during relaxation (end diastolic volume). Therefore, there are two categories of factors that affect SV—those that act on systolic functions and those that act on diastolic filling. In general, systolic function is affected in myocardial failure and diastolic filling is limited by true congestive failure.

What hampers systolic function and results in increased end systolic volume (ESV)? Obviously the contraction can be described by the speed of the systolic action (speed of contraction) and the strength of the muscular activity (force of contraction). When taken together the speed and force of contraction define one aspect of systolic function called *contractility*. Decreased contractility decreases the heart's ability to pump blood or defines myocardial heart failure. Another reason for increased ESV is unusual deferents to blood flow such as stenoses or increased vascular resistance. These factors increase a quantity known as *afterload*, which requires the heart to overcome back pressure created by the opposition to blood flow.

The opposite of afterload is preload. Preload is the quantity that impairs diastolic filling because of increased end diastolic pressure and insufficient emptying during systole. Finally, EDV is also determined by the ability of the heart to stretch during relaxation. This property is called *compliance*. If the ventricles are not compliant, then it is difficult for the blood to flow from the atria into the ventricles at the beginning of systole, and in turn, this increases the pressure needed in the atria and thus in the venous system, which leads to venous congestion and CHF.

In conclusion, we have described several components of the effects of cardiovascular disease and the initiation of heart failure. However, none of these exists in isolation. Myocardial and congestive failure can only be distinguished through etiology. This is the case because chronic myocardial failure due to decreased contractility, for instance, results in increased residual blood volume and pressure (preload) and becomes congestive failure. In addition, the increased strain caused by high preload in congestive failure chronically takes its toll on the myocardium and becomes myocardial failure. Thus both are referred to as CHF. The last realization that has to be made is that in time all of the diseases that have been presented lead to CHF. For this reason CHF can be considered "end stage cardiac disease." It can be treated and tolerated for many years, but eventually it is the true cause of most cardiac deaths.

Bibliography

Cohn PF: Clinical Cardiovascular Physiology. Philadelphia, W.B. Saunders, 1985
Gray H: Gray's Anatomy. New York, Bounty Books, 1977
Levine J: Clinical Cardiovascular Physiology. New York, Grune and Stratton, 1976
Netter H: Heart. Summit, NJ, Ciba-Geigy, 1978
Vogel S: Life in Moving Fluids. Boston, Willard Grant Press, 1981
Willerson T, Sanders CA: Clinical Cardiology. New York, Grune and Stratton, 1977
Bergen J: Aneurysms: Diagnosis and Treatment. New York, Grune and Stratton, 1982
Boucek J et al: Coronary Artery Disease: Pathologic and Clinical Assessment. Baltimore, Williams and Wilkins, 1984
Norman C: Coronary Artery Medicine: Concepts and Controversies.

Chapter 3
Cardiovascular Pharmacology

Lynn Bronson

This chapter is designed to give the reader an overview of cardiac drugs and their effects. It is impossible to cover all such drugs in depth, since technology is changing constantly and new medications are introduced daily.

Vasodilators

This group includes nitroglycerin and isosorbide dinitrate. Their effectiveness is based on the property of nitrates to relax smooth muscle, especially those muscles in the vascular beds.

Nitroglycerin: The preferred drug in the treatment of acute angina pectoris, because of its rapid onset, its ability to decrease cardiac oxygen demands, and to dilate coronary vessels.

Isosorbide dinitrate (Isordil): May be effective in terminating acute episodes of angina.

Sodium Nitroprusside (Nipride)

This is a vasodilating agent that acts directly on vascular smooth muscle independent of autonomic innervation. This drug is employed in the acute treatment of low cardiac output states and congestive heart failure, especially during myocardial infarction.

Hydralazine (Apresoline)

Directly relaxes vascular smooth muscle (arterioles to a greater degree than veins). As a result of vasodilatation, systemic vascular resistance decreases and renal, splanchnic, and hepatic blood flow increases. This drug is employed as an oral vasodilator to treat congestive heart failure and low cardiac output states.

Prazosin (Minipress)

Effects of this drug are similar to other vasodilators. Prazosin selectively blocks alpha adrenergic receptors to reduce peripheral vascular resistance. Studies suggest that the net effect is to dilate arterioles and venules equivalently, as does nitroprusside. A vasodilator to treat congestive heart failure and low cardiac outputs. Also used as an antihypertensive agent.

Antiarrhythmic Agents

This section outlines the features of each agent as applied to treatment of cardiac tachyarrhythmias.

Lidocaine: Preferred drug for emergency treatment of ventricular tachyarrhythmias and for the prevention of recurrent ventricular tachycardia and ventricular fibrillation, especially during acute myocardial infarction and digitalis toxicity.

Quinidine: An effective agent for a variety of ventricular and supraventricular arrhythmias. May be used to suppress or prevent serious ventricular arrhythmias during myocardial infarction, recurrent ventricular tachycardia, symptomatic premature ventricular complexes associated with chronic heart disease, recurrent atrial fibrillation or flutter, and recurrent paroxysmal supraventricular tachycardia.

Procainamide: A highly versatile antiarrhythmic agent. Used in oral form for chronic treatment of supraventricular and ventricular arrhythmias.

Disopyramide (Norpace): Popular agent for oral treatment of ventricular arrhythmias.

Phenytoin (Dilantin): Originally used as an anticonvulsive agent. Has antiarrhythmic effects in arrhythmias due to digitalis toxicity, and less commonly in arrhythmias associated with ischemic heart disease.

Bretylium (Bretylol): Currently approved for emergency administration to treat patients who have life-threatening ventricular tachycardia or fibrillation.

Mexiletine (Mexitil): An antiarrhythmic agent with structural and pharmacologic properties that resemble lidocaine. This agent effectively supresses ventricular arrhythmias associated with acute myocardial infarction.

Tocainide: Has produced significant reduction of premature ventricular contractions.

Slow Channel Blockers (Calcium Channel Blockers)

Calcium antagonists or slow channel blocking drugs affect electrophysiologic and mechanical properties of the heart and have vasodilator effects through action on vascular smooth muscle. Slow channel blockers have been used for the following: (a) to terminate and prevent recurrence of paroxysmal supraventricular tachycardia and to control ventricular rate during atrial fibrillation or flutter; (b) for treatment of coronary artery spasm; (c) for treatment of systemic hypertension; (d) for treatment of hypertrophic cardiomyopathy.

Verapamil (Isoptin, Calan, Iponeratril): Agent preferred to terminate acute episodes of paroxysmal supraventricular tachycardia. Also effective treatment of coronary artery spasm and hypertrophic cardiomyopathy.

Nifedipine (Procardia, Adalat): Acts by a mechanism different than verapamil to produce slow channel blockade. Major effect is vasodilatation and prolongation of AV nodal conduction time. Used as a vasodilator to treat coronary artery spasm, chronic stable angina pectoris, and systemic hypertension. Nifedipine does not have antiarrhythmic properties as does verapamil.

Diltiazem (Herebessor, Anginyl, Cardizem): Acts as a slow channel blocking agent with coronary vasodilating effects equal to those of verapamil. Also slows AV node conduction time to a lesser degree than verapamil. Agent used in the treatment of coronary artery spasm and chronic stable angina; also possesses antiarrhythmic properties.

Thrombolytic Agents

These agents act directly to lyse formed thrombi and appear to offer therapeutic advantages in certain situations.

Streptokinase: Derived from enzymes of the streptococcus that activates the fibrinolytic system. Intracoronary infusion of thrombolytic agents has been used to lyse coronary thrombi within the first few hours of myocardial infarction. Evidence has shown that streptokinase decreases and limits the extent of myocardial infarction.

Anticoagulants

Agents that inhibit the action or formation of one or more clotting factors; used to prevent or treat a variety of thromboembolic disorders.

Heparin: Predominantly affects blood coagulation and blood lipids by prolongation of clotting time, prothrombin time, and thrombin time. Heparin inhibits platelet aggregation induced by thrombin.

Coumadin: Acts in the liver to inhibit the synthesis of vitamin K-dependent clotting factors, especially prothrombin.

Adrenergic Pharmacology

This includes the study of the sympathetic nervous system with its principal neurotransmitter, norepinephrine; the naturally occurring catecholamines, epinephrine and norepinephrine, secreted by the adrenal medulla, and the effects of drugs that stimulate (agonist) or block (antagonist) the sympathetic receptors. The effects of drugs, hormones, or neurotransmitters on a specific end organ are mediated by the interaction of the agent with specific receptors on the end organ membrane. With regards to the cardiovascular system, alpha-receptors are located in the smooth muscles of arterioles, where stimulation results in arteriolar constriction. On the other hand, beta-receptors are located in the heart, arterioles, and lungs. Stimulation of beta-receptors increases heart rate and contractility, decreases AV nodal conduction time and refractoriness, dilates arterioles of skeletal muscle beds, and dilates bronchioles.

Beta-Adrenergic Blocking Agents

The cardioselective effects of beta-adrenergic blockade refer to the selective inhibition of beta-receptors, which produces a decrease in heart rate, contractility, myocardial oxygen demands, and cardiac output. The automatic discharge rate of the SA node is decreased and the refractory period and conduction time of the AV node are prolonged. Cardiac manifestations of beta-adrenergic blockade depend on the underlying level of beta-adrenergic tone so, in normal patients, resting heart rate and cardiac output change slightly, but the response to exercise is markedly reduced. Beta-adrenergic blocking agents are used most commonly in the treatment of angina, arrhythmias, and systemic hypertension. In addition, they can also be used for the treatment of hypertrophic cardiomyopathy, cardiovascular hyperthyroidism, and anxiety states. Common names of these drugs are:

Propranolol (Inderal)
Metoprolol (Lopressor)
Atenolol (Tenormin)
Timolol (Blocadren)

Alpha-Adrenergic Blocking Agents

These agents are most effective in peripheral vascular beds where vasoconstrictor responses are inhibited and vasodilatation results. Alpha-adrenergic agents also may accelerate heart rate by reflex effects from peripheral vasodilatation. Common names of these drugs are:

Dibenzyline
Regitine
Minipress

Alpha-Adrenergic Receptor-Stimulating Drugs

These agents vasoconstrict renal, splanchnic, cutaneous, and muscular vascular beds but generally do not change or slightly increase coronary blood flow. In essence, the increased mean arterial pressure reflexly increases vagal tone, which decreases heart rate. Common names of these drugs are:

Phenylephrine (Neosynephrine)
Methoxamine (Vasoxyl)

Beta-Adrenergic Receptor-Stimulating Drugs

Isoproterenol (Isuprel): This type of agent relaxes smooth muscles of bronchi, skeletal muscle, and alimentary tract. With regard to the heart, it increases the heart rate and contractility. It also lowers peripheral vascular resistance and decreases diastolic arterial pressure. The end result is to elevate cardiac output and systolic blood pressure and to decrease mean and diastolic arterial pressure. Other uses for this agent are:

1. To enhance pacemaker activity and improve AV conduction during bradycardia or AV block.
2. May be used to increase cardiac output and decrease peripheral vasoconstriction in cardiogenic shock.

Alpha- and Beta-Adrenergic Receptor-Stimulating Drugs

Ephinephrine (Adrenalin): Agent that acts on cardiac receptors to increase heart rate and contractility. Most often used during cardiac arrest to stimulate cardiac pacemaker activity and to increase contractility. Also drug most often used for anaphylaxis.

Norepinephrine (Levarterenol, Levophed): Norepinephrine has a greater stimulating effect than does epinephrine, but its cardiac-stimulating effect is approximately equivalent. This agent increases systolic and diastolic arterial pressure and total peripheral resistance. Usually, cardiac output remains unchanged or decreased because of the increased peripheral resistance and slowed heart rate, which results from reflex vagal activation. Coronary blood flow will increase whereas renal, cerebral, visceral, and skeletal muscle blood flow will diminish.

In summary:

Antianginal Agents

Beta-Adrenergic Blockers

Corgard	Inderal

Calcium Antagonists

Calan
Cardizem

Isoptin
Procardia

Nitrates

Cardilate
Dilatrate SR
Isordil
Nitro-Bid
Nitro-Bid IV
Nitro-Bid Ointment
Nitrodisc
Nitro-Dur
Nitrol Ointment

Nitrostat
Nitrostat IV
Nitrostat SR
Peritrate
Peritrate S.A.
Sorbitrate
Transderm-Nitro
Tridil

Other Antianginal Agents

Persantine

Antiarrhythmic Agents

Bretylol
Calan
Inderal
Isoptin
Norpace
Norpace CR
Procan SR

Pronestyl
Pronestyl-SR
Quinaglute
Quinidex
Tonocard
Xylocaine

Anticoagulants/Thrombolytic Agents/Other Blood Modifiers

Anticoagulants

Calciparine
Coumadin
Panwarfin

Thrombolytic Agents

Abbokinase
Abbokinase Open-Cath

Kabikinase
Streptase

Antifibrinolytic Agents

Amicar

Hemorrheologic Agent

Trental

Antihypertensive Agents
Beta-Adrenergic Blockers

Blocadren
Corgard
Inderal
Inderal-LA

Lopressor
Tenormin
Visken

Central Alpha$_2$-Adrenergic Agonists

Aldomet
Catapres
Wytensin

Peripheral Vasodilators

Apresoline
Hyperstat I.V.
Loniten
Minipress
Nipride
Nitro-Bid IV
Nitrostat IV
Tridil

Sympatholytics

Arfonad
Hylorel
Ismelin
Serpasil

Cardiac Pre- and Afterload Reducers/Cardiac Glycosides

Cardiac Pre- and Afterload Reducers

Capoten
Nitro-Bid IV
Nitrostat IV
Tridil

Cardiac Glycosides

Crystodigin
Lanoxicaps
Lanoxin

Other Cardiac Clycosides

Cedilanid-D
Digitalis
Purodigin

Bibliography

Andreoli, Fowkes, Zipes, Wallace: Comprehensive Cardiac Care. St. Louis, C.V. Mosby, 1983

The Cardiologist's Compendium of Drug Therapy. New York, Biomedical Information Corporation, 1985–1986

Chapter 4

Cardiovascular Terminology

Lynn Bronson

The terms used to describe the location and position of various body parts are extremely relevant in our studies. Generally, when using these terms, we must always consider the body to be in the anatomic position, or standing erect, facing forward, with the upper extremities at the sides and palms turned forward.

Superior: Above or toward the head. (The chest is superior to the abdomen.)
Inferior: Below or toward the tail end. (The neck is inferior to the head.)
Anterior/Ventral: Nearer the front or belly side of the body. (The navel is anterior on the abdomen.)
Posterior/Dorsal: Nearer the back side of the body. (The shoulder blades are on the posterior side of the chest.)
Medial: Nearer the midline of the body. (The nose is medial to the eyes.)
Lateral: Farther from the midline of the body. (The ears are lateral to the eyes.)
Internal: Deep within the body. (Organs within the body.)
External: Nearer the outer surface of the body. (The external surface of the face is covered with skin.)
Proximal: Nearer to the body or the origin of a part. (The arm is proximal to the forearm.)
Distal: Farther from the body or from the origin of a part. (The hand is distal to the elbow.)
Central: The principal part or related to center.
Peripheral: Toward the surface of the body.
Parietal: Pertaining to the walls of a cavity.

Visceral: Pertaining to the organs within a cavity.
Midsagittal: Passes through the midline of the body lengthwise and divides it exactly into even right and left halves.
Transverse or Horizontal: Passes through the body dividing it into superior and inferior portions.

In order to assure an understanding of terminology, the most commonly used roots, prefixes, and suffixes are listed below.

Roots

bio: Life
cardi: Heart
cephal: Head
cost: Rib
crani: Skull
cyst: Sac
cysto: Bladder
cyte: Cell
derm: Skin
encephal: Brain
gastro: Stomach
gynec: Woman
hem: Blood
hepa: Liver
hydra: Water
hyster: Uterus
lip: Fat
meno: Mouth
metr: Uterus
myo: Muscle

neph: Kidney
oophor: Ovary
osteo: Bone
ot: Ear
ovar: Ovary
path: Disease
ped: Children
phlebo: Vein
pneum: Lung
proct: Anus
psych: Mind
pyo: Pus
pyre: Heat
rach: Spine
rhin: Nose
salpin: Tube
septic: Poison
therm: Temperature
tox: Poison
trache: Trachea

Prefixes

a or an: Absence of, without
ab: From, away
ad: To, near, toward
ambi: Both
ante: Before
auto: Self
bi: Two
brady: Slow
contra: Opposed, against
di: Two
dys: Difficult, painful
endo: Within

epi: On, upon
erythro: Red
eu: Well
ex: From
exo: Outside
hemi: Half
hyper: Above, excessive
hypo: Below
inter: Between
intra: Within
leuco: White
macro: Large

40 Cardiovascular Terminology

micro: Small
neuro: Nerve
norm: Normal
peri: Around
poly: Many
pre: Before
pro: Before, in front
pseud: False

retro: Backward
semi: Self
sub: Under
super: Above
tachy: Fast, rapid
trans: Across
vaso: Vessel

Suffixes

-algia: Pain
-asis: Condition, state
-asthenia: Weakness
-cyte: Cell
-eatrics: Healing
-ectasis: Dilation
-ectomy: Excision
-emia: Blood
-esthesia: Feeling, sensation
-genic: Causing, origin
-itis: Inflammation
-logy: Science of, study of
-lysis: Reduction, destruction
-oma: Tumor
-oscopy: To view
-osis: State, condition

-ostomy: Forming an opening
-otomy: Cutting into
-pathy: Disease
-penia: Insufficiency
-plengia: Paralysis
-pnea: Breathing
-rrhagia: Excessive discharge
-rrhaphy: Suture of
-rrhea: Discharge
-rrhexis: Rupture
-rrhythmia: Rhythm
-sthenia: Region
-thrombo: Clot
-ulation: Act of
-uria: Urine

Systems Associated With the Body

Skeletal: Bones—the body's framework.
Muscular: Muscles, attached to bones, which make the body movements possible.
Circulatory: Heart, blood and blood vessels, lymph and lymph vessels. These organs carry food, H_2O and O_2, and wastes in the body.
Digestive: Mouth, salivary glands, pharynx, esophagus, stomach, intestines, liver, and pancreas. These organs take in food and convert it into substances the cells can use.
Respiratory: Nose, pharynx, trachea, bronchi, and lungs. These systems supply the body with O_2 and eliminate CO_2 as waste.
Urinary: Kidneys, ureters, urinary bladder, and urethra. They eliminate waste products from the body.
Reproductive: Ovaries, fallopian tubes, uterus, vagina, and mammary glands in women; testes, accessary glands, and penis in men.

Endocrine: *Ductless glands* (pituitary, thyroid, parathyroids, adrenals, testes, ovaries, thymus, pineal, and islands of Langerhans in pancreas). These glands secrete hormones that regulate various body processes, such as growth, cell metabolism, and so forth.

Nervous: Brain, spinal cord, and nerves. These control and coordinate the activities of the body.

Sensory: Eyes, ears, taste buds, organs of smell, touch, pain. These organs operate in special ways to bring stimuli from the outside to the brain.

Cardiovascular Terms and Definitions

Acrocyanosis: Mottled cyanosis of the hands and feet, associated with coldness and sweating.

Acute: Sharp or severe in nature, characterized by a rapid onset.

Adrenalin: One of the secretions of two small glands, called adrenal glands, located just above the kidneys. This secretion can be called epinephrine and, sometimes prepared synthetically, constricts the small blood vessels (arterioles), increases the rate of heart beat, and raises blood pressure. It is called a *vasoconstrictor* or *vasopressor substance*.

Allen Test: "Doppler Allen's Test" is used to check adequacy of palmar circulation.

Amaurosis Fugax: Temporary, partial, or total blindness, often resulting from transient occlusion of the retinal artery.

Amplitude: The maximal height of a wave form, either from baseline, or peak to peak.

Aneurysm: A spindle-shaped or saclike bulging of the wall of a vein or artery, due to weakening of the wall by disease or an abnormality present at birth.

Angina Pectoris: Literally means chest pain. A condition in which the heart muscle receives an insufficient blood supply, causing pain in the chest, and often in the left arm and shoulder. Commonly results when the arteries supplying the heart muscle (coronaries) are narrowed by atherosclerosis.

Angiocardiography: X-ray examination of the heart and great blood vessels that follows the course of an opaque fluid that has been injected into the blood stream.

Ankle-Arm Index: Comparison of the systolic blood pressure in the arm and ankle.

Anorexia: Lack or loss of appetite.

Anoxia: No oxygen. This condition occurs most frequently when the blood supply to a part of the body is completely cut off. This results in the death of the affected tissue. For example, a specific area of the heart muscle may die when the blood supply (and the oxygen supply) has been blocked, as by a clot in the artery supplying that area.

Antegrade Flow: Blood flowing towards the probe.

Anticoagulant: A substance that inhibits the action of the blood-clotting mechanism.

Antihypertensive Agents: Drugs that are used to lower blood pressure, such as thiazides.

Aorta: The main trunk artery that receives blood from the lower left chamber of the heart. It arises from the base of the heart, arches up over the heart like a cane handle, and passes down through the chest and abdomen in front of the spine.

Aortic Arch: Portion of the aorta leaving the heart, which curves up like the handle of a cane over the top of the heart.

Aortic Insufficiency: Improper closing of the valve between the aorta and the lower left chamber of the heart, admitting a back flow of blood.

Aortic Stenosis: Narrowing of the valve opening between the left ventricle and the aorta. The narrowing may occur at the valve itself or slightly above or below the valve. Aortic stenosis may be the result of scar tissue forming after rheumatic fever, or may have other causes.

Aortic Valve: Valve opening located between the left ventricle and the aorta. Formed by three cup-shaped membranes called semilunar valves, it allows the blood to flow from the heart into the artery and prevents back flow.

Aortography: X-ray examination of the aorta and its main branches.

Apex: Blunt rounded end of the heart, directed downward, forward, and to the left.

Apoplexy: Sometimes called *apoplectic stroke* or simply a *stroke*. A sudden interruption of the blood supply to the brain caused by the obstruction or rupture of an artery. Initially may be manifested by a loss of consciousness, sensation, or voluntary motion, and may leave a part of the body temporarily or permanently paralyzed.

Arrhythmia: An abnormal rhythm of the heart beat.

Arterial Blood: The blood is oxygenated in the lungs, passes from the lungs to the left side of the heart via the pulmonary veins. It is then pumped by the left side of the heart into the arteries that carry blood to all parts of the body.

Arterial Compliance: The ability of normal arterial walls to expand and contract with blood flow pulsations.

Arterial Occlusive Disease: Any disease process that closes the arteries.

Arterioles: The smallest arterial vessels resulting from repeated branching of the arteries. They conduct the blood from the arteries to the capillaries.

Arteriosclerosis: Commonly called *hardening of the arteries*. This is a generic term that includes a variety of conditions causing the artery walls to become thick and hard and lose elasticity.

Artery: Blood vessels that carry blood away from the heart to the various parts of the body. They usually carry oxygenated blood except for the pulmonary artery, which carries unoxygenated blood from the heart to the lungs for oxygenation.

Atheroma: A deposit of fatty substances in the inner lining of the artery wall, characteristic of atherosclerosis.

Atherosclerosis: A form of arteriosclerosis in which the inner layer of the artery wall is made thick and irregular by deposits of fatty substances.

Atrial Septum: Also called the interatrial septum. Muscular wall dividing left and right atria.

Atrioventricular Bundle: Also known as *auriculoventricular bundle*, *AV bundle*, or *bundle of His*. A bundle of specialized muscle fibers running from a small mass of muscular fibers between the upper chambers of the heart, down to the lower chambers. It is the only known direct muscular connection between the atria and the ventricle and serves to conduct impulses for the rhythmic heart beat from the atrioventricular node to the heart muscle.

Atrioventricular Valves: The two valves, one in each side of the heart, between the atria and the ventricles. The one in the right side of the heart is called the tricuspid valve, and the one in the left side is called the mitral valve.

Atrium: Upper chambers of the heart. Right atrium receives unoxygenated blood from the body. Left atrium receives oxygenated blood from the lungs.

Augmentation: Sounds of venous flow upon compression distal to the Doppler probe or release of compression proximal to the probe.

Auscultation: The act of listening to sounds within the body, usually with a stethoscope.

Autonomic Nervous System: Sometimes called *involuntary nervous system*. It controls tissues not under voluntary control that is, glands, heart, and smooth muscles.

Back Pressure: The increase pressure, engorgement, and dilatation proximal to a narrowed blood vessel.

Bacterial Endocarditis: Inflammation of the inner layer of the heart caused by bacteria. The lining of the heart valves is most frequently affected. It is most often associated with complications of an infectious disease, operation, or injury.

Barbiturate: A sedative. Drug used to produce a calming effect.

Basilar Artery: Artery formed by the union of two vertebral arteries, and terminating in the circle of Willis.

Benzothiadiazine: A diuretic. Drug used to increase the output of urine by the kidney.

Bifurcation: Division of two branches, as in an artery.

Bilateral: Pertaining to or affecting both sides of the body.

Biscuspid Valve: Another name for mitral valve.

Blood Pressure: The pressure of the blood in the arteries. *Systolic blood pressure:* Blood pressure when the heart muscle is contracted (systole). *Diastolic blood pressure:* Blood pressure when the heart muscle is relaxed between beats (diastole).

Blue Babies: Caused by insufficient oxygen in the arterial blood. Generally such babies have blueness of skin (cyanosis). This often indicates a heart defect, but may have other causes such as premature birth or impaired respiration.

Brachial Artery: Continuation of the axillary artery; terminally branches into the radial and ulnar arteries.

Bradycardia: Abnormally slow heart rate. Usually rate below 60 beats per minute is considered bradycardia.

Bruit: A sound heard on auscultation caused by turbulent blood flow.

Capillaries: Extremely narrow tubes forming a network between the arterioles and the veins. The walls are composed of a single layer of cells through which oxygen and nutritive materials pass out to the tissues, and carbon dioxide and waste products are admitted from the tissues into the bloodstream.

Cardiac Cycle: One total heartbeat, one complete contraction and relaxation of the heart.

Cardiac Output: The amount of blood pumped by the heart per minute.

Cardiovascular: Pertaining to the heart and blood vessels.

Cardiovascular-Renal Disease: Disease involving the heart, blood vessels, and kidneys.

Carditis: Inflammation of the heart.

Carotid Arteries: Left and right common carotid arteries are the principle arteries supplying the head and neck. Each has two main branches, external and internal carotid arteries.

Carotid Body: Small oval mass of cells and nerve endings located in the carotid sinus, that is, at the bifurcation of the internal and external carotid artery. These cells respond to chemical changes in the blood by causing changes in the rate of breathing, and certain other body changes. When the oxygen content of the blood is reduced, the carotid body causes an increase in respiration rate.

Carotid Sinus: Slight dilation at the point where the internal and common carotid artery branches. The carotid sinus contains special nerve endings that respond to changes in blood pressure by causing a change in rate of the heartbeat. By stimulating some of the nerves in the sinus external pressure on the carotid sinus can also cause a drop in blood pressure and/or faintness.

Catheter: A diagnostic device for taking samples of blood or pressure readings within the heart chambers that might reveal defects in the heart. A thin tube of woven plastic or other material to which blood will not adhere, which is inserted in a vein or artery, usually in the arm or leg, and threaded into the heart. The catheter is guided by the physician who watches its progress by means of a fluorescent screen.

Catheterization: A process of examining the heart by means of introducing a catheter into a vein or artery and passing it into the heart.

Cauterization: By the application of chemicals or heat, coagulation of blood is made possible.

Central Venous Pressure: The pressure representative of the filling pressure of the right ventricle.

Cerebral Vascular Accident: Sometimes called *stroke*. An impaired blood supply to some part of the brain, generally caused by one of the following three conditions: (a). A blood clot forming in the vessel (cerebral thrombosis). (b). A rupture of the blood vessel wall (cerebral hemorrhage). (c). A piece of a clot or other material from another part of the vascular system that flows to the brain and obstructs a cerebral vessel (cerebral embolism).

Chemotherapy: The treatment of disease by administering chemicals. Frequently used in the phrase "chemotherapy of hypertension", that is, the treatment of high blood pressure by the use of drugs.

Cholesterol: A fatlike substance found in animal tissue. A high level of cholesterol is often associated with high risk coronary atherosclerosis.

Chordae Tendineae: Fibrous chords that serve as guards to hold the valves between the atria and ventricles secure when forced closed by pressure of blood in the ventricles. They stretch from the cusps of the valves to muscles called papillary muscles in the walls of the ventricles.

Circle of Willis: Arterial circle of the cerebrum composed of the anterior, middle, and posterior communicating arteries.

Circulatory: Pertaining to the heart, blood vessels, and the circulation of the blood.

Claudication: Pain, limping, and or lameness caused by defective circulation of the blood in the vessels of the limbs.

Coagulation: The formation of a clot. Process of changing from a liquid to a thickened or solid state.

Coarctation of the Aorta: A narrowing or pressing together of the aorta, which is the main trunk artery conducting blood from the heart to the body. One of several types of congenital heart defects.

Collateral Circulation: Circulation of the blood through nearby small vessels when a main vessel has been blocked.

Commissurotomy: An operation to widen the opening in a heart valve that has become narrowed by scar tissue.

Compensation: A change in the circulatory system made to compensate for some abnormality. Often used specifically to describe the maintenance of adequate circulation in spite of the presence of heart disease.

Congenital Anomaly: An abnormality present at birth.

Congestive Heart Failure: Generally occurs when the heart is unable to pump out adequately all the blood that returns to it. There is a backing up of blood in the veins leading to the heart. A congestion or accumulation of fluid in the various parts of the body (lungs, legs, abdomen) may result from the heart's failure to maintain satisfactory circulation.

Constriction: Narrowing, as in vasoconstriction, which is a narrowing of the internal diameter of the blood vessels, caused by contraction of the muscular coat of the vessels.

Constrictive Pericarditis: A shrinking and thickening of the outer sac of the heart that prevents the heart muscle from expanding and contracting normally.

Contractile Proteins: A protein substance within the heart muscle fibers responsible for the heart contraction by shortening the muscle fibers.

Contralateral: Pertaining to the opposite side of the body.

Coronary Arteries: Two major arteries, arising from the ascending aorta above the aortic valve cusps and supplying blood to the heart muscle. Right coronary artery and left anterior descending.

Coronary Atherosclerosis: Commonly called *coronary heart disease*. An irregular thickening of the inner layer of the walls of the arteries that conduct blood to the heart muscle. The internal channel of these arteries becomes narrowed and the blood supply to the heart muscle is reduced.

Coronary Occlusion: Generally a blood clot in a branch of one of the coronary arteries that hinders the flow of blood to some part of the heart muscle. This part of the heart muscle then dies because of lack of blood supply.

Coronary Thrombosis: Formation of a clot in a branch of one of the coronary arteries.

Cor Pulmonale: Heart disease resulting from disease of the lungs or the blood vessels in the lungs. Due to resistance to the passage of blood through the lungs.

Coumarin: A chemical substance that delays clotting of the blood. An anticoagulant.

Decompensation: Inability of the heart to maintain adequate circulation, usually resulting in waterlogging of tissues.

Defibrillator: Any agent or measure, such as an electric shock, that stops an incoordinate contraction of the heart muscle and restores a normal heart beat.

Dextrocardia: Congenital phenomenon in which the heart is slightly rotated and lies almost entirely in the right (instead of the left) side of the chest. Another congenital abnormality is a condition in which there is a complete transposition—the left chambers of the heart being on the right side, and the right chambers of the heart on the left side, so that the heart presents a mirror image of the normal heart.

Diastole: In each heartbeat, the period of relaxation is called *diastole*. Atrial diastole is the period of relaxation in the atria and ventricular diastole is the period of relaxation in the ventricles.

Digitalis: A drug (prepared from leaves of foxglove plant) that strengthens the contraction of the heart muscle, slowing the rate of contraction by improving the efficiency of the heart. May also promote the elimination of fluid from body tissues.

Dilation: Stretching or enlargement of the heart or blood vessels beyond the norm.

Diuresis: Increased excretion of urine.

Diuretic: Any drug that promotes the excretion of urine.

Distal: Farthest from the midline or point of origin.
Dorsum: The back or analogous to the back, dorsal.
Ductus Arteriosus: Small duct in the heart of the fetus between the aorta and the pulmonary artery. Normally this duct closes soon after birth. If it does not close, the condition is known as *patent ductus arteriosus*.
Dysfunction: Impairment of function.
Dyspnea: Difficult or labored breathing.
Echocardiography: A diagnostic method by which pulses of sound are transmitted into the body and the echoes returning from the surfaces of the heart and other structures are electronically plotted and recorded.
Edema: Swelling associated with abnormally large amounts of fluid in the tissues of the body.
Electrocardiogram: Can be referred to as ECG or EKG. This is a graphic recording of the electrical currents produced by the heart.
Electrocardiograph: Machine used to record electrical currents produced by the heart.
Electric Cardiac Pacemaker: A small device that can control the beating of the heart by a rhythmic discharge of electrical impulses.
Electrolyte: Any substance that is capable of conducting electricity by means of its atoms or groups of atoms. Examples are sodium or potassium. These occur naturally in the body fluids.
Embolism: A blood clot (or other substance such as air, fat, tumor) inside a blood vessel, which is carried in the blood stream to a smaller vessel where it becomes an obstruction to circulation.
Endarterium: Also called intima. The innermost layer of an artery.
Endocarditis: Inflammation of the inner layer of the heart (endocardium).
Endocardium: A thin, smooth membrane forming the inner surface of the heart.
Endothelium: The thin lining of the blood vessels.
Enzyme: Enzymes are universally present in living organisms and are a complex organic substance capable of speeding up specific biochemical processes in the body.
Epicardium: Also known as the visceral pericardium; it is considered the outer layer of the heart wall.
Epidemiology: The science dealing with the study of factors that determine the frequency and distribution of disease in human population.
Epinephrine: Secretions of the adrenal glands, located just above the kidneys. This is also known as adrenalin and is capable of constricting the small blood vessels, increasing heart rate, and raising blood pressure. It is called a *vasoconstrictor* or *vasopressor* substance.
Erythrocyte: Also called red blood cell. Oxygen carrying blood cell.
Essential Hypertension: Commonly known as *high blood pressure* and often called *primary hypertension*. An elevated blood pressure not caused by kidney or other evident disease.
Etiology: The sum of knowledge about the cause of a disease.
Extracorporeal Circulation: Circulation made possible by a mechanical

pump-oxygenator. This often is done while surgery is being performed inside the heart.

Extrasystole: A premature contraction of the heartbeat, interrupting the normal rhythm.

False Negative Rate: Statistical term indicting the rate of negative results on a diagnostic test when disease actually was present.

False Positive Rate: Term indicating the rate of positive results on a diagnostic test when no disease actually was present.

Femoral Artery: Main blood vessel supplying blood to the leg.

Fibrillation: Uncoordinated contractions of the heart muscle occurring when the individual muscle fibers develop independent irregular contractions.

Fibrin: Forms the essential portion of a blood cot; it is composed of elastic protein.

Fibrinogen: A soluble protein in the blood that, by the action of certain enzymes, is converted into the insoluble protein of a blood clot.

Fibrinolysin: Enzyme that can cause coagulated blood to return to a liquid state.

Fibrinolytic: Having the ability to dissolve a blood clot.

Fluoroscope: An instrument used for observing structures deep within the body. X-rays are passed through the body onto a fluorescent screen where the shadow of deep-lying organs can be seen.

Fistula: An abnormal communication between an artery and a vein.

Fluoroscopy: The examination of structures deep within the body.

Foramen Ovale: In the fetus, a hole between the left and right atrium of the heart. Normally closes shortly after birth and is then called the *fossa ovalis*.

Gallop Rhythm: When the heart rate is fast, its rhythm resembles a horse's gallop.

Gangrene: Tissue death due to failure of blood supply, disease, or direct injury.

Genetics: The study of heredity.

Graft: The replacement of a defect in the body with a portion of a suitable material, either organic or inorganic.

Heart Block: Interference with the conduction of the electrical impulses of the heart that can be either partial or complete.

Hemangioma: A tumor composed of blood vessels.

Hemiparesis: A slight paralysis or incomplete loss of muscular power on one side of the body.

Hemodynamics: The study of the flow of blood and the forces involved.

Hemoglobin: Oxygen-carrying red pigment of the red blood corpuscles. When it has absorbed oxygen in the lungs, it is bright red and called *oxyhemoglobin*. After it has given up its oxygen load in the tissues, it is purple in color.

Hemorrhage: Loss of blood from a blood vessel. External hemorrhage blood escapes from the body. Internal hemorrhage blood passes into the tissues surrounding the ruptured blood vessel.

Heparin: An anticoagulant that tends to prevent blood from clotting.
Hypertrophy: The enlargement of a tissue or organ due to an increase in the size of the constituent cells. This may result from a demand for increased work.
Hypotension: Known as *low blood pressure*.
Hypothermia: The lowering of the body temperature in order to slow the metabolic processes during heart surgery. In the cooled state, body tissues require less oxygen.
Hypovolemia: Decrease in blood volume usually due to blood or plasma loss in trauma.
Hypoxia: Abnormal content of oxygen in the organs and tissues of the body.
Iliac Artery: A large artery that conducts blood to the pelvis and legs.
Impedance Plethysmograph: A device used to sense changes in a minute electric current sent through a portion of the body by means of separate electrodes proximal and distal to the sending electrode.
Incompetent Valve: Any valve that does not close tightly and leaks blood back in the wrong direction. Also known as *valvular insufficiency*.
Infarct: An area of tissue that is damaged or dies as a result of not receiving a sufficient blood supply. Also called *myocardial infarct*, referring to an area of the heart muscle damaged or killed by an insufficient flow of blood through the coronary arteries.
Innominate Artery: Also known as the *brachiocephalic artery*. One of the largest branches of the aorta. It arises from the arch of the aorta and divides to form the right common carotid artery and right subclavian artery.
Interventricular Septum: Sometimes called *ventricular septum*. Muscular wall dividing the right and left ventricles.
Intima: The innermost layer of a blood vessel.
Ipsilateral: Pertaining to structures on the same side of the body.
Ischemia: Usually temporary deficiency of blood in some part of the body, often caused by a constriction or an obstruction in the blood vessel supplying the part.
Jugular Veins: Veins that return blood from the head and neck to the heart.
Lipid: Fatlike substance.
Lipoprotein: Complex substance of fat and protein molecules.
Lumen: The passageway inside a tubular organ. Vascular lumen is the passageway inside the blood vessel.
Malignant Hypertension: Severe high blood pressure caused by damage to the blood vessel walls in the kidney, eye, and so forth.
Metabolism: A term assigned to all chemical changes that occur to substances within the body.
Mitral Insufficiency: An improper closing of the mitral valve between the left atrium and left ventricle.
Mitral Stenosis: A narrowing of the valve between the left atrium and the left ventricle.
Mitral Valve: Bicuspid valve located between the left atrium and left ventricle.

Mitral Valvulotomy: An operation to widen the opening of the valve. Usually performed when the valve opening is so narrowed as to obstruct blood flow.

Murmur: An abnormal heart sound that is heard between the normal "lubb-dupp" heart sound.

Myocardial Insufficiency: The inability of the heart muscle (myocardium) to maintain normal circulation.

Myocarditis: Inflammation of the heart muscle (myocardium).

Myocardium: The muscular wall of the heart. The thickest layer of the heart wall, it lies between the inner layer (endocardium) and the outer layer (epicardium).

Nitrites: A group of chemical compounds, many of which cause dilation of the small blood vessels, and thus lower blood pressure. They are vasodilators. Examples are amyl nitrite, sodium nitrite, and others.

Occlusion: Venous or arterial occlusion is a state of being closed or shut.

Ophthalmic Artery: Major artery of the eye, arising as a branch of the internal carotid.

Organic Heart Disease: Heart disease caused by some structural abnormality in the heart or circulatory system.

Pacemaker: Sinoatrial node, a small mass of specialized cells in the right atrium of the heart that give rise to the electrical impulses initiating contraction of the heart. The term pacemaker or electric cardiac pacemaker is applied to an electrical device that can substitute for a defective natural pacemaker and control the beating of the heart by an electrical discharge.

Palpation: Examination by touch for diagnostic purposes.

Palpitation: A fluttering of the heart or an abnormal rhythm of the heart.

Pancarditis: Inflammation of the whole heart including all layers.

Papillary Muscles: Small bundles of muscle in the walls of the ventricles. Attached to these muscles are cords leading to the cusps of the valves (chordae tendineae). When the valves are closed, these muscles contract and tighten the cords that hold the valve firmly shut.

Parasympathetic Nervous System: A part of the autonomic or involuntary nervous system. Stimulation of this system slows the heartbeat.

Parietal Pericardium: A thin, membranous sac that surrounds the heart and roots of the great vessels. It is the outer layer of the pericardium.

Paroxysmal Tachycardia: A period of rapid heartbeats that begins and ends suddenly.

Patency: The condition of blood flow through an opening.

Pericarditis: Inflammation of the thin, membranous sac (pericardium) that surrounds the heart.

Peripheral Resistance: The resistance offered by the arterioles and capillaries to the flow of blood from the arteries to the veins. An increase in peripheral resistance causes a rise in blood pressure.

Phlebitis: Inflammation of a vein.

Plasma: The cell-free liquid portion of uncoagulated blood.

Cardiovascular Terms and Definitions

Pressor: A substance that raises the blood pressure and accelerates the heartbeat.

Pulmonary Artery: The large artery that conveys unoxygenated blood from the right ventricle to the lungs. It is the only artery in the body that carries unoxygenated blood.

Pulmonary Circulation: The circulation of blood through the lungs and back to the left atrium.

Pulmonary Valve: Also known as the semilunar valve, located at the junction of the right ventricle and pulmonary artery.

Pulmonary Veins: Four veins (two from each lung) that conduct oxygenated blood from the lungs into the left atrium.

Pulse: The expansion and contraction of an artery that may be felt with the fingers.

Pulse Pressure: The difference between the blood pressure in the arteries when the heart is in systole and in diastole.

Purkinje's Fibers: Specialized muscular fibers forming a network in the walls of the ventricles and believed to be involved in conducting electrical impulses to the muscular walls. These electrical impulses are responsible for the contraction of the heart.

Regurgitation: The backward flow of blood through a defective valve.

Renal Circulation: The circulation of blood through the kidneys. Important in heart disease because of its function in the elimination of water, certain chemical elements, and waste products.

Rheumatic Fever: A disease usually occurring in childhood that may follow a few weeks after a streptococcal infection. It is sometimes characterized by one or more of the following: fever, sore, swollen joints, skin rash, occasionally by involuntary twitching of the muscles and small nodes under the skin. In some cases the infection affects the heart and may result in scarring the valves, weakening the heart muscle, or damaging the sac enclosing the heart.

Sclerosis: Hardening usually due to an accumulation of fibrous tissue.

Secondary Hypertension: An elevated blood pressure caused by certain specific disease or infection.

Shunt: A passage between two blood vessels or between the two sides of the heart, as in cases where an opening exists in the wall that normally separates them. In surgery, the forming of a passage between blood vessels to divert blood from one part of the body to another.

Sinuses of Valsalva: Pouchlike structure behind the aortic semilunar valve.

Stethoscope: A device for listening to sounds within the body.

Stokes-Adams Syndrome: Sudden attacks of unconsciousness, sometimes with convulsions that may accompany heart block.

Stroke Volume: The amount of blood that is pumped out of the heart at each contraction.

Sympathetic Nervous System: A part of the autonomic nervous system that speeds the rate of the heartbeat.

52 Cardiovascular Terminology

Syncope: Fainting. One cause for syncope can be an insufficient blood supply to the brain.

Systemic Circulation: The circulation of the blood through all parts of the body except the lungs, the flow being from the left ventricle, aorta, and through the body, back to the right atrium.

Systole: In each heartbeat, the period of contraction of the heart.

Tachycardia: Abnormal fast heart rate. Usually over 100 beats per minute.

Tetralogy of Fallot: Congenital malformation of the heart involving four distinct defects: (1) abnormal opening in the wall between the ventricles; (2) misplacement of the aorta "overriding" the abnormal opening, so that it receives blood from both ventricles instead of only the left; (3) narrowing of the pulmonary artery; (4) enlargement of the right ventricle.

Thrombus: Blood clot that forms inside a blood vessel or cavity of the heart.

Transcutaneous: Performed through the skin.

Transducer: A device that transforms one kind of energy into another.

Transient Ischemic Attack: An episode of transient cerebral symptoms including visual disturbances, memory loss, and so forth, which are brief in duration and resolve with no residual dysfunction.

Tricuspid Valve: Valve consisting of three cusps or triangular leaflets located between the right atria and ventricle.

Vasoconstrictor: The vasoconstrictor nerves are one part of the involuntary nervous system. When these nerves are stimulated, they cause the muscles of the arterioles to contract, thus narrowing the passage, increasing the resistance to the flow of blood, and raising the blood pressure.

Vasodilator: Vasodilator nerves are nerve fibers of the involuntary nervous system that cause the muscles of the arterioles to relax, thus enlarging the arteriole passage, reducing the resistance to the flow of blood, and lowering the blood pressure.

Vasoinhibitor: Agent or drug that inhibits the action of the vasomotor nerves. When these nerves are inhibited, the muscles of the arterioles relax, the vessel becomes enlarged, and the blood pressure is lowered.

Vasopressor: A chemical substance that causes the muscles of the arterioles to contract, narrowing the vessel, and thus raising blood pressure.

Vectorcardiography: Determination of the direction and magnitude of the electrical forces of the heart.

Vein: Series of vessels of the vascular system that carries blood from various parts of the body back to the heart. All veins in the body carry unoxygenated blood except the pulmonary veins that distribute the blood from the lungs back to the heart.

Vena Cava: Superior and Inferior vena cava are large veins conducting blood from the upper and lower extremities or the right atrium.

Venous Blood: Unoxygenated blood.

Venule: A very small vein.

Bibliography

Webster's Third New International Dictionary. Springfield, MA, G. & C. Merriam Company, 1981

U.S. Department of Health, Education, and Welfare: A Handbook of Heart Terms, DHEW Publication No. (NIH) 78-131. Bethesda, MD, National Institutes of Health, 1977

Taber's Cyclopedic Medical Dictionary. Philadelphia, F.A. Davis, 1981

Anderson: Clinical Anatomy and Physiology for Allied Health Sciences. Philadelphia, WB Saunders, 1976

Chaffee EE, Lytle IM: Basic Physiology and Anatomy, 4th ed. Philadelphia, JB Lippincott, 1980

Huszar RJ: Emergency Cardiac Care. Bowie, MD, Robert J. Brady Company, 1974

Chapter 5

The Heart and Electrical Hazards

Lynn Bronson

The achievement of electrical safety in the hospital requires the cooperation of all personnel and all departments. To ensure a comprehensive safety program, the entire staff must be aware of potential hazards, both to patients and to personnel. This chapter, essentially on "electrical safety primer," deals with four topics basic to understanding hospital safety. *Basic Electricity* introduces the fundamentals of electricity. *Electric Shock* is described in general, then the nature of *Electric Shock in the Hospital* gives specific examples of that problem. Finally, *Precautions in Patient Care Areas* describes the procedures to be taken by all members of the hospital staff.

Basic Electricity

Short of knowing not to touch a fallen high tension wire or telling children not to stick their fingers into a wall outlet, we seldom consider the hazards of electricity in our daily lives. However, electricity and its dangers take on keen significance in the hospital. When patients are physically connected to electronic devices, or are confined to electrically operated beds, they may be highly susceptible to electric shock and injury.

It is not necessary to be an electricity "wizard" in order to use electrical medical equipment safely. All that is required to help ensure safety is some understanding of the basic principles.

To begin at the beginning, all matter is made up of atoms. Atoms, in turn, are composed of a positive and a neutral core surrounded by electrons that are negatively charged. Electricity is thought of as the movement of these electrons. Moving electrons (*i.e.*, electricity) blindly follow a simple rule that Georg Simon Ohm discovered in trying to describe their behavior. Ohm's law states that the voltage (V) between any two points is equal to the current flowing (I) times the resistance to that flow between those two points (R). The equation is shown as $V = I \times R$.

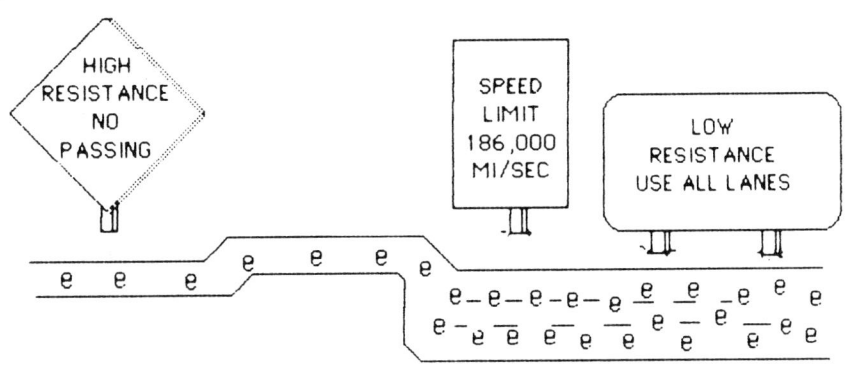

OHM'S LAW
$V = I \times R$ (VOLTAGE = CURRENT × RESISTANCE)

Every object has resistance (R) or a tendency to prevent passage of electrons. Conductors such as metals and ionic solutions (blood, saline, most body tissue, *etc.*) have a relatively low resistance. Hence electrons flow easily through conductors. Nonconductors (rubber, plastic, and air) have high resistance to direct current flow, thus preventing electrons from flowing.

Voltage (V) is the push that makes electrons flow. It is not a measure of the amount of electrical flow but rather the force pushing electrons through a point of resistance. A battery is a chemical source of voltage. The wall outlet is another source of voltage that is derived from thermal, nuclear, gravitational, or other types of energy. A voltage can exist between any two conductive points. Whether or not electric current (I) actually flows and how much current flows will depend on the voltage (V) and resistance (R) between two points. *According to Ohm's Law, if voltage and resistance are known, Ohm's Law will permit a person to predict the current traveling through a conductor.* By this means we can predict the current that could flow through a hospital patient or staff member and produce a shock.

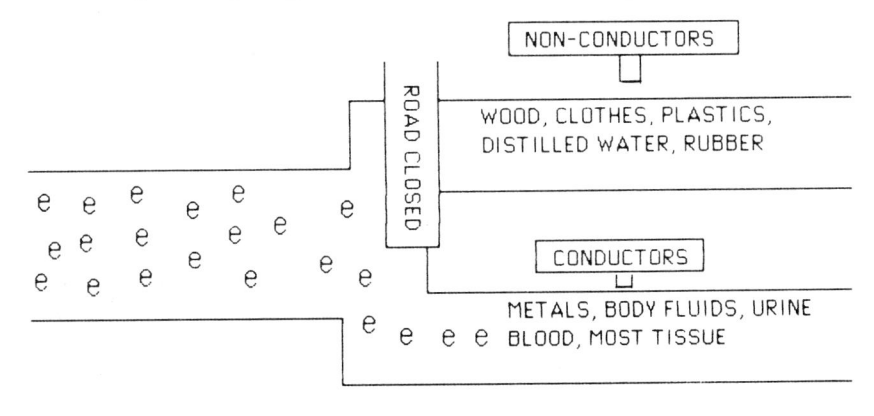

56 The Heart and Electrical Hazards

A corollary to Ohm's Law requires that a completely circular path be provided in order for current to flow. When a voltage is developed between two poles of a battery and a low-resistance path is provided between them, the current that flows must start at one pole and flow around to the other. *Electrons always return to their source.* An electron pushed from the Niagara Falls Power Plant must return to Niagara Falls. Usually it returns through the power lines, but given the chance, it will return through any conductive path it can find. The earth is a good conductor and often provides the necessary return route. We term this path, appropriately, "ground."

ELECTRICITY RETURNS TO SOURCE

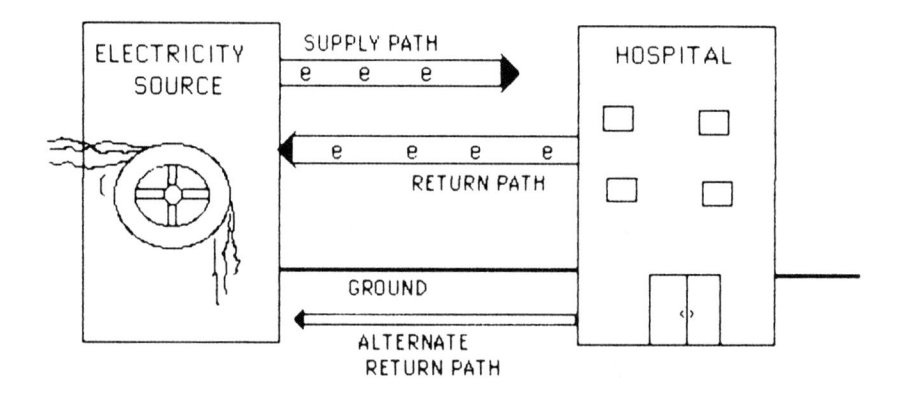

Electric Shock

The effects of electrical current flowing over and through people have been determined experimentally. Two degrees of electrical shock have been loosely defined. These are "macroshock" and "microshock."

"Macroshock" occurs when relatively large amounts of current flow across a person's body. Burns, open wounds, cardiac arrest, and ventricular fibrillation can be produced by these large currents. Painful stinging, muscle contraction, reflex movements, or a slow burn can be caused by lesser degrees of macroshock. Typical responses to electrical current flow of various amounts are presented in Figure 5-1. The meaning of these measurements of current will be discussed later; the relative degrees of electrical shock and its consequences are indicated.

"Microshock" is a hazard produced when small currents pass internally near a patient's heart. We must return to Ohm's Law to understand this phenomenon. Dry skin has a very high electrical resistance. The skin serves as a substantial barrier to electrons. Moist skin or living tissue is a good conductor of electric current and a poor barrier to electrons. Under these conditions the resistance is less than 1000 ohms. Thus, if a small voltage (battery, power outlet, *etc.*) is applied to the dry skin, very little current will flow through the skin. But, if the voltage is applied to wet skin

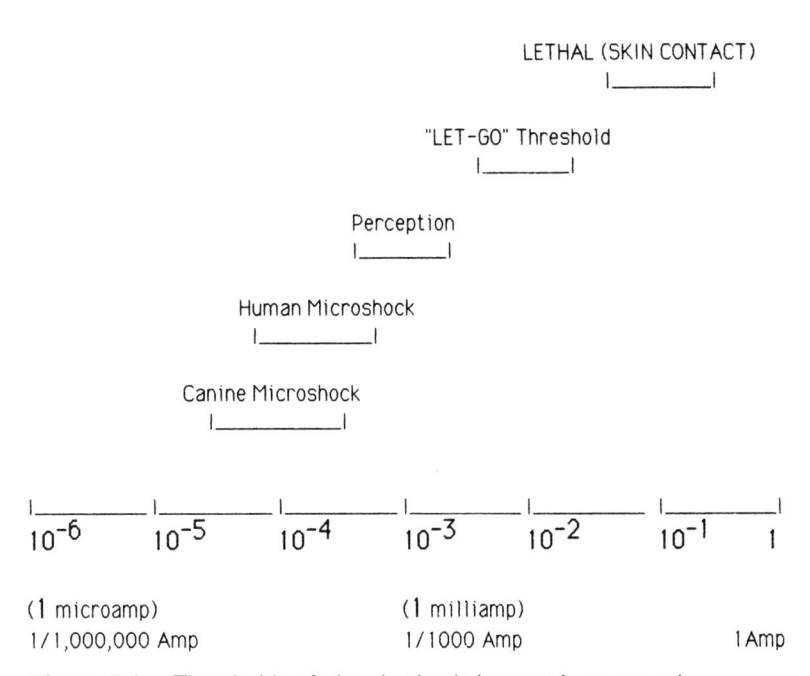

THRESHOLDS OF ELECTRIC SHOCK
CURRENT IN AMPERES

```
                                    LETHAL (SKIN CONTACT)
                                    |_____|

                          "LET-GO" Threshold
                          |_____|

                  Perception
                  |_____|

          Human Microshock
          |_____|

    Canine Microshock
    |_____|

|_____|_____|_____|_____|_____|_____|
  $10^{-6}$   $10^{-5}$   $10^{-4}$   $10^{-3}$   $10^{-2}$   $10^{-1}$   1

(1 microamp)              (1 milliamp)
1/1,000,000 Amp           1/1000 Amp                    1 Amp
```

Figure 5-1 Thresholds of electric shock (current in amperes).

inside the low-resistance thorax, a great deal of current can flow and some of it may go through the heart. The cardiac response to electric current is dependent on the amount and concentration of the current. If a current is concentrated through a needle, wire, or catheter, it can have a greater effect on the heart than if it were diffused through a large plate. The principal result of current of different magnitude being concentrated on the heart is a depolarization of the heart cells and a resultant contraction. Timed properly, electric current can be used for cardiac pacemaking, but if no account is taken of the duration and timing of the current being applied, then ventricular fibrillation can occur.

Electrical Shock in the Hospital

Electrical accidents in the hospital are probably not commonplace. The potential for these accidents is often present, however, and when circumstances permit an accident, the consequences are often harmful.

Macroshock accidents usually occur from major, though often avoidable, changes in electrically powered devices or the electrical environment. As discussed before, macroshock requires a substantial voltage to drive electrons through a high-resistance skin path. The power line voltage is

58 The Heart and Electrical Hazards

nominally 110 volts* with respect to the earth. Remembering that electrons must have a completely circular path, any low-resistance path between the power line and the earth will allow a substantial current to flow. If, for some reason, the power line voltage contacts the carrying case of a device, or other conductive surface, and a connection to the ground is available through the building structure, power system, or plumbing, then a patient or staff member who inadvertently completes the electrical path from the device carrying case to the ground will conduct current and can suffer "macroshock." There are three requirements for this type of accident: a high voltage, the ground, and the resistance path. Each must be examined in the hospital environment.

Voltages in the order of 110 volts with respect to the ground are available at every hospital. Each line-operated device uses this potential. Fortunately, the voltage is usually insulated from our contact by virtue of rubber or plastic around the power cord and by the case of the instrument. Occasionally, though, a frayed power cord or damage or alteration of the components of an electronic device makes a large voltage accessible to a patient or staff member. Spilling saline or coffee into a monitor or dropping a hemostat into the inside of an ECG machine can cause the line voltage to contact the case of the instrument. A radio with no backing can be a sudden source of high voltage to the nurse who leans on it. The old gooseknecked lamp that has been bent one too many times may contain a broken power wire inside that touches the lamp case and can be a source of high voltage.

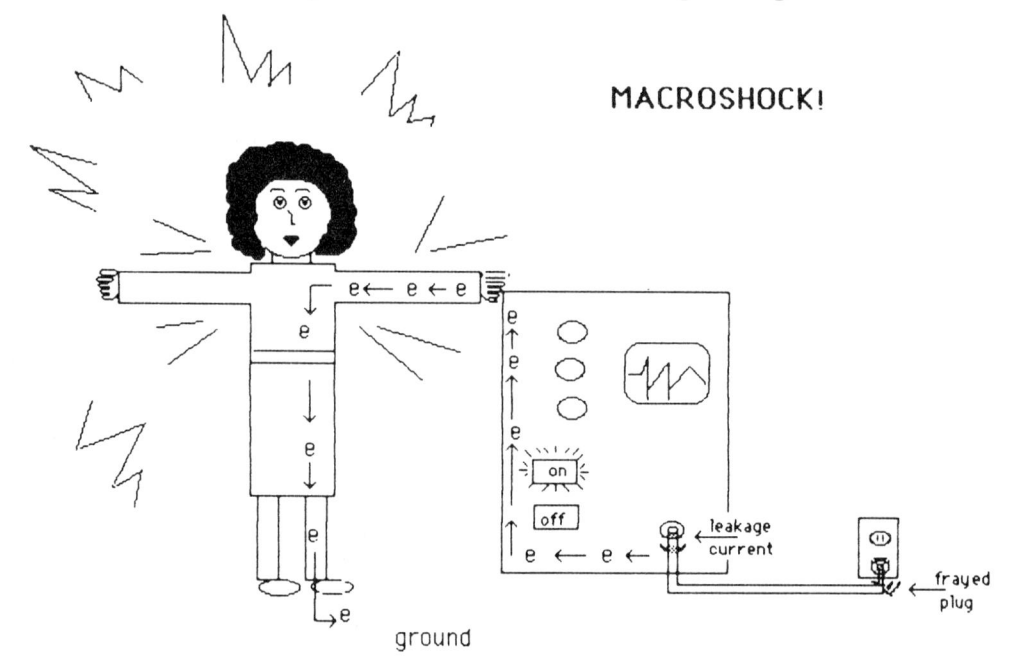

MACROSHOCK!

*Power line current is 60-cycle alternating current (AC). This means that instead of supplying a steady stream of electrons, the power is provided by alternately pushing and pulling electrons 60 times a second.

The ground forming the return path for electrons to a voltage source is built into the hospital itself. The girders, plumbing, and so forth are all conductive avenues to the earth. Electrons, which start at Niagara Falls or the local power station and are delivered to the hospital wall outlet, are drawn from the earth and must return to the earth if current is to flow. In each and every electrical outlet in the hospital there is a direct connection to the building ground. Each electrical device plugged into these sockets should have a three-pronged plug. One flat prong is to be connected to the power source and this is called the *"hot" prong*. The other flat prong is called the *neutral pin* and this provides a direct wired path back to the generating station. Normally, current flows in through the "hot" prong, through the electronics of the device, and then back to the power station via the neutral line. The third prong is U-shaped and fits into the ground hole in the wall socket. This prong is called the *ground prong*, since it simply connects the chassis or outer covering of the instrument to the building ground. Most of the time there are almost no electrons flowing through the ground line. However, under certain circumstances, the ground does serve a safety function. In the situation where the hemostat was dropped into the ECG machine, the 110-volt power source comes in contact with the instrument case. If a ground connection is properly made from the case through the U-shaped plug to the earth, a path is established for the electrons to return to their source. Since this path is of very low-resistance and the voltage is 110 volts, a substantial current will flow. One of the important safety tests is to validate that the ground wire is conductive (offers a low-resistance path to electrons). Since no person is in the major current path, despite the fact that the chassis is directly connected to 110 volts, no real harm is done and the ground connection has served a useful purpose. *Every electrical or nonelectrical large metal object in the vicinity of the patient must be connected to the building ground with a wire.* Each instrument or object in the hospital room (the monitor, the bed, the lamps, the radiator, the doorframe, the defibrillator case, the ophthalmoscope) must be joined to the building ground and can serve as a return path for current whose source is the wall outlet. There are two implications to this rule. First, the ground path serves as a harmless return for current that results from the accidental direct contact of the power source and grounded object. Second, the ground serves as the return for an inadvertent connection of the power source and the object through a route that might involve the patient or staff person. This situation can be hazardous, but since the ground connection serves as protection, we choose, in many cases, to ground everything securely. A patient in a wet bed will be grounded as well as someone leaning against a radiator. The green right-leg lead (RL) of an ECG often serves as a connection to ground.

The actual resistance path that might connect the high voltage source and the ground return is the key element in the macroshock hazard. Because of the number of conductive surfaces and ground connections in the patient environment, the resistance path that might initiate an accident can be complex. As a general rule, remember: Ohm's Law says that the higher the resistance path becomes, the less current will flow. It follows that when

60 The Heart and Electrical Hazards

electrons come to a "fork in the road" and must decide which path to take, they can split up as long as both routes eventually lead back to the source. Ohm's Law will not be violated, though, and this electric current will split proportionately. More current will follow the low-resistance path than the high-resistance path.

Let us consider these resistance paths when involving a patient. The patient is being monitored and his right leg is grounded by the means of the right lead. One hand is grasping the bedrail. The U-shaped prong on the electric bed power cord was broken off when the bed was last moved. The patient reaches up and moves the nightstand closer so that he can see the old TV set with the frayed cord that his family brought to him. The frayed cord touches the bedrail and current flows through the rail to the patient's hand, across his body, out the right lead through the monitor, into the ground hole in the wall outlet, down a girder, into the ground, and back to the power station. The extent of the injury depends on the resistance of the path. If the patient's body were wet (lower resistance), more current would flow and the injury would be greater. If we replaced the bedrail in our example with an ungrounded saline infusion pump that made a low-resistance connection with the interior of the patient's body, still greater damage could have resulted. On the other hand, if the bed or the infusion pump were grounded as they should be, almost all of the current would return to Niagara Falls, harmlessly. *When macroshock occurs, it is important to realize that the three components of a macroshock accident must be considered: (1) the voltage*

MICROSHOCK!

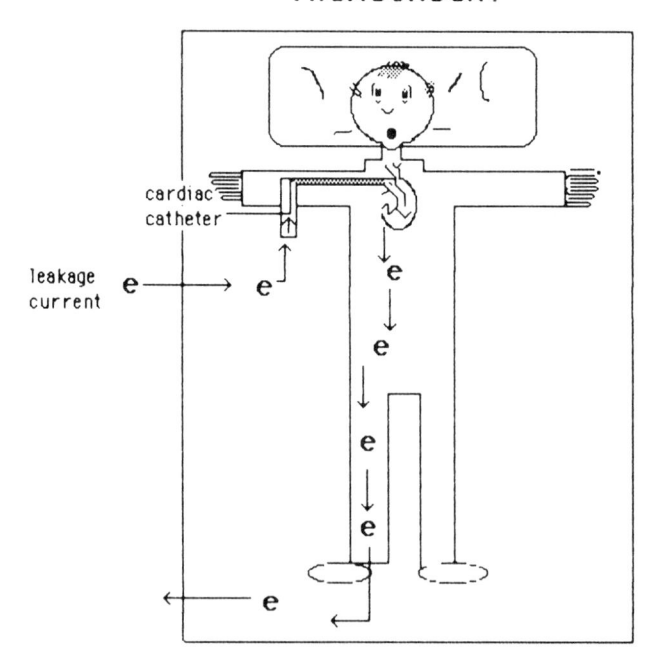

source; (2) the return (ground); and (3) the low-resistance path involving the accident victim.

The microshock hazard is more subtle than the macroshock danger. While the macroshock accident usually arises from a gross failure of the equipment or patient environment, microshock can occur from normally undetectable malfunctions. Microshock currents must have a low-resistance path which involves the heart in order to do damage. Because of the proximity of the electronic components in a device to its instrument case, a small voltage with respect to ground exists on the equipment chassis. Normally, a small "leakage current" is produced that flows down the groundline through the U-shaped prong of the power cord. If an alternative path develops that connects the equipment chassis to ground via a patient's heart, some of the current can be diverted from the groundline. Usually this current is extremely small because the resistance of the path involving the patient is much greater than the resistance of the ground wire. If the ground wire breaks, however, all of this "leakage current" follows the patient path and if it is sufficiently concentrated at the heart, fibrillation can result.

Consider a patient whose central venous pressure (CVP) is being monitored with a fluid-filled catheter and a glass monometer. The glass monometer has a metal stopcock at its base. The ECG is being monitored so that the right leg is grounded. The electric bed power plug has seen better days, the ground prong is bent, and the wire inside the plug has pulled loose from the prong. An old electric bed can push several hundred microamperes of "leakage current" through a conductive catheter, through the heart, down the body, and out through a firmly attached ECG electrode that is grounded. Under the proper conditions, this small amount of current can produce ventricular fibrillation. This might result if the metal stopcock connecting the monometer to the catheter should accidentally contact the rail of the "leaky," ungrounded bed.

Many circumstances produce a potentially dangerous microshock situation but they all have common characteristics. Like macroshock, a voltage must be available, a low-resistance path through the patient must be present, and a return path, usually ground, must be provided. Unlike macroshock, though, the voltage may be very small, but the low-resistance path must involve a connection directly to the neighborhood of the heart.

Precautions in Patient Care Areas

Assessment of patient risk is an easy but often overlooked task. Every patient's electrical risk potential should be classified according to his medical and physical condition. Once you have established standards for electrical equipment, regular testing is required to ensure that these standards are met. OSHA requirements and inspections insist on documentation of these tests. The most important electrical tests are for leakage current, ground wire resistance, and cord, plug, and receptacle inspections. (Isolated power systems are explained later in this chapter.)

1. Inspect the power cord and plug before every use. The plug should be physically intact and no metal wires or screws should be accessible. The U-shaped prong should be secure and unbent. The power cord insulation should be unbroken and uniform throughout its length. Special attention should be given to the point where the cord and plug join, as well as to the point where the cord enters the device.
2. If an auxiliary ground system is available (critical care locations), then a conscious effort must be made to attach each device to the ground sockets.
3. Do not use equipment on which liquids have been spilled or into which objects have been dropped. Do not place equipment in wet locations.
4. Never stack objects on or behind electrical equipment so that they might interfere with proper ventilation of the device. Remove the power cord, then report any burning or unusual odors that come from a device.
5. Note the condition of patient-owned electrical appliances if they are allowed in your hospital. They should not be used if they are suspected of being faulty.
6. Extension cords, adapters, or two-pronged plugs should never be used.

Patient Environment

1. Check the condition of the wall outlets whenever plugs are inserted or removed. Outlets should not be cracked or damaged. It is important that firm tension be provided by the outlet for the plug. An outlet which holds a plug loosely should be reported.
2. Whenever possible, keep equipment as far from the patient's bedside as possible. Do not rest electrical appliances against a bed.
3. The patient vicinity should be kept as free from wetness as possible when electrical devices are being used.
4. Try not to touch the patient and an electrical appliance at the same time because *you* can conduct current.

The third aspect of electrical safety is knowledge and care by the staff. The rules and suggestions made previously may be inadequate when unusual circumstances prevail. In these cases it is the understanding of some of the basic principles that will ensure safety.

The important points to remember are as follow:

1. Electric current originating from a device that is plugged into the wall will seek a return path to ground.
2. Recognize the possible sources of high voltage and attempt to keep them out of patient reach and contact.
3. Electric current must follow a completely circular path and it is important to keep the patient out of that path.
4. Many fluids and all metals are conductive.

Special Precautions: Anesthetizing and Critical Care Areas

Operating Room

The operating room is an electrical world unto itself. The OR is equipped with an electrical power system that is different from any other system in the hospital. It is called an *isolated power system*.

Historically, the use of flammable anesthetizing agents such as ether and cyclopropane required special precautions to prevent explosion and fire. Measures to prevent electrical sparking were employed and most are still in use today. To eliminate small sparks that may occur when plugging and unplugging power cords and operating switches, heavy steel "explosionproof" plugs and switches were used. By using conductive shoes for personnel and conductive casters or chains for equipment, static electricity was harmlessly dissipated to the special conductive floor. To further inhibit electrical accident, a special "isolated power system" was added. This device changes the introduction of power into the operating room so that current flowing down the power line returns only through the power line and does not seek ground. In this case the neutral and groundlines are not connected.

A "line isolation monitor" or "ground fault detector" measures the degree of affinity for ground of the electrons in the OR system. With the introduction of nonflammable anesthetic agents such as halothane, Ethrane, and parenteral agents, the need for explosion protection has diminished substantially. However, there are electrical safety benefits from the isolated power system making it useful even in ORs that do not employ any explosive anesthetic agents.

Most line isolation monitors or ground fault detectors use a red or green light and audible alarm to alert staff. Newer line isolation monitors employ a meter that demonstrates the degree of isolation the system possesses. When an alarm sounds or a red light illuminates, or the meter movement denotes an unsafe condition, the monitor is signifying that *if an accident were to occur*, an unsafe amount of electrical current could be involved. This situation can result from a defect in a particular device, thus defeating the isolation system, or the combined "leakage paths" from all of the devices in a room. When the alarm sounds, it is usually not advisable to interrupt any part of an operative procedure. Since the alarm signifies a *potential* danger, it is best to unplug the nonlife support devices in the room one at a time. If the alarm ceases when a particular device is unplugged, then that instrument should be inspected by a qualified person before it is used again.

The presence of explosionproof plugs and sockets in operating rooms presents other electrical safety problems for the OR staff. In most institutions, flammable agents are not used, so many ORs use conventional plugs with adapters or extension cords for connection to the explosionproof outlets. The use of these adapters increases the chance for damaged wiring, fluids in the extension plugs, and tripping over wires. They are not allowed under most jurisdictions, though the design of some OR suites makes them necessary.

Intensive or Coronary Care

Critical care areas require special attention to electrical safety. Because of the multitude of electrical and mechanical instruments, the condition and location of the patient, and the deluge of concerns with which the staff must be cognizant, some critical care units have isolated power systems much like those in the operating room. The section on special precautions in the OR describes such systems in some detail.

All critical care areas are equipped with special grounding connectors for the attachment of auxiliary ground wires. This system allows for the connection of a green grounding wire that is attached to the chassis of all portable instruments and large stationary metal objects (beds, tables, etc.). The ground plugs should be connected to the special grounding system to allow accidental electrical currents to flow harmlessly out of the room. Patient-owned equipment such as TVs and radios should never be allowed in critical care units. The risk of accident is too great to allow an untested device in the vicinity of the patient.

Section 2

Diagnostic Techniques or Directions in Cardiovascular Technology

Chapter 6

Electrophysiology

Stephen D. Kaniecki

This chapter provides a basic understanding of the way in which the cardiac cell functions and establishes a foundation to enhance an understanding of the remaining chapters in this text.

It should be emphasized that the area of cardiac electrophysiology is undergoing constant research. With the advent of modern procedures such as endocardial mapping, intracardiac electrophysiologic testing, and electron microscopy, existing theories are continually being modified or even discarded. The areas covering anatomy are fairly well established. However, research conducted while this text was being published may have invalidated some of its concepts. Indeed, some of the information presented is based, in part, on theory, and may be subject to argument—particularly those sections dealing with impulse formation and excitation-contraction coupling. The information contained herein is felt to be the most widely accepted at this time.

Conduction System of the Heart

The heart is endowed with a system of specialized fibers whose primary purpose is that of electrical impulse formation and conduction. A brief review of their gross anatomy would be helpful in understanding some of the concepts presented in this chapter. The anatomy about to be described follows the normal pathways of conduction as a wave of electrical stimulation follows its course from beginning to end.

Cardiac electrical impulses normally arise from the sinoatrial or *sinus node* of the heart (Figure 6-1). The sinus node lies in the superior portion of

68 Electrophysiology

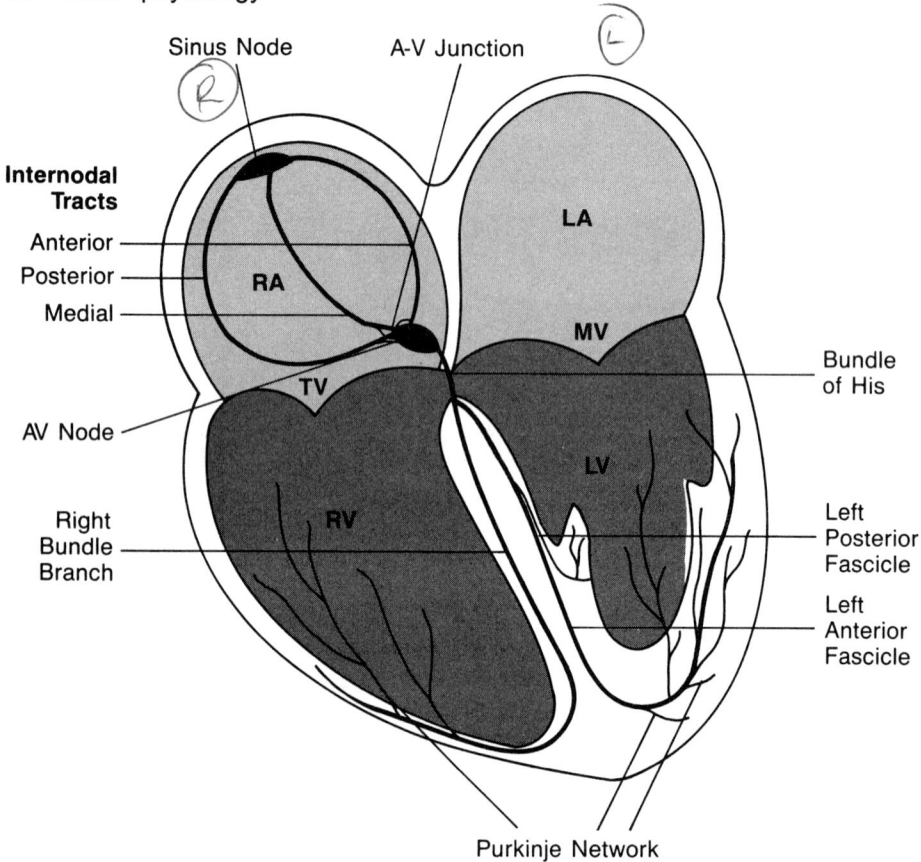

Figure 6-1 Gross anatomy of the specialized conduction system of the heart.
TV = Tricuspid Valve; **MV** = Mitral Valve; **RA** = Right Atrium; **RV** = Right Ventricle; **LA** = Left Atrium; **LV** = Left Ventricle.

the right atrium proximal to the superior vena cava. The impulse travels through the right atrium via three tracts of specialized fibers called *internodal pathways* or tracts. These three pathways are the medial, posterior, and anterior internodal pathways. The anterior internodal tract has a branch called *Bachmann's Bundle* that courses along the intra-atrial septum and penetrates it. As the internodal tracts come in close proximity to the atrioventricular node or *AV node*, they intertwine to form a complex set of fibers called the *AV junction*. The AV junctional fibers enter the AV node at various points. The AV node itself lies on the floor of the right atrium along the outer edge of the septal leaflet of the tricuspid valve. The impulse is delayed as it travels through the AV node for a period of about 0.04 of a second before it is passed along to the remainder of the conduction system. This allows time for the atria to contract and eject their contents into the ventricles before they are stimulated. In addition to facilitating atrial ejection, this delay also "shields" the ventricles from excessively high rates of stimulation sometimes found in the atria. This is accomplished by allowing a limited number of impulses to be transmitted to the ventricles in a given time period. The AV node passes the impulse to the *bundle of His* that penetrates the *anulus fibrosus*. The anulus fibrosus serves an important function in electrical conduction. It acts as an electrical insulator between the atrial and ventricular myocardial tissue. The bundle of His forms the only normal pathway of conduction through the anulus fibrosus (discussed later). Next in the conduction system are the bundle branches. The bundle of His follows a short course around the posterior aspect of the membranous interventricular septum where it reaches the beginning of the muscular interventricular septum. The bundle of His then gives rise to the *right bundle branch* that continues toward the apex of the heart. The *left bundle branch* is formed by the continuation of the original bundle of His and fans out over the interventricular septum as it heads toward the apex. As the left bundle branch begins to branch out, it divides into two major fascicles called the *anterior* and *posterior fascicles* or *bundle branches*. These fascicles course approximately two thirds of the lower length of the interventricular septum. Near the apex all three of these fascicles begin branching into the *Purkinje network*, which fans out over the ventricular myocardium.

Certain accessory pathways exist that are worth mentioning since they are believed to contribute to abnormal conduction.

Kent's bundle forms a connection between the AV junctional area and the distal portion of the AV node or the bundle of His. This tract is believed to be responsible for bypassing the AV node, with its inherent delay, resulting in early stimulation (pre-excitation) of the ventricles. Numerous other tracts which surround the AV valves and connect the atrial and ventricular musculature have been identified recently. These may also be possible sites of abnormal atrial-to-ventricular conduction.

Cellular Anatomy and Electrophysiology

The myocardium, or heart muscle, is comprised of four basic types of cells. These may be divided into two subgroups according to their function. The first subgroup of cells are those of the ordinary contractile cells of the atria and ventricles. These are the actual "working" cells of the heart and comprise a majority of cardiac tissue. The second subgroup of cells are those of the previously described specialized conduction system. These cells function as the specialized electrical network within the heart and perform little, if any, contractile work.

Contractile Cells

The contractile cells of the heart are all basically the same in structure. As will be discussed later, even though the contractile cells are concerned mainly with the mechanical activity of the heart, they are found within the specialized conduction pathways.

The contractile cells are arranged in a parallel fashion and are joined end to end. Each of the cells is surrounded by a cell membrane known as the *sarcolemma* (Figure 6-2).

The sarcolemma encases all of the cells' internal structures. These internal structures are suspended in a substance known as the sarcoplasm. This may be compared to the skin of a grape which encases the fruit; in this comparison, the grape skin would be the sarcolemma and the fruit of the grape would be the sarcoplasm. The sarcolemma is comprised of two layers. The innermost layer is a plasma membrane that totally surrounds each cell. The outermost layer is a basement membrane that is situated along the sides of the cell and continues from one cell to the next. This basement membrane binds the cells into muscle fibers. The contractile cells are separated one from the other by structures known as *intercalated disks*. The intercalated disks are found exclusively in cardiac muscle. They are not flat structures, but are more like a geometrical zigzag in three dimensions, with each cell meshing like a jigsaw puzzle. The intercalated disks are structures of extremely low electrical resistance. This characteristic feature facilitates rapid conduction of electrical impulses from one cell to the next.

The basic contractile structure of the cell is a system of filaments known as the *sarcomere*, shown in Figure 6-3.

There are many sarcomeres joined end to end within each cell; they form a continuous line stretching from one end of the cell to the other and are anchored into the intercalated disks. The sarcomeres are banded together

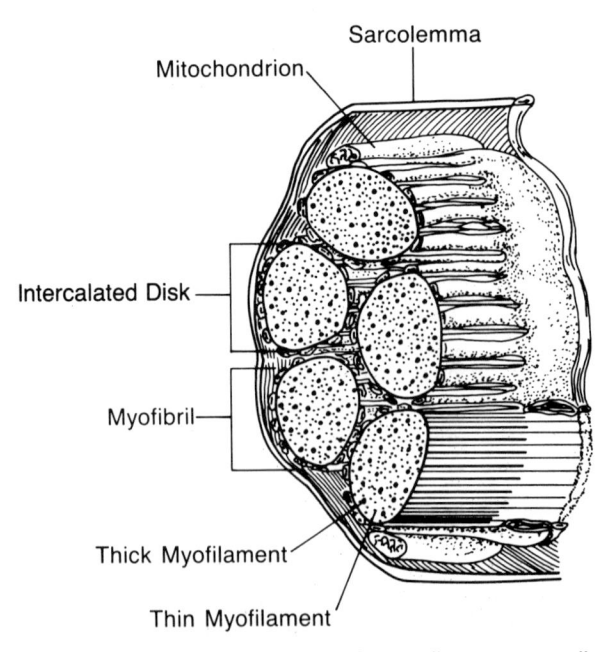

Figure 6-2 Cellular anatomy of an ordinary contractile cell.

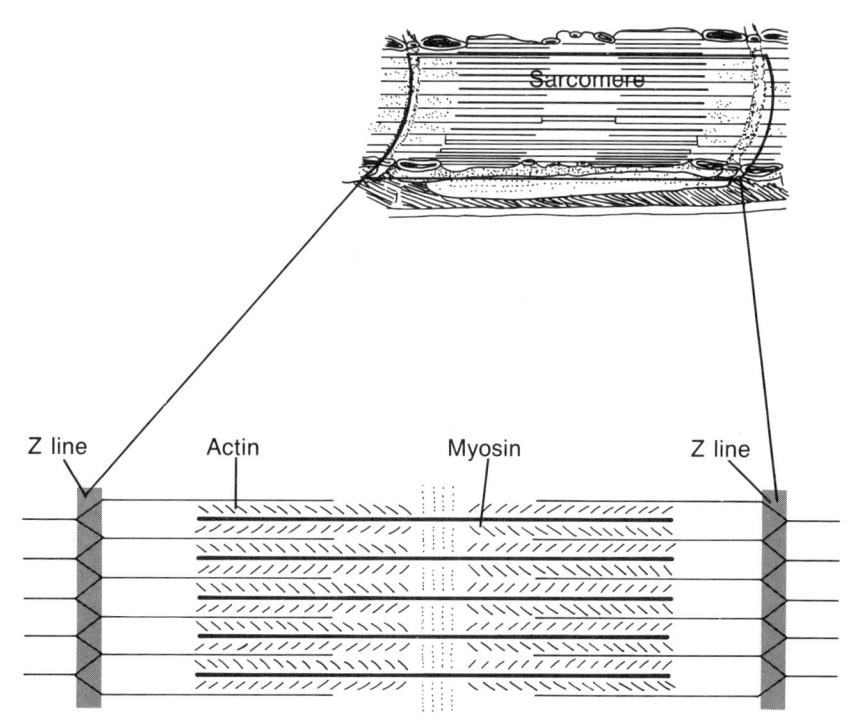

Figure 6-3 Detailed anatomy of the sarcomere—the basic contractile unit of the cardiac muscle cell. Each sarcomere is bordered by the Z line and is composed of thin (actin) and thick (myosin) myofilaments.

side by side. These bands of sarcomeres within the cells are known as *myofibrils*. Each contractile cell is packed with many myofibrils.

The filaments that comprise each sarcomere are composed of two types of myofilaments called *actin* (thin filaments) and *myosin* (thick filaments). These are referred to as such since the thin filaments are comprised principally of actin proteins and the thick filaments are comprised of myosin protein.

The actin filaments are attached at one end to the *Z line* and extend inward toward the center of each sarcomere. As Figure 6-3 demonstrates, the Z line is the border that separates each sarcomere. The cell's sarcolemma is indented regularly at the point where the Z lines lie in close proximity to it. This gives the sarcolemma a fine, bumpy appearance. The myosin filaments are suspended between the actin filaments. They are thicker than the actin and display a nodular thickening at their center. As Figure 6-3 demonstrates, the actin and myosin filaments overlap each other. The actin filaments appear smooth, whereas the myosin filaments have projections that come in contact with the surface of the actin. On cross section, each myosin filament is surrounded by six actin filaments in a geometric fashion, as is seen in Figure 6-4.

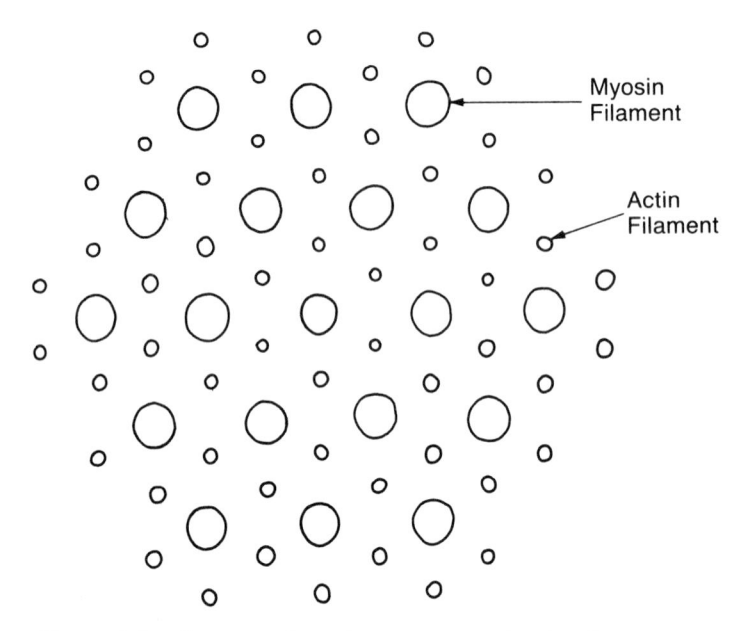

Figure 6-4 Cross section of a sarcomere showing the geometrical arrangement of the actin and myosin myofilaments. Note that each myosin filament is surrounded by six actin filaments.

During contraction, these filaments interdigitate, or slide between each other, thus shortening the length of the sarcomere and, consequently, the cell. The exact mechanism of this "interdigitation" will be covered in detail in the section on "Excitation-Contraction Coupling" at the end of this chapter.

Sandwiched between the myofibrils are structures called *mitochondria*, or *sarcosomes*. These structures provide the necessary energy required to carry on the metabolic and physiologic functions of the cells. The mitochondria convert carbohydrates, lipids, and protein into adenosine triphosphate (ATP) for use by the cell. The contractile cell has the greatest number of mitochondria as compared with the other types of cells within the heart. This is logical, considering the need for the tremendous amount of energy required to feed the continually contracting myocardium. These mitochondria are so numerous as to actually comprise between 25% and 50% of the muscle mass.

The basic function of contraction is initiated by electrical stimulation of the sarcolemma. Since each cell contains many myofibrils, there must be a structure allowing electrical current to reach the deepest myofibrils. This structure is known as the *sarcoplasmic reticulum*, illustrated in Figure 6-5.

The sarcoplasmic reticulum is a network of tubes that penetrate the cell and surround the myofibrils. These tubes may be divided into two systems,

Cellular Anatomy and Electrophysiology 73

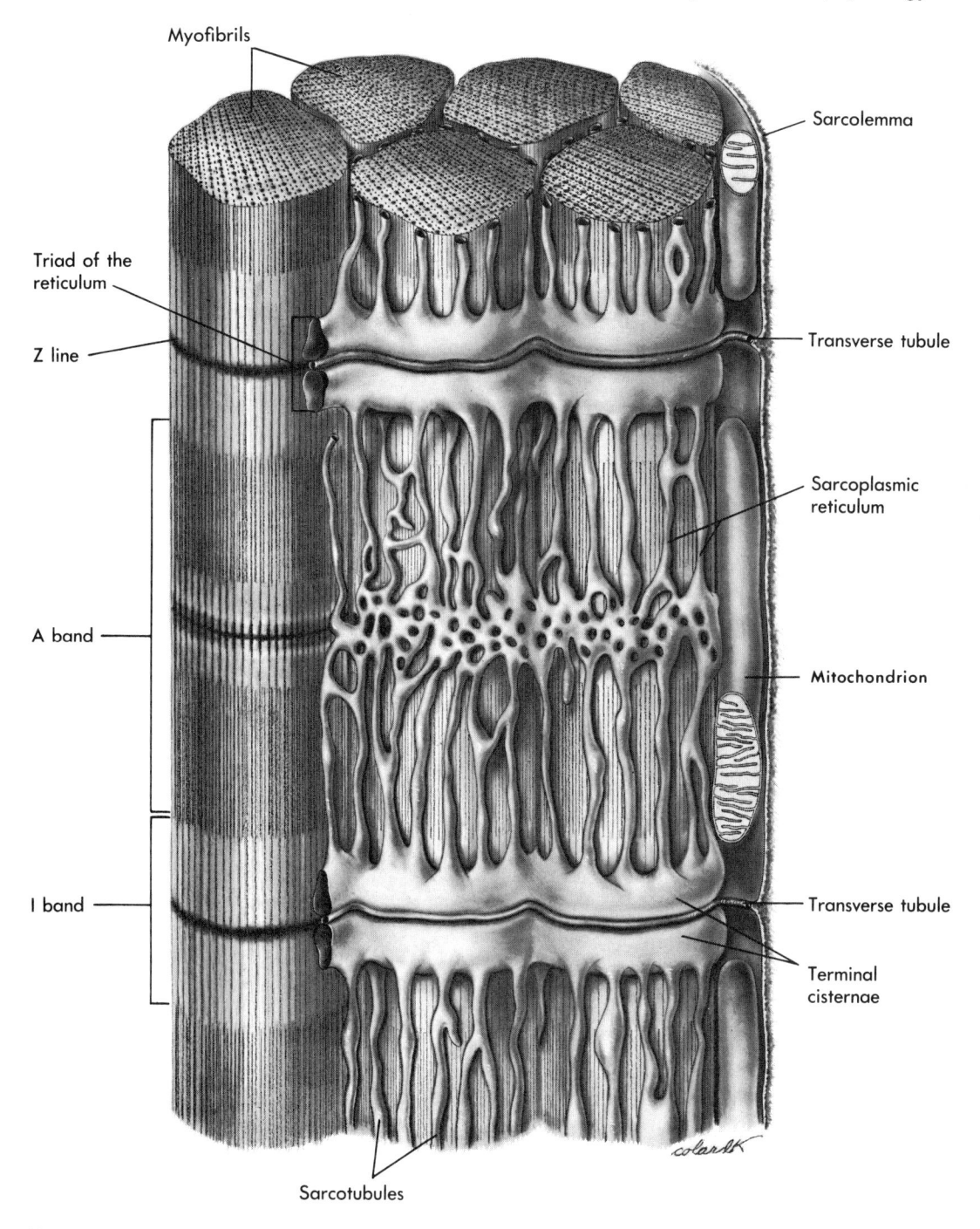

Figure 6-5 Structure of the sarcoplasmic reticulum. Note the T tubules that communicate with the extracellular area and the L system that surrounds the sarcomere. Also note the size and number of mitochondria.

the first of which is called the *T system*. The T system runs transversely across the cell at the level of the Z lines. This T system is a tubular network that penetrates the sarcolemma and opens to the extracellular space, thus permitting extracellular substances to come in close proximity to the deepest of myofibrils.

The sarcoplasmic reticulum also consists of a lateral and longitudinally oriented system of tubules known as the *L system*. These tubules run the length of the sarcomeres, surrounding them in a netlike fashion. There is no known direct connection between the transverse (T) and longitudinal (L) systems of the sarcoplasmic reticulum. The T system is thought primarily to be involved in conducting electrical impulses from the extracelluar area to the sarcomeres, in addition to storing calcium. The L system is thought to be more concerned simply with moving and storing the calcium ion reserve.

Finally, the cell nucleus is located in a central position between the other structures of the cell. However not much is known about its function.

Specialized Cells

The second subgroup of cardiac cells is concerned with impulse formation and conduction of cardiac electrical activity. These cells are referred to as the *specialized conduction cells*. They differ from the ordinary contractile cell not only in function, but in structure as well. There are three types of such cells—the *P cells*, the *transitional cells*, and *Purkinje's cells*.

P Cells

P Cells are located in the central portions of the sinus node, the AV node, and the internodal pathways. They are most densely concentrated in the sinus node, followed by the AV node, then the internodal tracts. It is thought that their main function is that of impulse formation and their location adds weight to this assumption.

P cells have no intercalated disks. Their junctions are formed by plasma membrane to plasma membrane junctions and they are clustered in groups surrounded by a single basement membrane.

Internally, the P cells contain few, if any, myofibrils, demonstrating a relatively "empty" appearance compared to the myofibril-packed contractile cell. The P cells have a poorly developed sarcoplasmic reticular network, although there are occasional tubules here and there of varying length and internal caliber. This is presumably due to the lack of contractile sarcomeres and their need for a reticular network within the cells.

The plasma membrane of the sarcolemma exhibits a more profound set of indentations as compared to the contractile cell.

The P cells have fewer mitochondria than the previously described contractile cell since the metabolic demand for contractile processes is absent. The mitochondria are randomly distributed within the cell.

The nucleus of the P cell comprises a greater bulk of the cell than that found in the contractile cells.

Transitional Cells

The second type of specialized cells, the transitional cells, are located along the margins of the P cells and surround them. They are the sole link between the P cells and the rest of the heart.

Transitional cells have a structure similar to that of the P cells and those of the rest of the heart. They are more elongated and may resemble the P cell at one end and a contractile cell at the other end. Both the sinus node and the AV node are comprised primarily of transitional cells; however, the percentage of transitional cells to P cells is much greater in the AV node than the sinus node.

The sarcoplasmic reticulum becomes more developed as the transitional cell intermingles with the contractile cells. Their myofibrils increase in number for the same reason as they become arranged in their more usual parallel fashion, as compared to the contractile cell.

Purkinje's Cells

The last of the three types of specialized cells and the final of the four types of cardiac cells to be described are the Purkinje's cells. It is important to note that the *Purkinje's cell* is not to be confused with *"Purkinje's network."* The Purkinje's cells are not named because of their location within the heart, but rather are named for their functional properties. Purkinje's cells comprise a majority of the specialized fibers. They are structurally similar to the P cells with some minor differences. The Purkinje's cells contain a few scattered myofibrils but, unlike the P cells, the myofibrils are arranged in a parallel fashion, as opposed to the unorganized myofibrils of the P cells. Additionally, the Purkinje's cells have fully developed intercalated disks—much the same as the contractile cells of the working myocardium, whereas the P cells have a plasma membrane-to-plasma membrane connection. Since the intercalated disks are areas of low resistance, this supports the role of the Purkinje's cells in rapid electrical conduction. The Purkinje's cells have a centrally located nucleus with a majority of their mitochondria located proximally. The final difference to be mentioned is their location within the specialized conduction system. This lends to their classification as a separate cell of the heart since they are located outside the central regions of the sinus and AV nodes and are generally (under normal circumstances) not involved in pacing the heart, though they have the functional capability of doing so when necessary.

Cellular Electrophysiologic Properties

Excitability and Conduction

All cardiac myocardial tissue is said to be excitable. Excitability is the ability of a cell to respond to an external stimulus. Cardiac tissue is responsive to three basic types of stimuli—chemical, mechanical, and electrical.

Chemical. Myocardial excitability may be enhanced or depressed by exposure to certain chemicals. For example, exposure to higher-than-normal levels of potassium will cause the cardiac cell to depolarize.

Mechanical. Myocardial cells may be depolarized by mechanical stimulation. This is the principle behind the "precordial thump" delivered to patients experiencing cardiac standstill while being monitored. More commonly, though, mechanical stimulation may be witnessed during cardiac catheterization when the catheter strikes the heart wall, causing an extrasystole or premature complex.

Electrical. This is by far the most common means by which the myocardium is stimulated. Electrical stimulation is initiated by a spontaneous impulse arising from an automatic cell somewhere within the heart (usually the sinus node).

It is important to understand the functional syncytial nature of myocardial tissue. A mass of cells functions as a syncytium when it displays what may be termed an all-or-nothing principle. That is, what happens to one cell of this mass of cells happens also to all the other cells of that same mass. This applies to cardiac depolarization. The two syncytiums to be concerned with are the atria and the ventricles. As one cell in either group is stimulated, the impulse will be conducted from that cell to the next, and so on, until all the cells are depolarized. If the AV node is intact, the impulse will be transmitted to the ventricles where the all-or-nothing principle is repeated. These two syncytiums are insulated from each other by a structure previously described as the *anulus fibrosus*. Again, the only normal conduction pathway between the atria and the ventricles is the AV node.

All cardiac cells conduct impulses. However, the majority of the specialized conduction system cells conduct these impulses at a much faster rate of speed than other cardiac cells. Ventricular myocardium transmits impulses at a speed of approximately 13 feet per second, while the Purkinje's fibers propagate impulses at a speed of 130 feet per second—10 times faster. On the other hand, propagation of impulses through the AV junction may be as slow as 6 feet per second. The depressed rate of conductivity through this area prevents the transmission of excessively high rates of impulses sometimes found in the atria, such as that of atrial flutter. If these impulses were conducted to the ventricles, they would not have sufficient time to fill with blood, thereby reducing the cardiac output and resulting in probable death.

As mentioned earlier, there are contractile cells found within the specialized conduction system of the heart, intermingled with the Purkinje's cells. This may suggest that though the specialized fibers are charged with rapidly conducting electrical impulses, some of the working myocardial cells may also be capable of rapid conduction.

Automaticity

Automaticity may be defined as the ability of a cell to initiate a depolarization impulse *without* external stimulation. Many of the cells of the specialized conduction system possess automatic capabilities. The intrinsic rate of any one given cell is dictated by its relative position in the specialized conduction system. For example, automatic cells of the sinus node possess an intrinsic or inherent rate of approximately 60 to 100 impulses per minute. The AV junctional cells possess an inherent rate of approximately 40 to 60 impulses per minute, while the Purkinje's network cell possesses an inherent rate of approximately 40 or less impulses per minute.

Stimulation of automatic cardiac cells at a rate higher than the inherent rate of that cell produces an inhibitory effect. If an AV junctional cell (with an inherent rate of 40 to 60 impulses per minute) were stimulated at a rate of 72 impulses per minute by the sinus node, the AV junctional cell would be inhibited or prevented from initiating its own impulse. This hierarchy of automaticity serves to maintain orderly cardiac electrical activity. Additionally, it also maintains a "fail-safe" mechanism to provide stimulation when needed should any one group of cells farther up in this hierarchy of cells fail to stimulate the lower conduction system. Indeed, if conduction were blocked at the AV node, the ventricles would receive no stimulation from the atria. Once the automatic cells of the ventricles are no longer inhibited by the higher atrial rate, they begin to discharge at their own inherent rate and take over the pacing responsibilities of the ventricles. This phenomenon is classically demonstrated in the patient with complete heart block. The atrial-to-ventricular conduction is blocked somewhere in or near the AV node. The atria continue to discharge at a rate of 75 impulses or so per minute while the ventricles, receiving no inhibitory stimulation from the atria, discharge at their inherent rate of 40 impulses per minute or less. (See Chapter 7.)

Refractory Period

Refractory periods occur immediately following depolarization of the cardiac cell. The cell will only respond to stimuli when it is in the polarized or resting state. Once the cell has been stimulated, it is said to be in a depolarized state. While the cell is in this depolarized state, it is refractory, or unresponsive, to external stimuli. This is an important characteristic of cardiac tissue and will be discussed in greater detail in the following section.

The Action Potential

The action potential is a wave form recorded on an instrument similar to the electrocardiograph itself. It represents the measure of electrical potential differences between the interior (intracellular) and exterior (extracellular) areas of the myocardial cell. This tracing is obtained by placing one electrode inside a cell and one electrode outside of the cell. In order to understand more easily the nature of the action potential of the specialized fibers, it would be helpful to first review the action potential recording of an ordinary contractile myocardial cell.

Figure 6-6 represents a typical action potential recording through a single, complete phase of cardiac depolarization and repolarization. Note that the action potential has five different phases:

Phase 4: This is the stage when the cell is *polarized*—that is, there is a

78 Electrophysiology

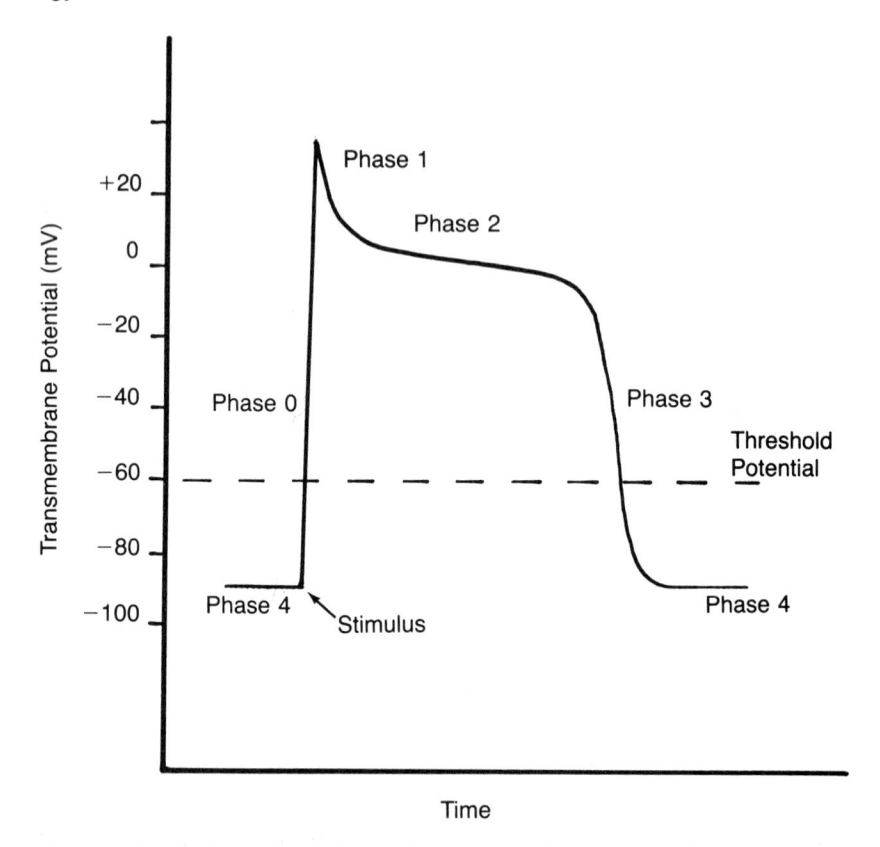

Figure 6-6 Action potential recording of an ordinary contractile cell, obtained by placing one electrode inside the cell and one electrode outside the cell, then recording the electrical activity. Phase 4: Resting; Phase 0: Depolarization; Phase 1: Return to 0 mV; Phase 2: Plateau; Phase 3: Repolarization.

potential difference measured between the interior and exterior of the cell. The actual potential difference is measured at about −90 millivolts (mV). At this point, the cell is in an excitable state, awaiting a stimulus to cause it to depolarize.

Phase 0: During this phase, note that the cell is actively undergoing *depolarization*. Phase 0 begins when the cell receives an impulse. This is a *rapid* upstroke. In fact, the upstroke is so rapid that the voltage actually overshoots the zero potential line.

Phase 1: During this short phase, the potential difference comes to rest near 0 mV.

Phase 2: During this phase, the potential difference remains near 0 mV. Logically, since the potential difference is relatively zero, this is the time period when the cell is said to be in a *depolarized* state. At the end of this phase, the cell beings to *repolarize* as Phase 3 of the action potential begins.

Phase 3: This is the *repolarization* phase. During this phase, the cell moves to restore itself to the original polarized state from a potential difference of 0 mV back to its resting, excitable state of -90 mV and Phase 4. Note that Phase 4 remains stable at -90 mV.

These processes now make evident the origin of the terms depolarization, polarization, and repolarization.

Now that the cardiac action potential has been reviewed, concepts previously mentioned in the text can be related directly to the action potential recording.

Excitability. When the cell is polarized (Phase 4), it can respond to external stimulation. The stimulation must be of sufficient magnitude to push the potential above a point known as the *threshold* potential. Whenever the threshold potential is reached, the cell depolarizes. If the arriving stimulus does not reach the threshold potential, the cell will not depolarize. The normal threshold potential for the ordinary myocardial cell is around -60 mV.

Refractory Period. As the cell can only respond to external stimulation when it is polarized, it likewise will not respond to external stimulation while it is depolarized. This is refractoriness and occurs during Phase 1, Phase 2 and part of Phase 3. See Figure 6-7.

The refractory period may be divided into two parts: the *absolute refractory period* and the *relative refractory period*. During the absolute refractory period, the cell will not respond to external stimulation of any magnitude. Since the cell is unresponsive to stimulation during the absolute refractory period, this time period serves to protect the cell against excessively high rates of stimulation. During the relative refractory period, however, the cell will respond to external stimulation but only of higher magnitudes than normal. Additionally, the resulting action potential generated after stimulation during the relative refractory period will be slurred and of lower magnitude. The relative refractory period is a time of transition, very short in duration, between absolute refractoriness and the excitable state.

Ionic Basis for the Action Potential

The changes in electrical potential just described are a result of the movement of certain ions across the sarcolemma of the cell. The sarcolemma is a selective membrane that either admits, bars, or transports certain ions between the intracellular and extracellular areas of the cardiac cell. This accomplishes the required changes in electrical potential necessary to propagate, or advance, an electrical charge to the next cell.

The principle ions responsible for this activity are potassium (K^+), sodium (Na^+), and calcium (Ca^{2+}).

Figure 6-8 outlines the ionic activity present during the different phases of the action potential. During Phase 4, the cell is polarized and in a resting,

80 Electrophysiology

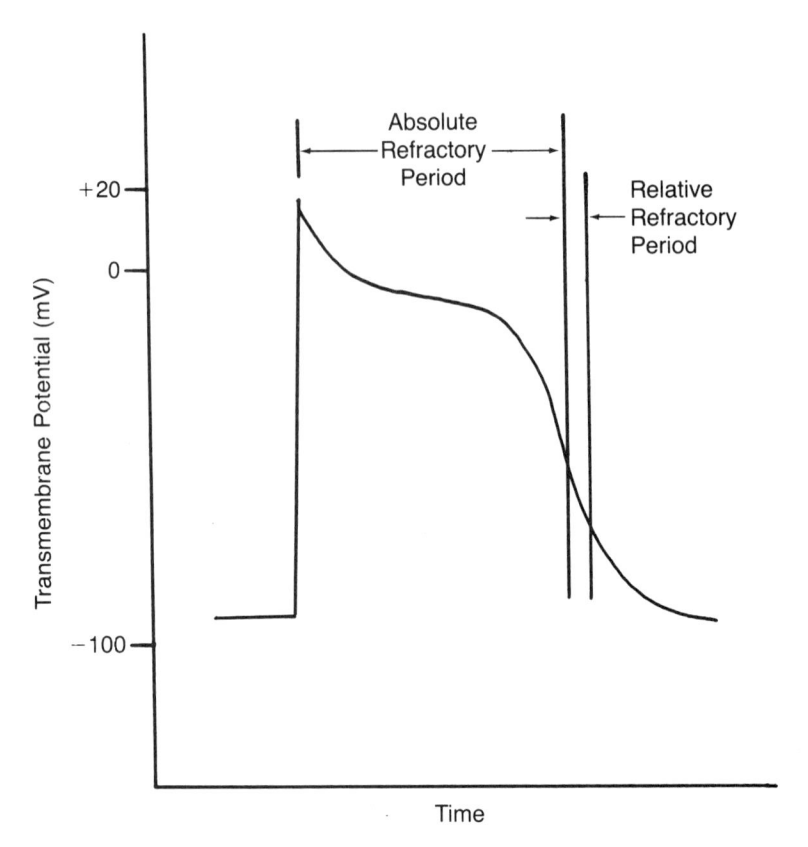

Figure 6-7 Refractory periods during the action potential. The cell is unresponsive to stimuli during the absolute refractory period, but is responsive to stimuli of higher magnitudes during the relative refractory period.

excitable state. There is a relatively high concentration of potassium (K^+) ions inside the cell and a relatively high concentration of sodium (Na^+) ions outside the cell. This ionic imbalance is responsible for the potential difference of -90 mV. When a stimulus above threshold potential strikes the cell, the sarcolemma instantly becomes permeable to Na^+ ions and the cell *depo*larizes. The Na^+ ions rush into the cell, causing the potential difference to race toward zero. This is Phase 0 of the action potential. This inward rush is so rapid that the potential difference goes beyond the 0 mV potential.

Phases 1, 2, and 3 of the action potential are not yet completely understood. The following text summarizes recent research supporting the ionic activity that is believed to be at least partially responsible for these phases.

Near the end of Phase 0, as the potential value reaches an area near

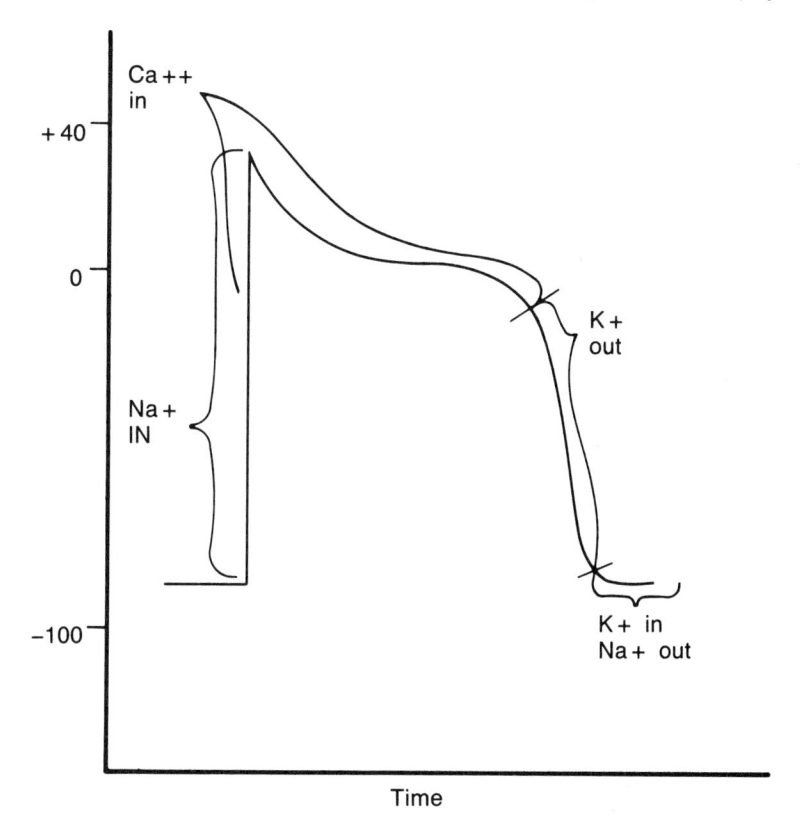

Figure 6-8 Ionic movement across the sarcolemma during each phase of the action potential. Phase 4: Resting; Phase 0: Sodium rapidly in; Late Phase 0: Slow calcium in; Phases 1 and 2: Calcium slowly in; Phase 3: Potassium out; Phase 4: Sodium out, potassium in.

−20 mV or so, the sarcolemma begins to allow a slow inward movement of calcium (Ca^{2+}) ions. When the rapidly rising Phase 0 ends (near +20 mV), the potential difference falls to the plateau near 0 mV (Phase 1). This happens because of the cessation of Na^+ ions' inward flow. The "plateau" phase (Phase 2) is named due to its relative appearance. During Phase 2 there is a continued slow inward movement of Ca^{2+} ions (which had begun during the latter half of Phase 0) that causes the potential difference to remain close to 0 mV. Phase 3 of the action potential occurs as the cell begins to extrude K^+ ions across the sarcolemma to the extracellular area. This is the repolarization phase of the cell. As the cell's potential difference reaches Phase 4 and −90 mV, a process occurs that exchanges the Na^+ still inside the cell (left from Phase 0) for the K^+ just pushed out. This is done so that the concentrations present before the initial stimulus arrived are restored. This process is referred to as the *sodium-potassium pump* and should not be considered an anatomical structure.

Action Potential of the Specialized Cells

P Cells. Since the P cells are responsible for the pacemaking activity of the heart, their action potential differs from the ordinary myocardial cell previously described. Referring to Figure 6-9, the most important difference noted is the lack of a stable resting potential during Phase 4. The upward sloping of Phase 4 is a diastolic depolarization of the cell membrane. The P cell displays automaticity characteristics previously described and this diastolic depolarization is responsible for the pacemaking activity.

The ionic activity responsible for the Phase 4 diastolic depolarization is not understood. However, as diastolic depolarization continues, it eventually reaches the threshold potential and begins Phase 0. The overall potential differences encountered in the P cell are generally above those of the ordi-

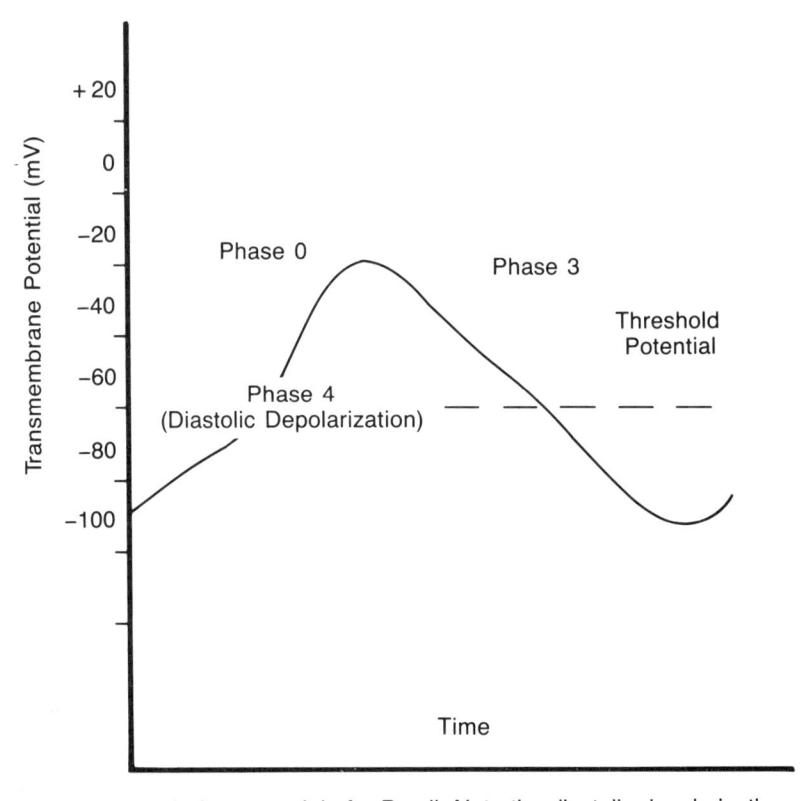

Figure 6-9 Action potential of a P cell. Note the diastolic depolarization during Phase 4 that is responsible for the pacemaking activity. As the transmembrane potential reaches threshold, the cell depolarizes.

nary contractile cell. This includes the threshold potential, as Figure 6-9 depicts. Phase 1 is indistinguishable from Phase 2, which is much less of a plateau. The Phase 3 slope is less steep and merges gracefully with Phase 4, where the diastolic depolarization process begins once again.

It is interesting to note that the relative slope of the diastolic depolarization phase will determine the inherent impulse formation rate or discharging rate of the cell. As the heart rate slows, the slope of Phase 4 of the pacemaking cell begins to flatten so that it takes longer for the cell to reach threshold potential. Therefore, a P cell located in the sinus node will have a faster rate of diastolic depolarization than a P cell located in the AV node, which has a slower inherent rate.

Transitional and Purkinje's Cells. The action potential of the transitional and Purkinje's cells is similar to that of both the P cell and the contractile cell.

As Figure 6-10 demonstrates, Phases 0, 1, 2, and 3 are quite similar to

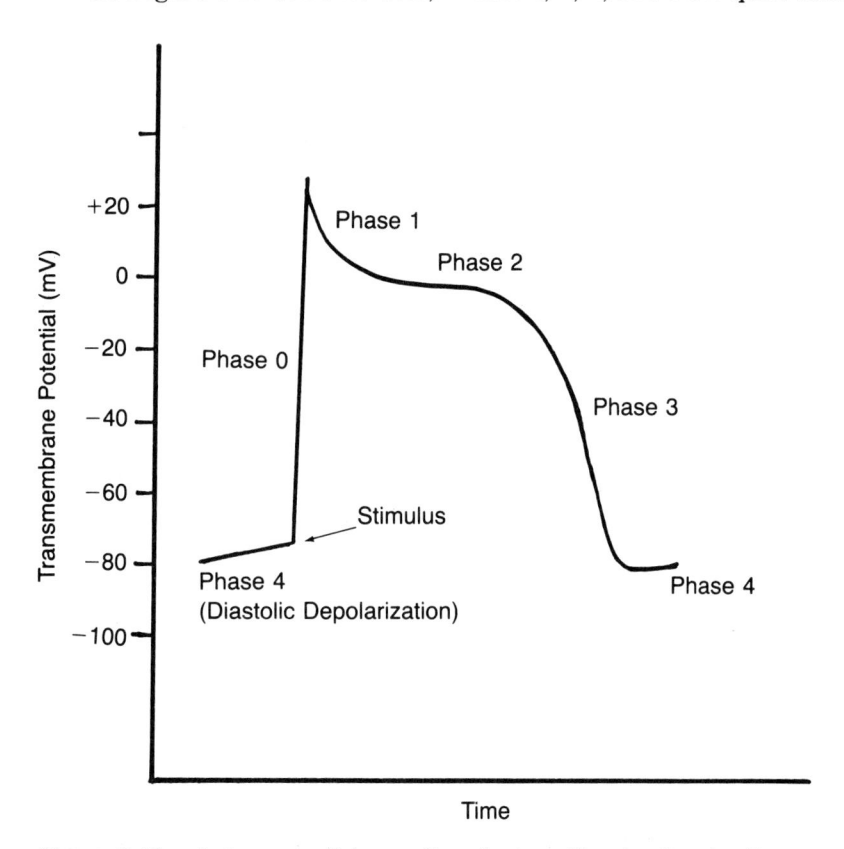

Figure 6-10 Action potential recording of a transitional cell and a Purkinje cell. These cells combine the characteristics of both the P cell (diastolic depolarization) and the ordinary contractile cell (rapid depolarization [Phase 0] and a plateau [Phase 2]).

the contractile cell. Phase 4, however, displays a slow diastolic depolarization more consistent with that of the P cells. This diastolic depolarization becomes more pronounced as the inhibitory effect of the higher rates of stimulation of the P cells are removed. This affords the transitional and Purkinje's cells with automatic properties.

Excitation-Contraction Coupling

Excitation-contraction coupling is the process by which the contractile cells contract once they have been stimulated. The contraction process is actually a function of the reaction between Ca^{2+} ions and the *actin/myosin* protein filaments rather than a result of electrical charges applied to these proteins. In Figure 6-11, the actin and myosin structures are shown in detail.

The myosin filaments have small projections called *cross-bridges*. These cross-bridges come in contact with the actin filaments. The actin filaments have small binding sites along their length.

When the cell is in the relaxed (stretched) state, a protein known as *troponin-tropomyosin* covers the binding sites of the actin filaments which inhibits their binding ability. When the sarcolemma is stimulated, Ca^{2+} is released from the L system and T tubules of the sarcoplasmic reticulum into the intracellular areas adjacent to the sarcomeres. The Ca^{2+} acts to neutralize the inhibitory effect of the troponin-tropomyosin protein and the cross-

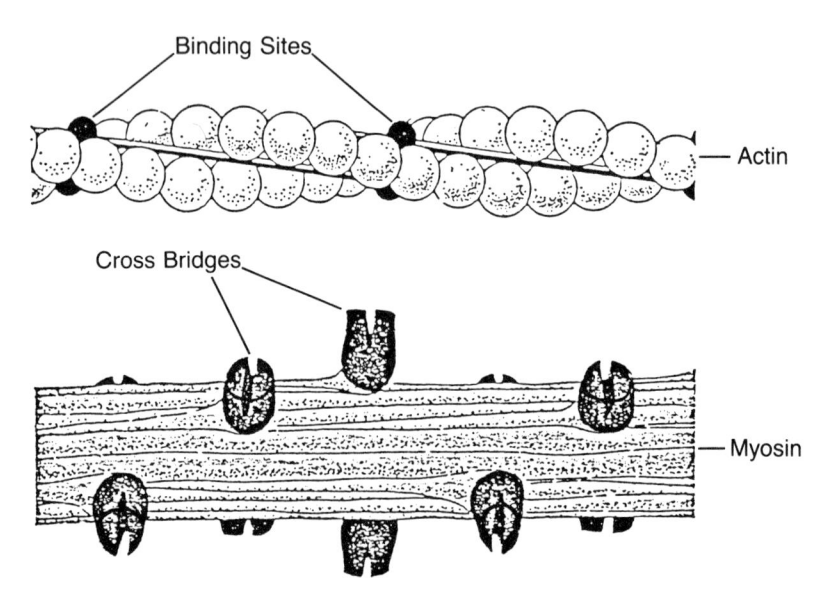

Figure 6-11 Ultrastructure of the actin and myosin myofilaments. Demonstrating the cross bridges of the myosin and the binding sites of the actin. (Adapted from Ham AW, Cormack DH: Histology, 8th ed. Philadelphia, JB Lippincott, 1979.)

bridges of the myosin filaments are attracted to the binding sites of the actin filaments. The cross-bridges bend and pull the myosin filaments along the shaft of the actin filaments, causing the filaments to interdigitate and the cell to shorten.

After a short period of time, the intracellular Ca^{2+} is pumped back into the sarcoplasmic reticulum and the troponin-tropomyosin protein again inhibits the attraction between the cross-bridges of the myosin and the binding sites of the actin, and the cell relaxes.

Bibliography

Bloom W, Fawcett DW: A Textbook of Histology, 9th ed. Philadelphia, WB Saunders, 1965

Chung EK: Electrocardiography: Practical Applications with Vectorial Principles, 2d ed. Hagerstown, Harper and Row, 1980

Ciba Collection of Medical Illustrations: The Heart, Vol. 5. Summit, NJ, Ciba Pharmaceutical Company, 1978

University of Maryland School of Pharmacy: Cornell Postgraduate Course on Cardiac Arrhythmias. New York, Medcom, 1981

Guyton AR: Textbook of Medical Physiology, 6th ed. Philadelphia, WB Saunders, 1981

Helfant RH: Bellet's Essentials of Cardiac Arrhythmias, 2d ed. Philadelphia, WB Saunders, 1980

Hurst WJ, et al: The Heart, Arteries and Veins, 4th ed. New York, McGraw-Hill, 1978

Keung ECH, Aronson RS: Physiology of calcium current in cardiac muscle. Prog Cardiov Dis 25 (4): 279–296, 1983

Little RC: Physiology of the Heart and Circulation, 3d ed. Chicago, Year Book Medical Pub, 1985

Phillips RE, Feeney MK: The Cardiac Rhythms—A Systematic Approach to Interpretation, 2d ed. Philadelphia, WB Saunders, 1980

Tortora GJ, Anagnostakos NP: Principles of Anatomy and Physiology, 3d ed. New York, Harper and Row, 1981

Wellens HJJ: The Conduction System of the Heart—Structure, Function, and Clinical Applications. Philadelphia, Lea and Febiger, 1976

Chapter 7

Electrocardiography and Arrhythmias

Dale Davis

An electrocardiogram (ECG) is a graphic recording of the electrical activity of the heart each time it contracts. To make a recording, electrodes are placed on the four limbs and designated areas of the chest and, by the use of various combinations of these electrodes, 12 different electrical views of the heart are recorded on ECG graph paper. Each electrical view is considered an *ECG lead*.

Standard Leads

The standard leads are called *bipolar leads* because they are composed of two electrodes—one that is positive and one that is negative. The ECG records the difference in electrical potential between them.

Lead I is derived from an electrode on the right arm that is designated as negative and an electrode on the left arm that is considered positive. *Lead II* is composed of an electrode on the right arm that is considered negative and one on the left leg that is considered positive. *Lead III* is made up of an electrode on the left arm that is designated as negative and one on the left leg that is designated as positive. A fourth electrode is placed on the right leg but is used only to stabilize the ECG and takes no part in ECG lead formation. Figure 7-1 demonstrates these standard leads.

Augmented Leads

The same three electrodes used for standard lead formation are used for the augmented leads, but in different combinations. The augmented leads are *unipolar leads* because they are composed of one positive electrode—either

LEAD I **LEAD II** **LEAD III**

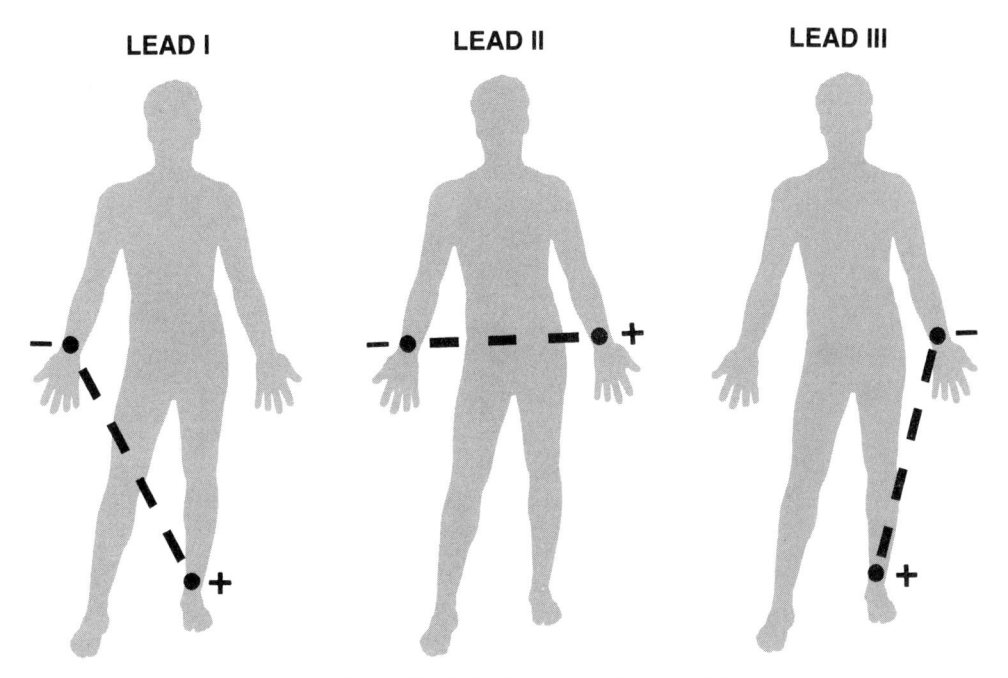

Figure 7-1 Standard leads. (From Davis D: How to Quickly and Accurately Master ECG Interpretation. Philadelphia, JB Lippincott, 1985)

the left arm, right arm, or left leg—recording the electrical potential at that one point with reference to the other two remaining leads. Because of the manner in which these leads are arranged, the voltage is extremely low and must be augmented in order to equal the voltage of the remainder of the ECG. This augmentation is accomplished by the ECG machine.

AVR (augmented voltage of the right arm). The right arm is the positive electrode in reference to the left arm and left leg. *AVL* (augmented voltage of the left arm). The left arm is considered as the positive electrode in reference to the right arm and left leg. *AVF* (augmented voltage of the left foot). The left leg is the positive electrode in reference to the left arm and right arm. (Figure 7-2 illustrates the augmented leads.)

Precordial Leads

The six precordial leads are *unipolar leads* and view the electrical activity of the heart in the horizontal plane. A suction cup is placed on six different positions on the chest in order to obtain the correct precordial recordings:

V_1 4th intercostal space to the right of the sternum
V_2 4th intercostal space to the left of the sternum
V_3 Directly between V_2 and V_4 on the diagonal

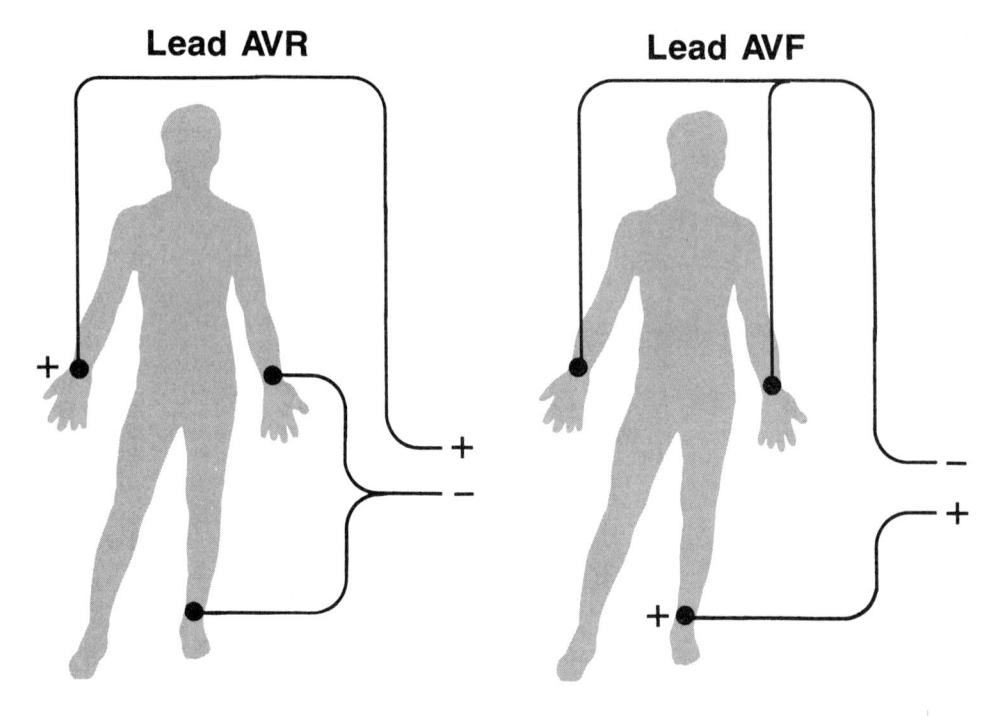

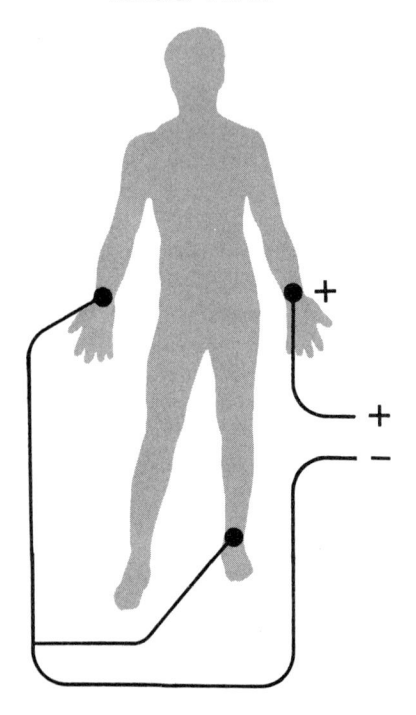

Figure 7-2 Augmented leads. (From Davis D: How to Quickly and Accurately Master ECG Interpretation. Philadelphia, JB Lippincott, 1985)

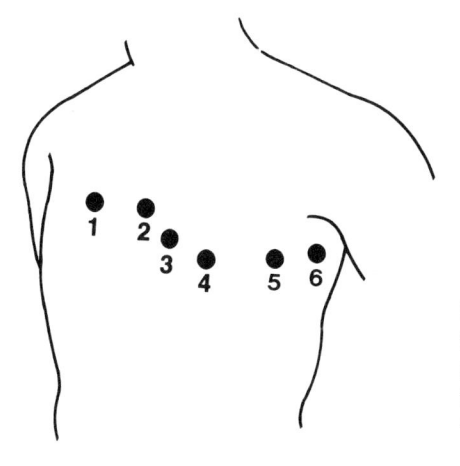

Figure 7-3 Precordial lead placement. (From Davis D: How to Quickly and Accurately Master ECG Interpretation. Philadelphia, JB Lippincott, 1985)

V_4 5th intercostal space—left midclavicular (midcollarbone) line
V_5 5th intercostal space—left anterior axillary (armpit) line
V_6 5th intercostal space—left midaxillary line

See Figure 7-3 for this precordial lead placement.

Depolarization and Repolarization

Each cardiac cell is surrounded by and filled with a solution that contains ions. In the resting period of the cell, the inside of the cell membrane is considered negatively charged and the outside of the cell membrane is positively charged. The movement of these ions inside and across the cell membrane constitutes a flow of electricity that generates the signals on the ECG.

When an electrical impulse is generated in the heart, the inside of the cardiac cell rapidly becomes positive in relation to the outside of the cell. The electrical impulse causing this excited state and change in polarity is called *depolarization*. The return of the stimulated cell to its resting state is called *repolarization*. The resting state is maintained until the next wave of depolarization (Figure 7-4).

Electrical Conduction System

In the normal heart, the cardiac impulse originates in the sinus or sinoatrial (SA) node called the *pacemaker of the heart*, located in the wall of the right atrium. The sinus impulses spread to both atria, causing them to depolarize. Atrial depolarization is represented on an ECG by a P wave (usually upright and slightly rounded).

When cardiac cells depolarize, they must also repolarize in order to regain their proper resting charge. Atrial repolarization is usually not visible

90 Electrocardiography and Arrhythmias

Figure 7-4 Depolarization and repolarization of the cardiac cell.

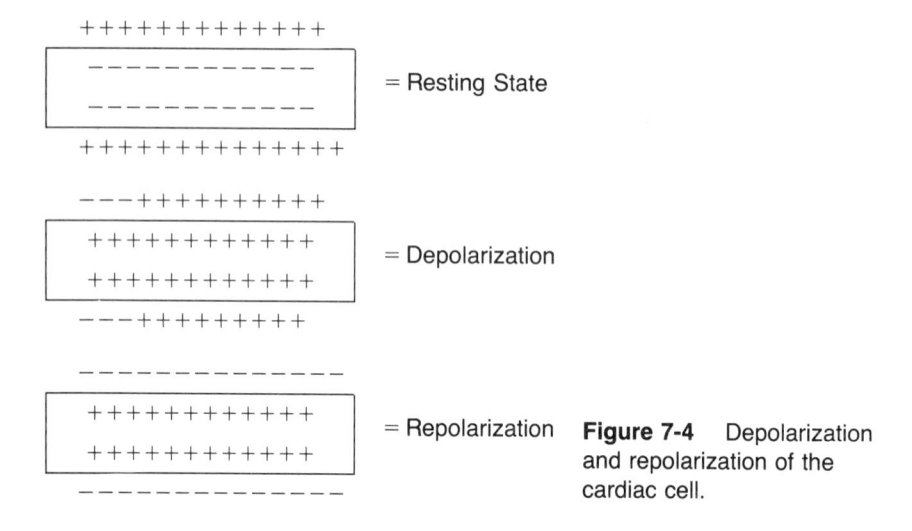

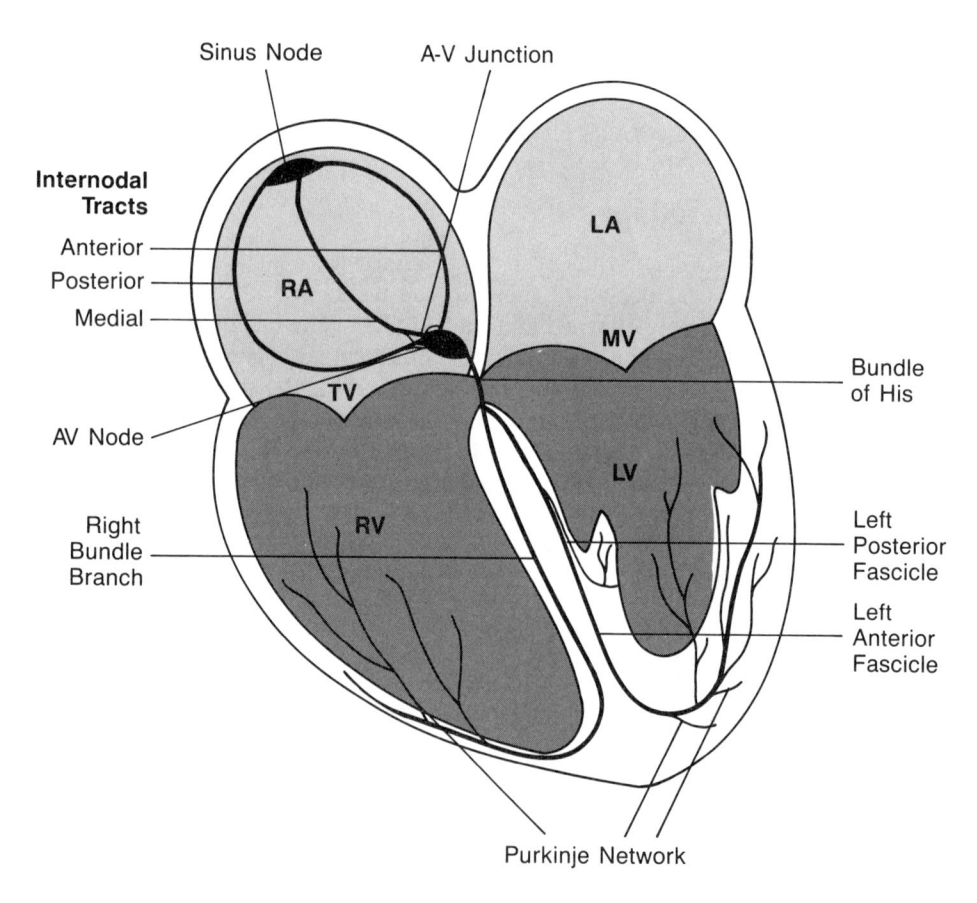

Figure 7-5 Electrical conduction system.

on the ECG. The electrical impulse then spreads from the atria to the atrioventricular (AV) node, which is located in the lower part of the intraatrial septum. The PR interval represents atrial excitation and contraction, the penetration of the AV node by the impulse.

From the AV node, the electrical impulse travels to the bundle of His, which is located in the interventricular septum. The bundle of His immediately divides into the left and right bundle branches. The right bundle branch supplies electrical impulses to the right ventricle, and the left bundle branch supplies the left ventricle. The left bundle divides almost immediately into the anterior fascicle, which supplies the anterior and superior portions of the left ventricle with electrical impulses, and the posterior fascicle, which supplies the posterior and inferior portions of the left ventricle with electrical impulses. Impulses travel down the bundle branches into the Purkinje's fibers located in the ventricular myocardium and cause ventricular depolarization. Ventricular depolarization is represented on an ECG by a QRS complex. Ventricular repolarization is represented on the ECG by a T wave.

The ST segment is a sensitive indicator of myocardial ischemia or injury. It is the distance from the point where the S wave of the QRS ends (J point) to the onset of the ascending limb of the T wave (Figures 7-5 and 7-6).

A QRS complex may be composed of a Q wave, an R wave, and an S wave, or various combinations of them.

R wave is a *positive* deflection of a QRS.

Q wave is a *negative* deflection of a QRS *before* an R wave.

S wave is a *negative* deflection of a QRS *after* an R wave.

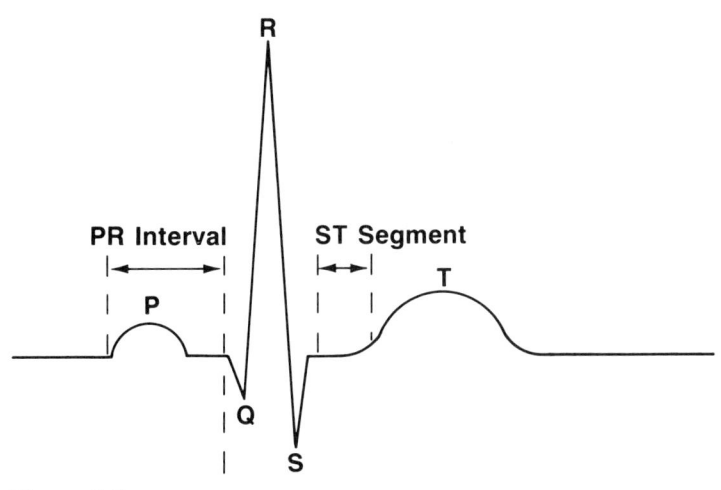

Figure 7-6

92 Electrocardiography and Arrhythmias

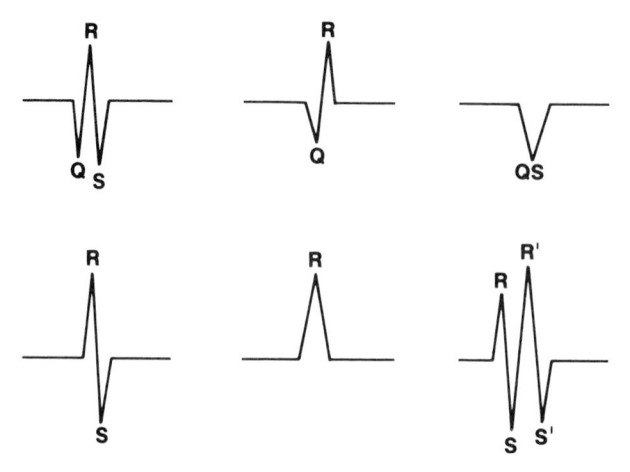

An R wave is a positive deflection.
A Q wave is a negative deflection before an R wave.
An S wave is a negative deflection after an R wave.

Figure 7-7   Various kinds of QRS complexes. (From Davis D: How to Quickly and Accurately Master ECG Interpretation. Philadelphia, JB Lippincott, 1985)

A ventricular depolarization complex is always called a QRS complex whether all three waves are present or not (Figure 7-7).

On an ECG, the point of reference is always the *isoelectric line*. This is the line before the P wave. Any stylus movement above this line is considered positive or elevated and any movement below this line is considered negative or depressed. Any P or T wave that is both above and below the isoelectric line is considered *diphasic* (Figure 7-8).

ECG Graph Paper and Measurements

On the horizontal axis of the graph paper, time is measured in seconds. Each small square is .04 second in duration and each large square is .20 second in duration. On the vertical axis voltage or height is measured in millimeters

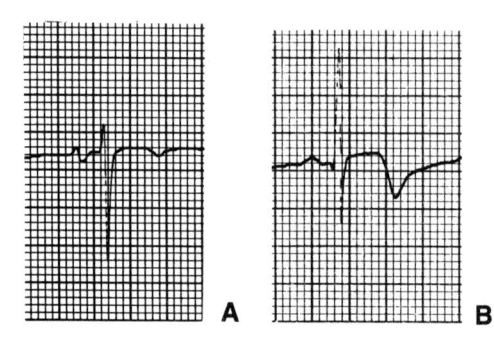

Figure 7-8   (*A*) Diphasic P wave. (*B*) Diphasic T wave.

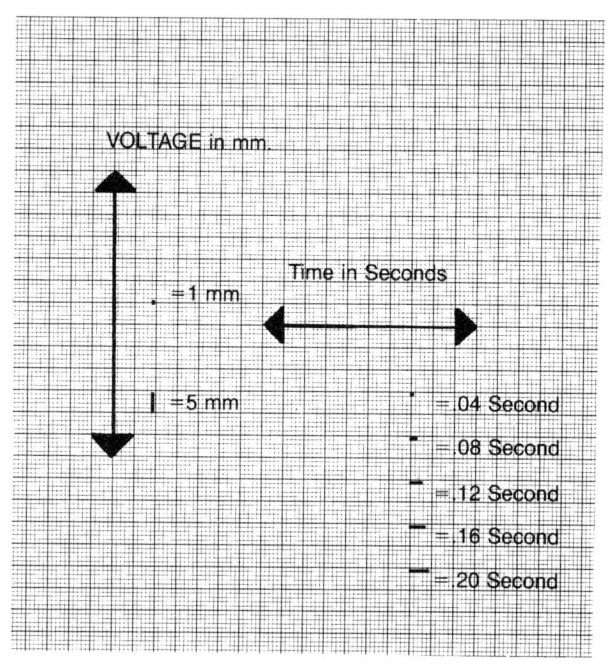

Figure 7-9 Measuring ECG graph paper.

(mm). Each small square is 1 mm high and each large square is 5 mm high (Figure 7-9).

PR Interval: Measure from the beginning of the P wave, where the P wave lifts off the isoelectric line, to the beginning of the first wave of the QRS complex. Count along the horizontal axis every .04 second (.04, .08, .12, .16, and .20 second, etc.) until you obtain the correct distance between the two points; this is the PR interval in seconds. The normal range for a PR interval is .12 to .20 second. If the PR interval is greater than .20 second, first degree AV block is present. If the PR interval is shorter than .12 second, accelerated AV conduction is present.

QRS Interval: Measure from the beginning of the first wave of the QRS, where it lifts off the isoelectric line, to the end of the last wave of the QRS. Count along the horizontal axis every .04 second until you obtain the correct distance between the two points; this is the QRS interval in seconds. The normal range for a QRS is .04 to .11 second (Figure 7-10).

ST Segment and T wave: The ST segment should be isoelectric. Possible pathological ST segment elevation or depression is 1 mm or more above or below the isoelectric line. The T waves should be upright and slightly rounded in most leads (Figure 7-10a).

Determination of Rate

Heart rate is the number of times the heart depolarizes and contracts in one minute. On an ECG, the ventricular rate is measured from R wave to R wave

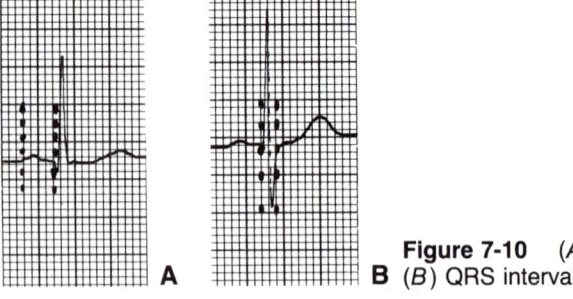

Figure 7-10 (A) PR interval of .16 second. (B) QRS interval of .08 second.

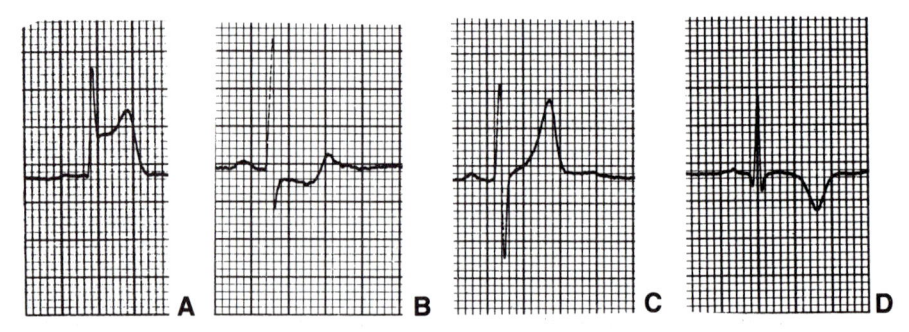

Figure 7-10a (A) ST elevation. (B) ST depression. (C) Normal T wave. (D) Inverted T wave.

and the atrial rate is measured from P wave to P wave. QRS complexes represent ventricular depolarizations and P waves represent atrial depolarizations. The ventricular and atrial rate are usually the same unless an arrhythmia is present. Use the calipers to check the regularity of the R to R and P to P cycles in the rhythm strip being observed.

Determining the heart rate by utilizing a rate ruler is easy and extremely accurate. The directions for use are printed on the rate ruler. Unfortunately, technicians do not always carry a rate ruler in their pockets so another way must be found to determine rate.

The 300–150–100–75–60–50 method is the easiest and quickest method of calculation. Choose an R wave that falls on or close to a heavy black line on the ECG paper. The first heavy black line to the right is the *300* line, the second is the *150* line, the third is the *100* line, the fourth is the *75* line, the fifth is the *60* line, and the sixth is the *50* line. If the next R wave falls on the fifth heavy black line to the right, the heart rate is 60 beats per minute (Figure 7-11).

QRS Axis

The QRS axis refers to the average direction of depolarization that spreads through the ventricles to stimulate the muscle fibers to contract. The QRS axis of the heart can be determined by using the hexaxial reference system.

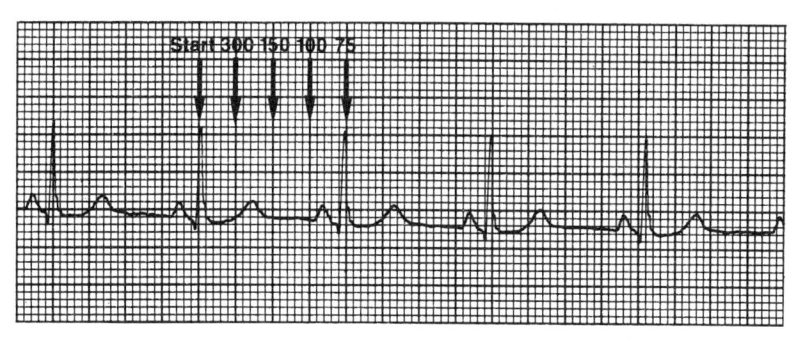

Figure 7-11 The heartbeat is slightly above the rate of 75 beats per minute. (From Davis D: How to Quickly and Accurately Master ECG Interpretation. Philadelphia, JB Lippincott, 1985)

This system is formulated by placing the six limb leads around a circle in their respective ECG lead positions and by their positive poles. The circle is then divided into 30 degree segments (Figure 7-12).

Axis from 0° to +90° is a normal axis deviation.

Axis from −1° to −90° is a left axis deviation.

Axis from +91° to +180° is a right axis deviation.

Axis from −90° to −180° is either an extreme left or extreme right axis deviation.

There is an easy way to calculate QRS axis on an ECG using leads I, II, III, aVR, aVL, and aVF. Find the lead in which the QRS complex has the most voltage. Determine where that lead lies on the hexaxial reference circle. If the voltage is positive, the axis points directly to that lead and the respective degrees in that position. If the voltage is negative the axis points directly to the opposite end of that lead and the respective degrees on the hexaxial reference circle (Figures 7-13 and 7-14).

12 Lead ECG Configurations

The P wave should be upright in lead I and negative in lead aVR, and the P wave in lead V_1 is often diphasic. The limb leads are open to some variability in their configuration. The chest leads must remain within a more standard format in order to be considered normal. The QRS should have a small R wave and a large S wave in V_1, with the R wave becoming progressively larger and the S wave becoming progressively smaller as it moves across the precordium. This is called a normal R wave progression (Figure 7-15).

Hypertrophy

Hypertrophy is an increase in the thickness of the muscular wall of one of the chambers of the heart. Either or both of the atrial or ventricular walls can display hypertrophy.

(Text continues on page 98)

96 Electrocardiography and Arrhythmias

HEXAXIAL REFERENCE SYSTEM

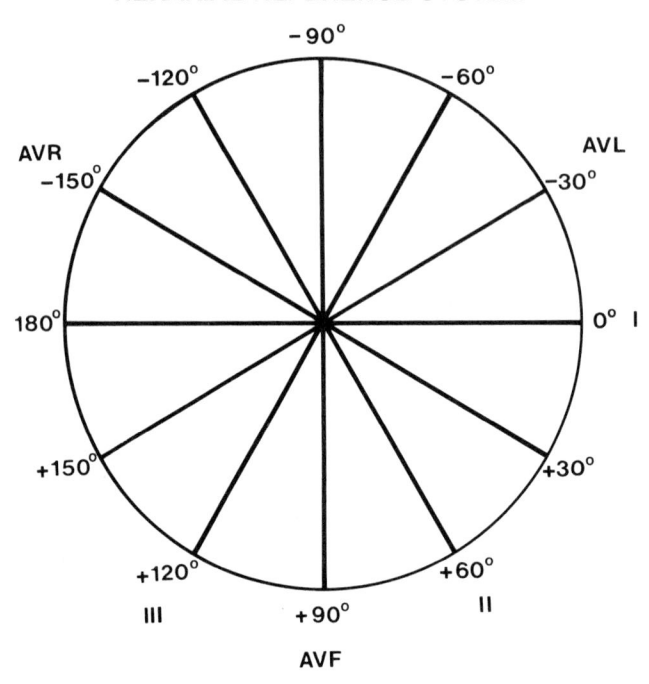

Figure 7-12 The axis is calculated using the hexaxial reference system. (From Davis D: How to Quickly and Accurately Master ECG Interpretation. Philadelphia, JB Lippincott, 1985)

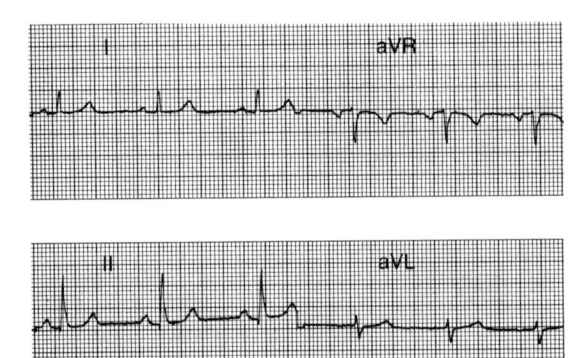

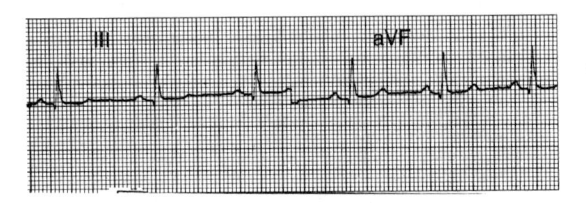

Figure 7-13 The QRS complex in lead II has the most voltage. The voltage is positive, so the axis is pointing directly toward lead II or at +60°.

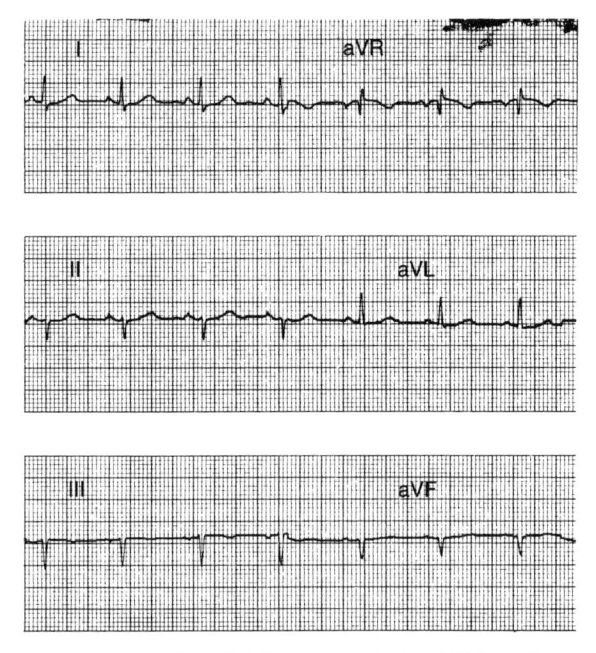

ECG Graph Paper and Measurements 97

Figure 7-14 The QRS complex in lead III has the most voltage. The voltage is negative, so the axis is pointing directly away from lead III or at −60°.

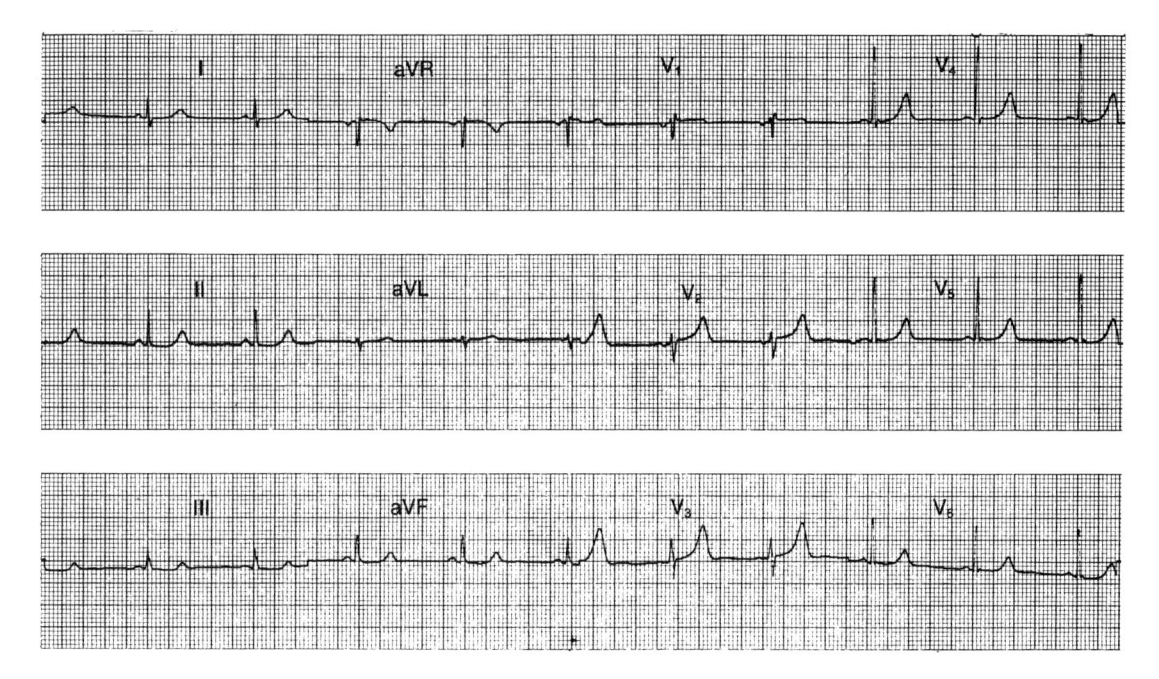

Figure 7-15 Normal 12 lead ECG configuration. The P wave should be upright in lead I and inverted in lead aVR. The chest leads demonstrate a normal R wave progression across the precordium.

Atrial Hypertrophy

This is an increase in the size of either the left or right atrial wall. Left atrial hypertrophy is best demonstrated in lead V_1. The terminal portion of the P wave in V_1, representing left atrial depolarization, will enlarge to 1 mm or more deep. Right atrial hypertrophy is best seen in lead II. The normal P wave in lead II is 2.4 mm or less in height. In right atrial hypertrophy the P wave height increases to 2.5 mm or greater (Figures 7-16 through 7-20).

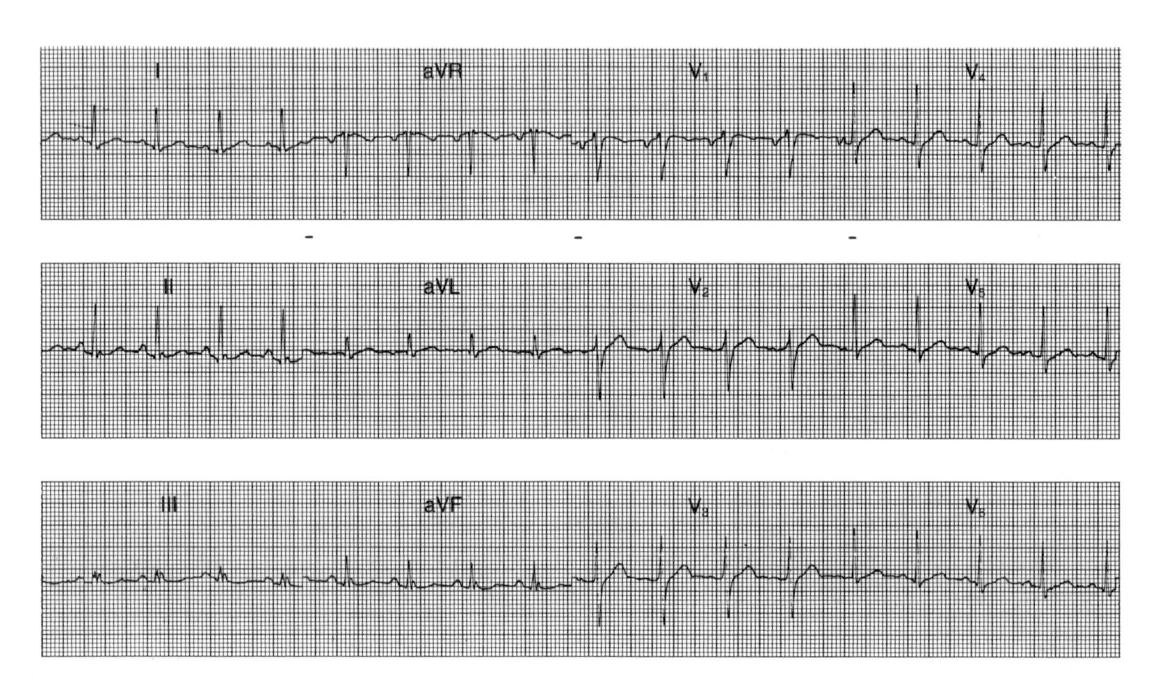

Figure 7-16 Left atrial hypertrophy.

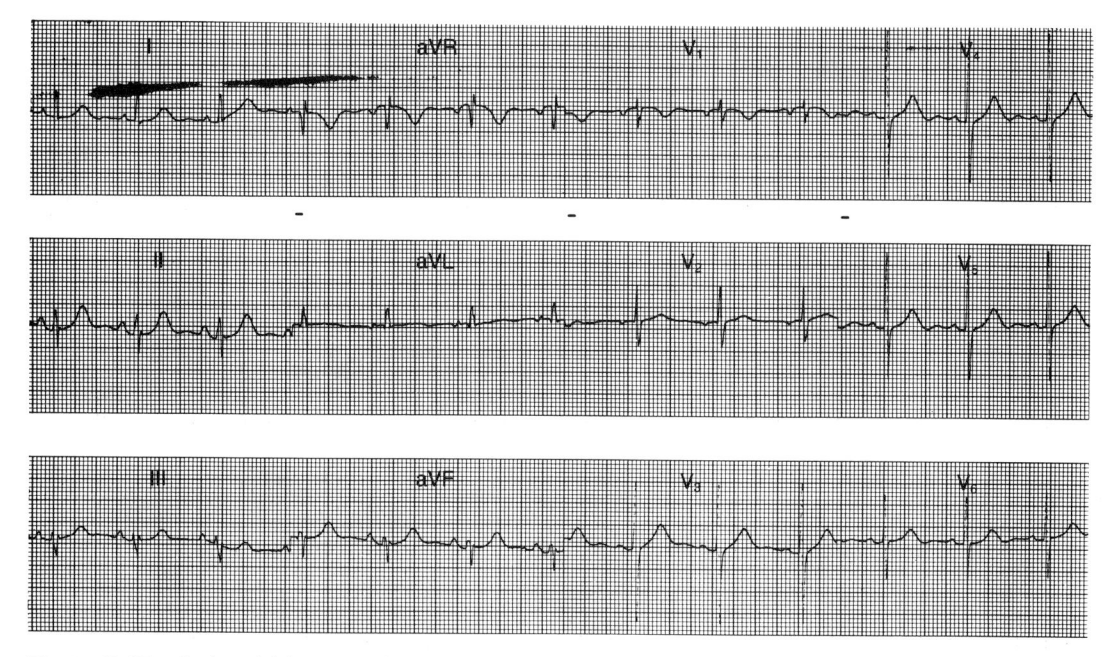

Figure 7-17 Left atrial hypertrophy and left axis deviation.

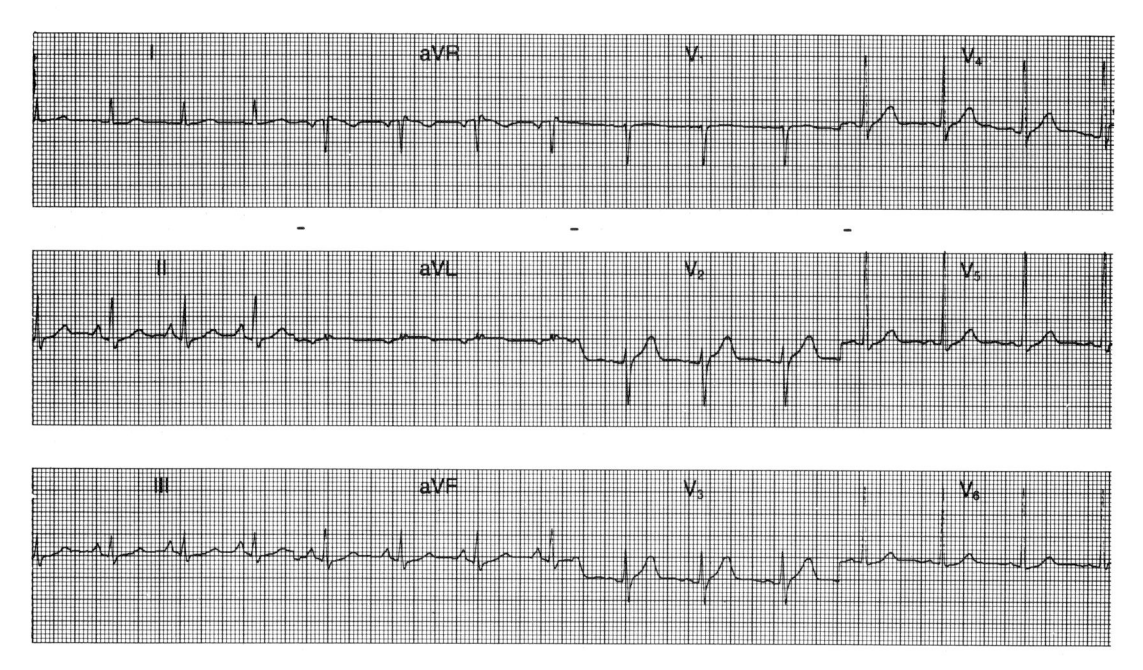

Figure 7-18 Right atrial hypertrophy.

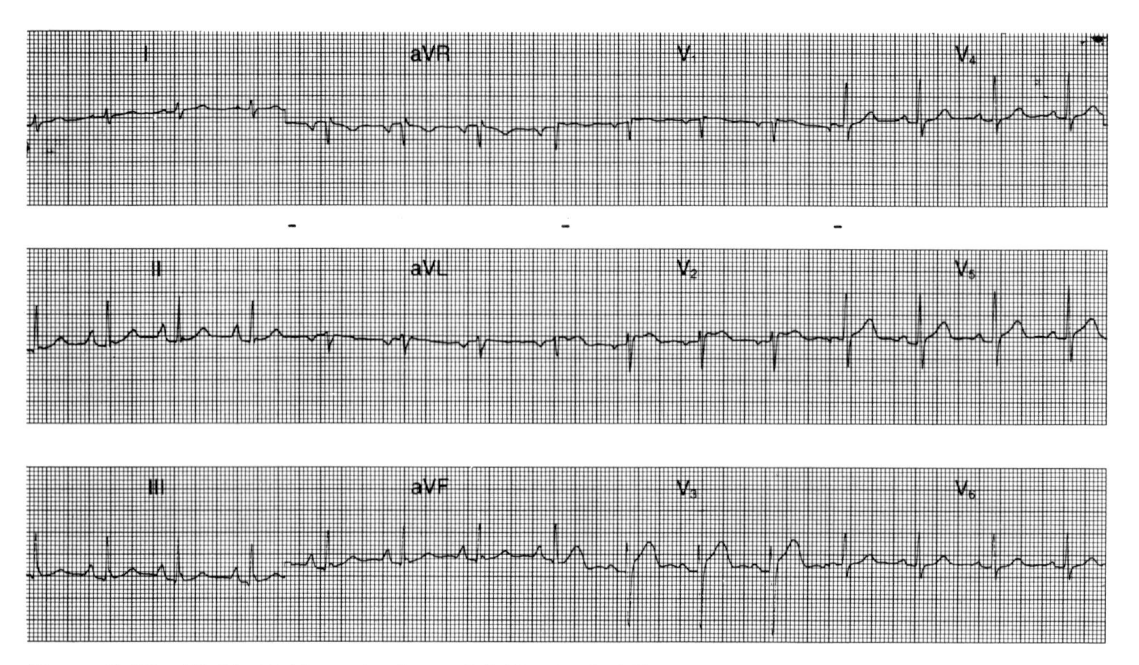

Figure 7-19 Right atrial hypertrophy and right axis deviation.

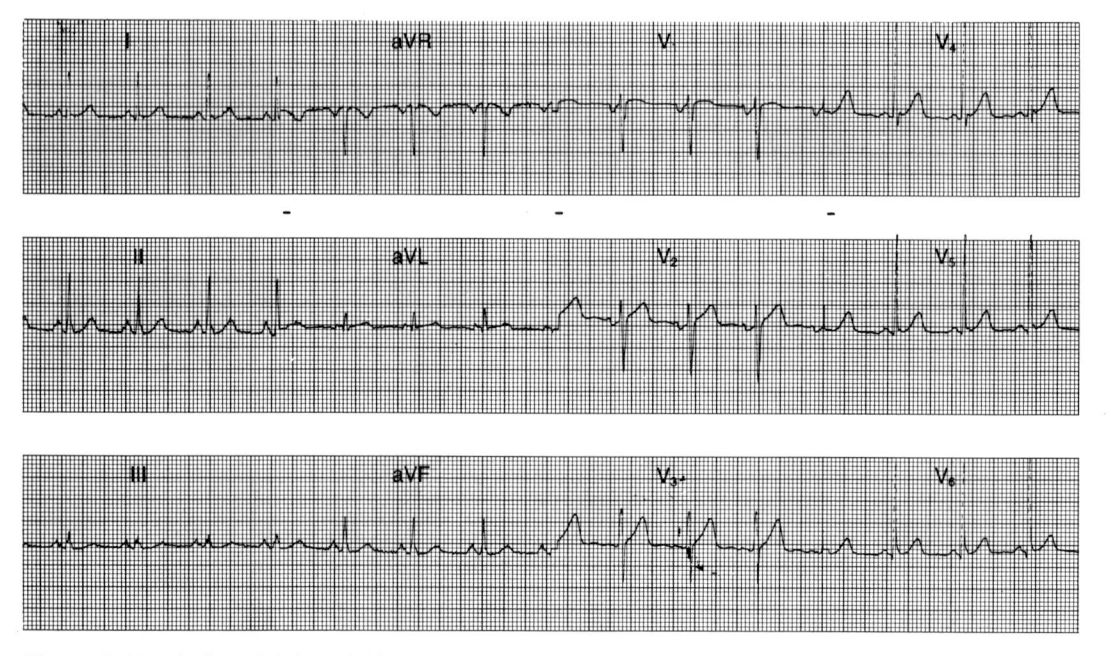

Figure 7-20 Left and right atrial hypertrophy.

Ventricular Hypertrophy

This condition is characterized by an increase in the size of either the left or right ventricular wall. When a ventricular wall increases in thickness, large voltages are recorded in the leads over the hypertrophied area. In left ventricular hypertrophy, voltage criteria are usually used for the diagnosis. Large voltages may be seen in leads I, aVL, V_5, or V_6.

$$S \text{ wave } V_1 + R \text{ wave } V_5 > 35 \text{ mm}$$
$$\text{or}$$
$$R \text{ wave } aVL > 11 \text{ mm}$$
$$\text{or}$$
$$R \text{ wave } V_5 \text{ or } V_6 > 27 \text{ mm}$$

Repolarization changes showing ST depression and asymmetrical T wave inversion are often present in the leads over the left ventricle—leads I, aVL, V_5, and V_6 (Figures 7-21 through 7-24).

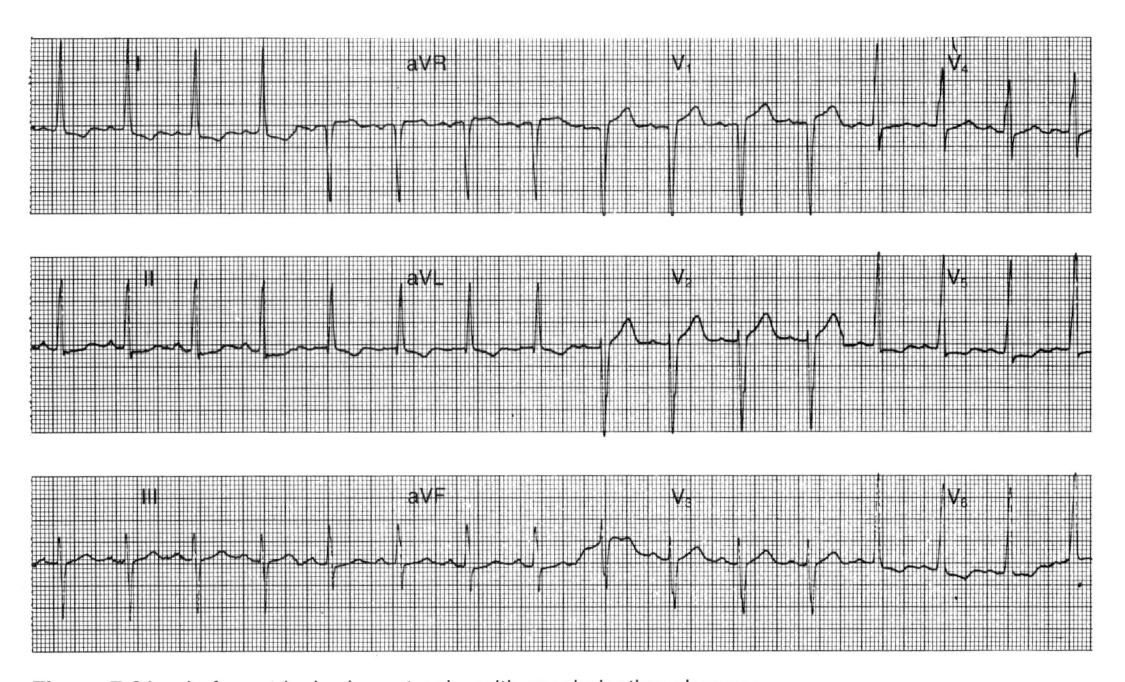

Figure 7-21 Left ventricular hypertrophy with repolarization changes.

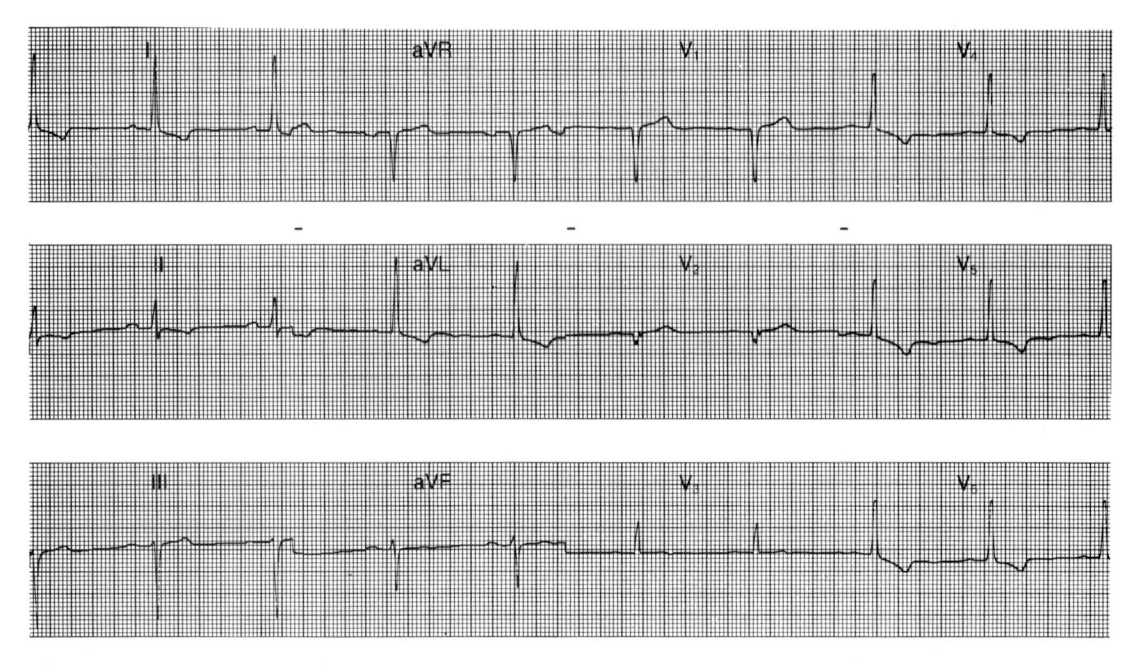

Figure 7-22 Left ventricular hypertrophy with repolarization changes and first-degree AV block.

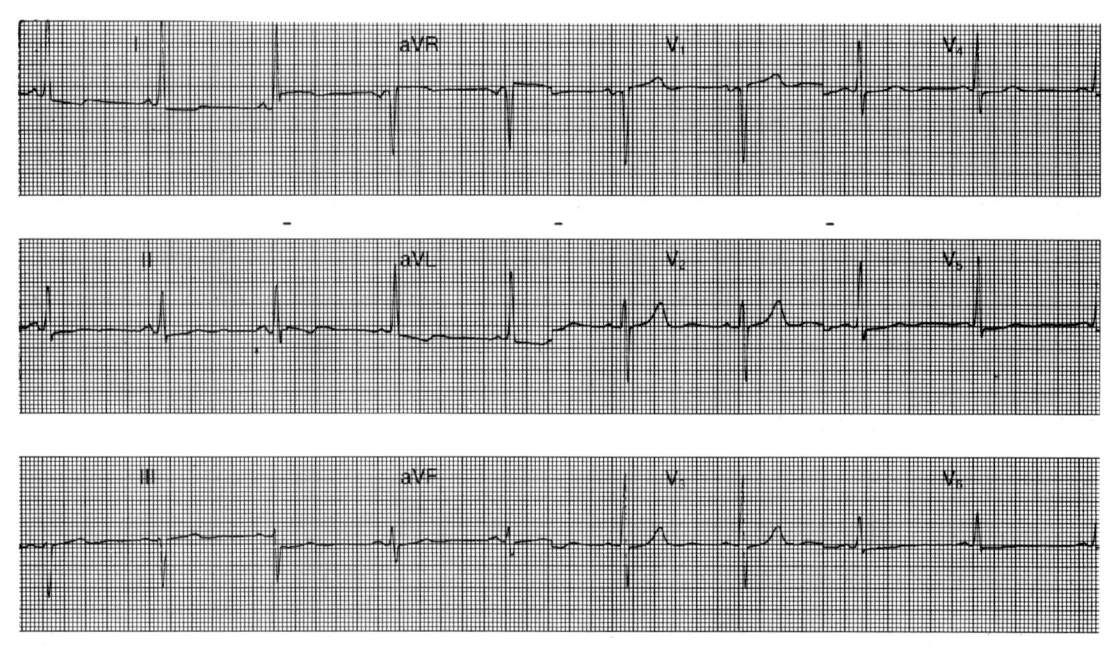

Figure 7-23 Left ventricular hypertrophy with repolarization changes and left atrial hypertrophy.

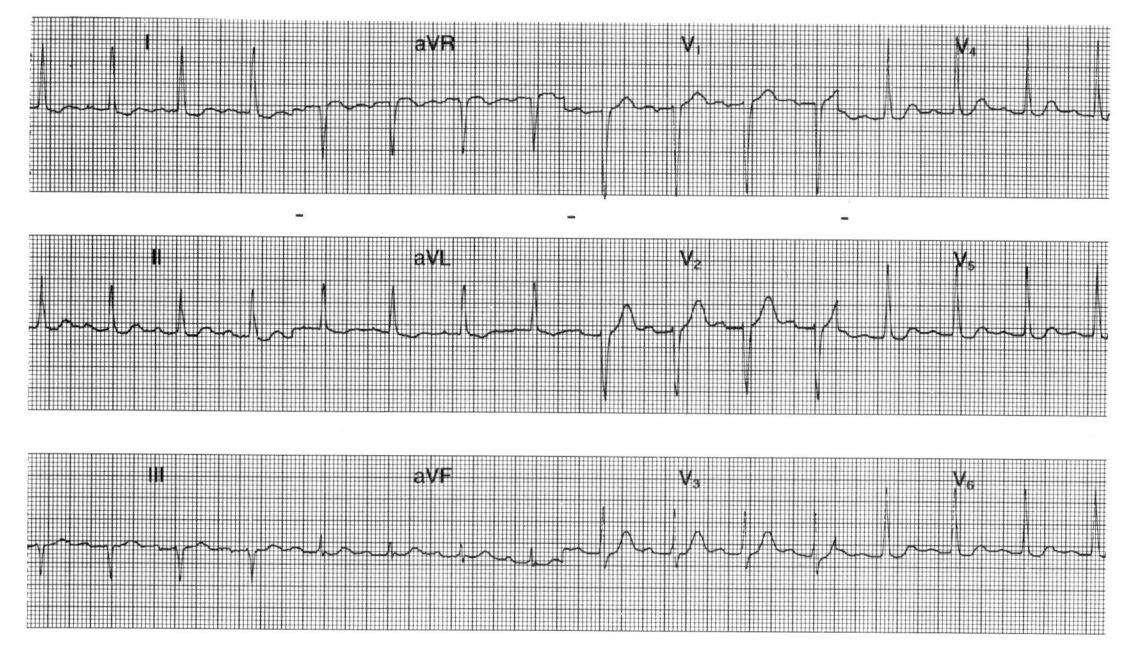

Figure 7-24 Left ventricular hypertrophy with repolarization changes and first-degree AV block.

In right ventricular hypertrophy, voltage is one of the two criteria needed for recognition. Large voltages may be noted in V_1 and V_2.

1. R wave > S wave V_1
2. Right axis deviation

Repolarization changes demonstrating ST depression and asymmetrical T inversion may be seen in V_1 and V_2 (Figures 7-25 through 7-28).

Intraventricular Conduction Disturbances

An intraventricular conduction disturbance is an abnormal conduction of an electrical impulse in one or more of the conduction pathways below the bundle of His: the right bundle branch, left bundle branch, left anterior fascicle, or left posterior fascicle.

Right Bundle Branch Block: This represents a delay or blockage of electrical conduction in the right bundle branch. The normal cardiac impulse travels down the normal conduction pathways until it reaches the right bundle branch. Upon finding the right bundle blocked, the electrical impulse advances to the left bundle branch and depolarizes the left ventricle and then proceeds across the septum into the right ventricle and initiates right ventricular depolarization.

(Text continues on page 106)

104 Electrocardiography and Arrhythmias

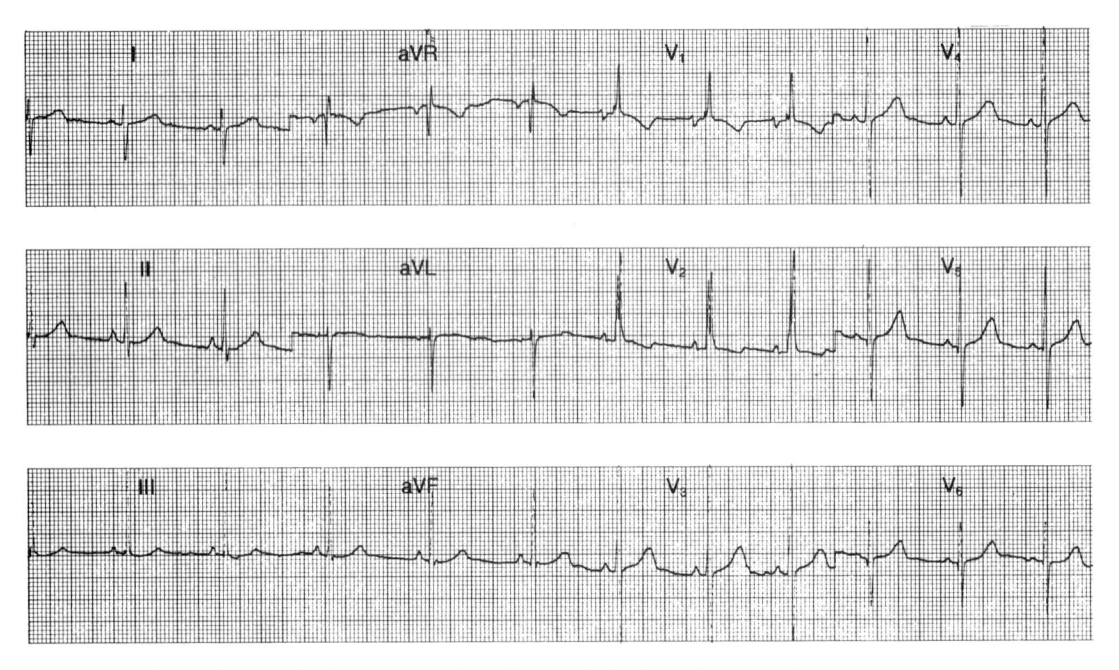

Figure 7-25 Right ventricular hypertrophy with repolarization changes, right axis deviation, and left and right atrial hypertrophy.

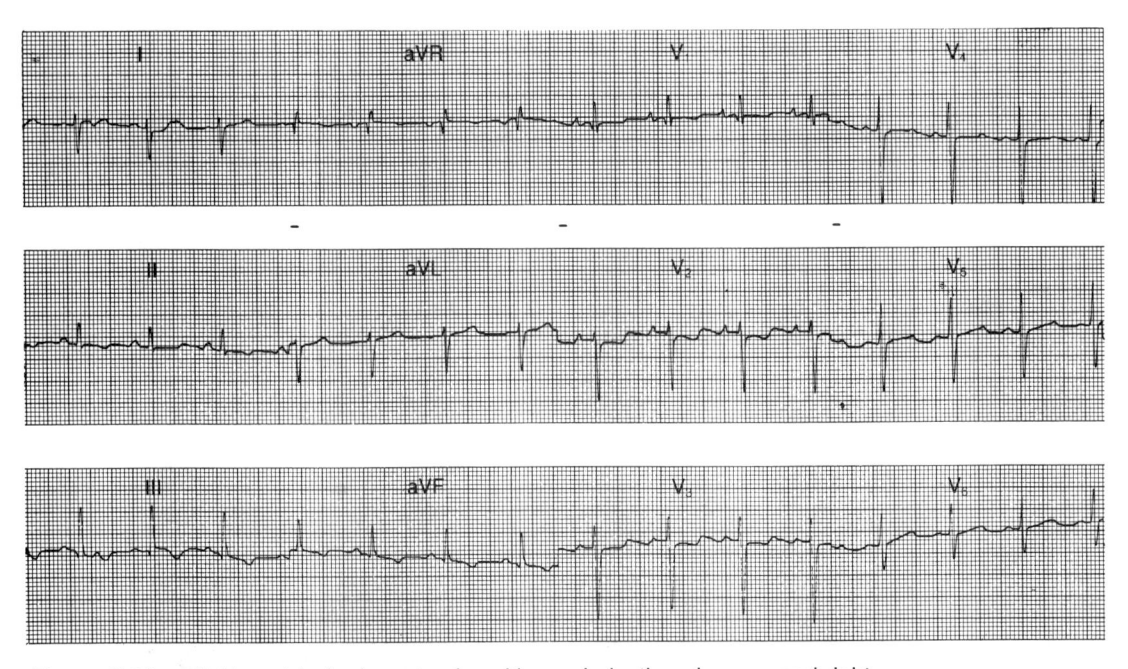

Figure 7-26 Right ventricular hypertrophy with repolarization changes and right axis deviation.

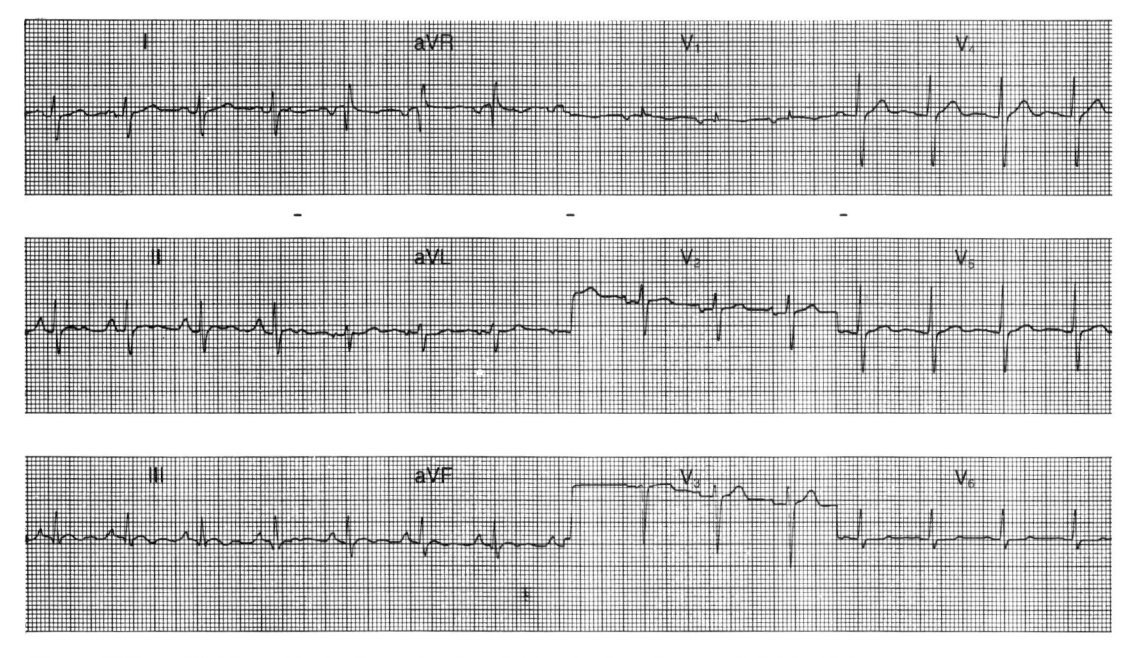

ECG Graph Paper and Measurements 105

Figure 7-27 Right ventricular hypertrophy, right axis deviation, and right atrial hypertrophy.

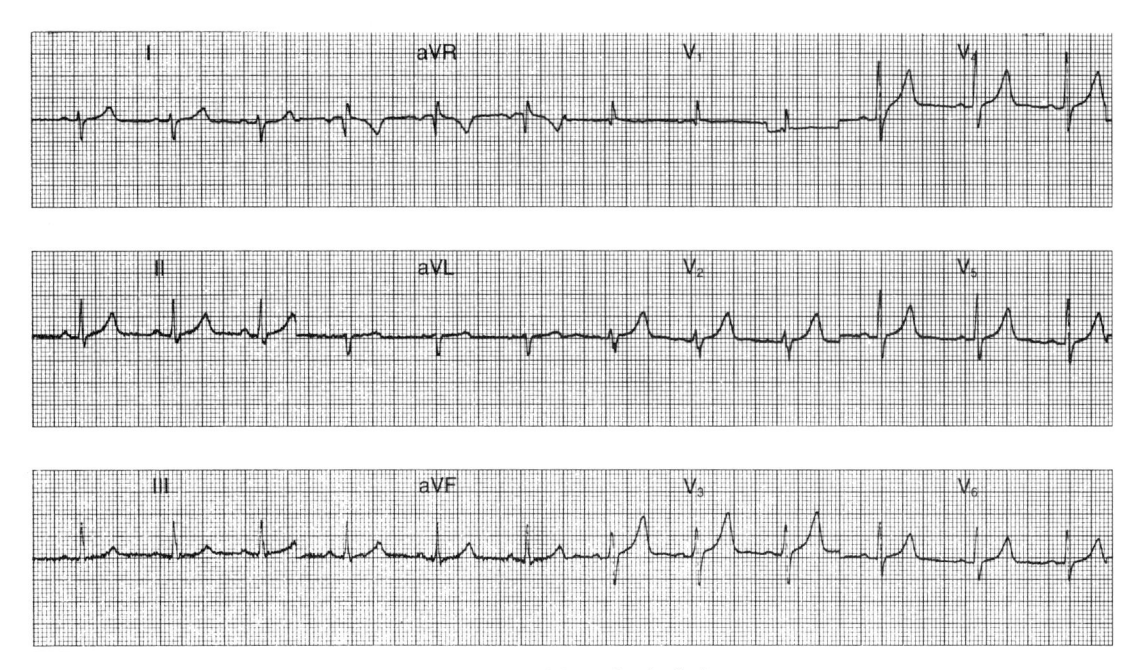

Figure 7-28 Right ventricular hypertrophy and right axis deviation.

Because of the delay in conduction, the QRS will be widened to .12 second or greater and there will be a predominantly positive QRS complex in V_1. Repolarization changes are often seen in V_1 and V_2. In the presence of right bundle branch block, right ventricular hypertrophy should not be diagnosed (Figures 7-29 through 7-32).

Left Bundle Branch Block: A delay or blockage in the left bundle branch is called *left bundle branch block*. The cardiac impulse begins normally and travels down to the left bundle branch. Upon finding it blocked, the electrical impulse advances to the right bundle branch and depolarizes it, then travels across the septum to depolarize the left ventricle.

Because of the delay in conduction, the QRS is widened to .12 second or greater and the QRS is predominantly negative in V_1. Repolarization changes are often seen in leads I, aVL, V_5, and V_6. In the presence of left bundle branch block, left ventricular hypertrophy should not be diagnosed (Figures 7-33 through 7-35).

(Text continues on page 110)

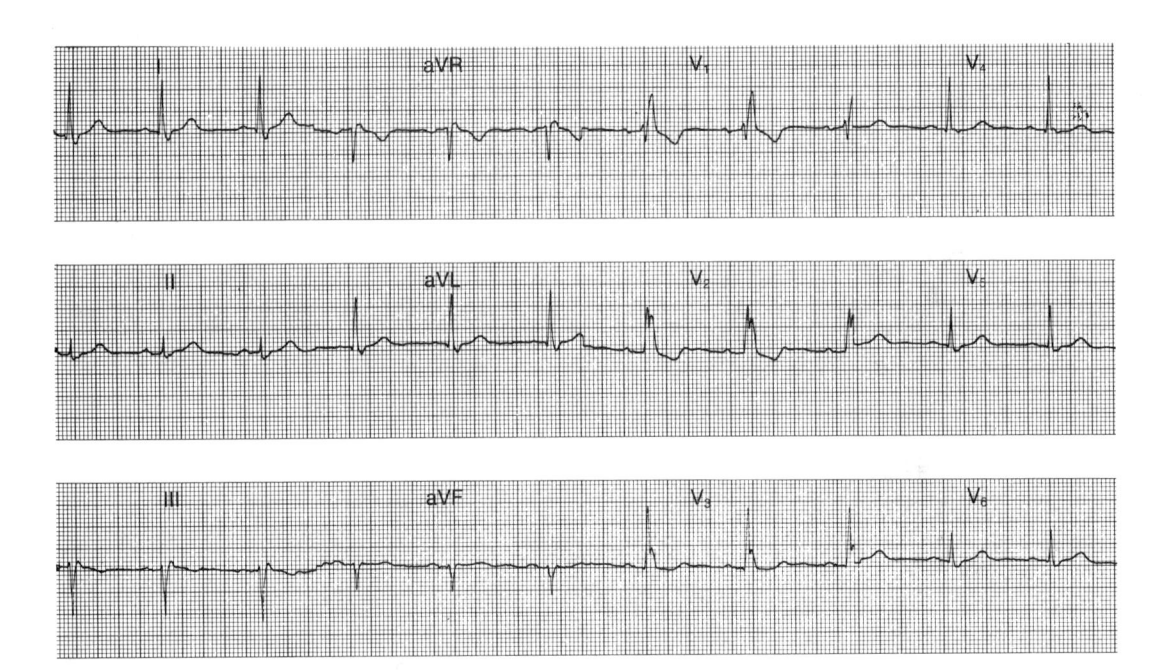

Figure 7-29 Right bundle branch block.

ECG Graph Paper and Measurements 107

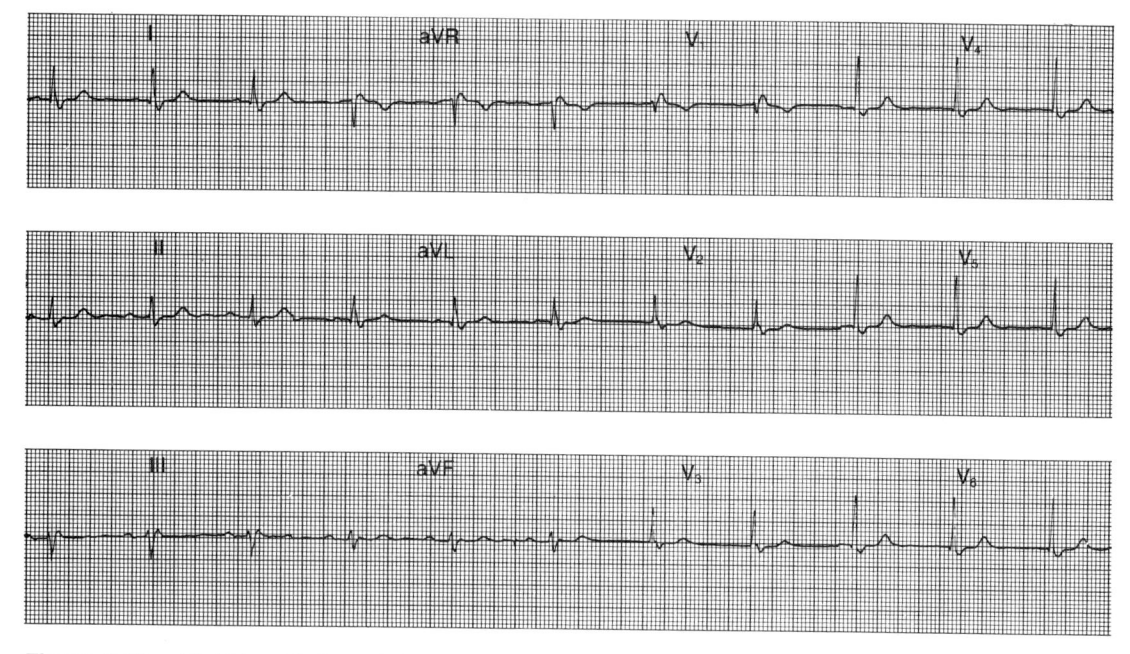

Figure 7-30 Right bundle branch block and first-degree AV block.

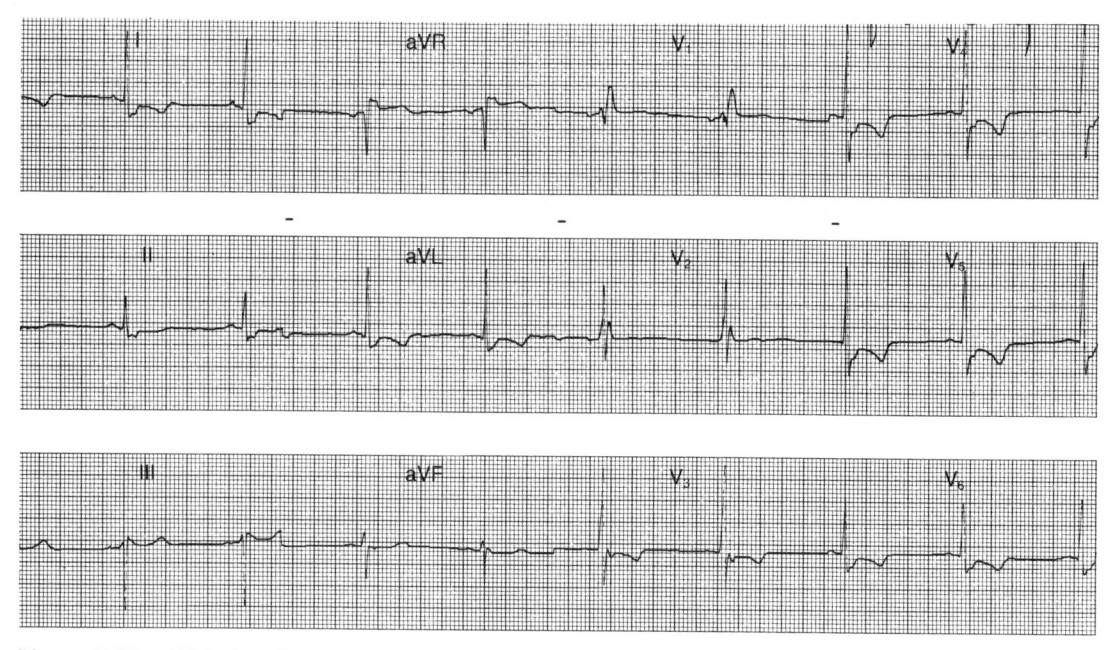

Figure 7-31 Right bundle branch block, left atrial hypertrophy, and left ventricular hypertrophy.

108 Electrocardiography and Arrhythmias

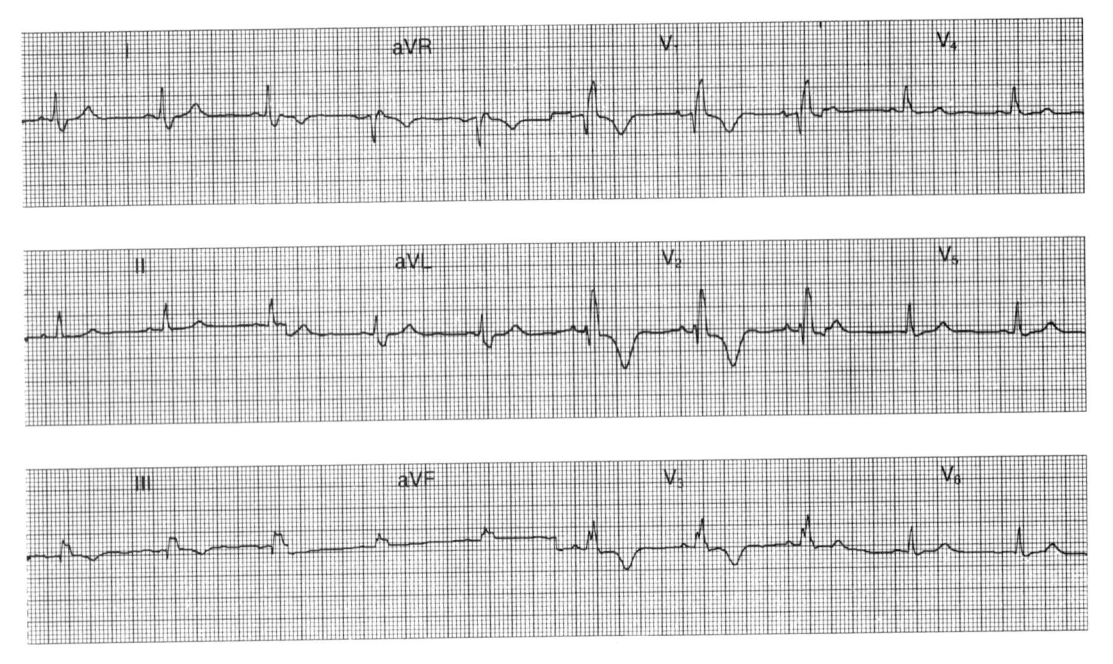

Figure 7-32 Right bundle branch block.

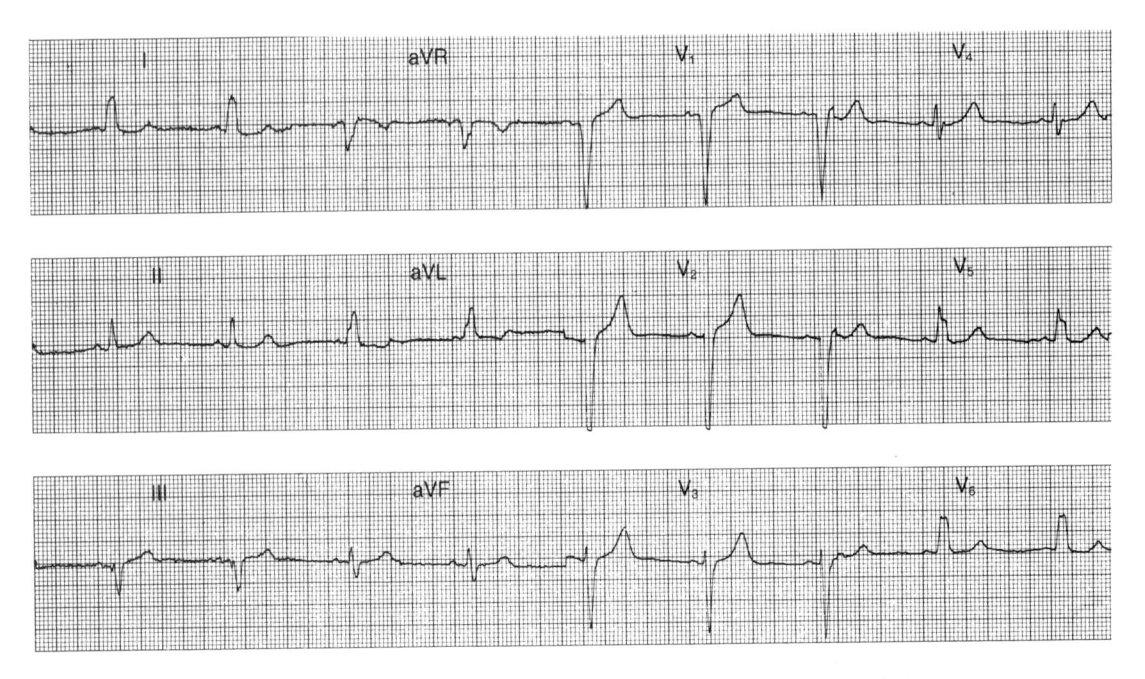

Figure 7-33 Left bundle branch block.

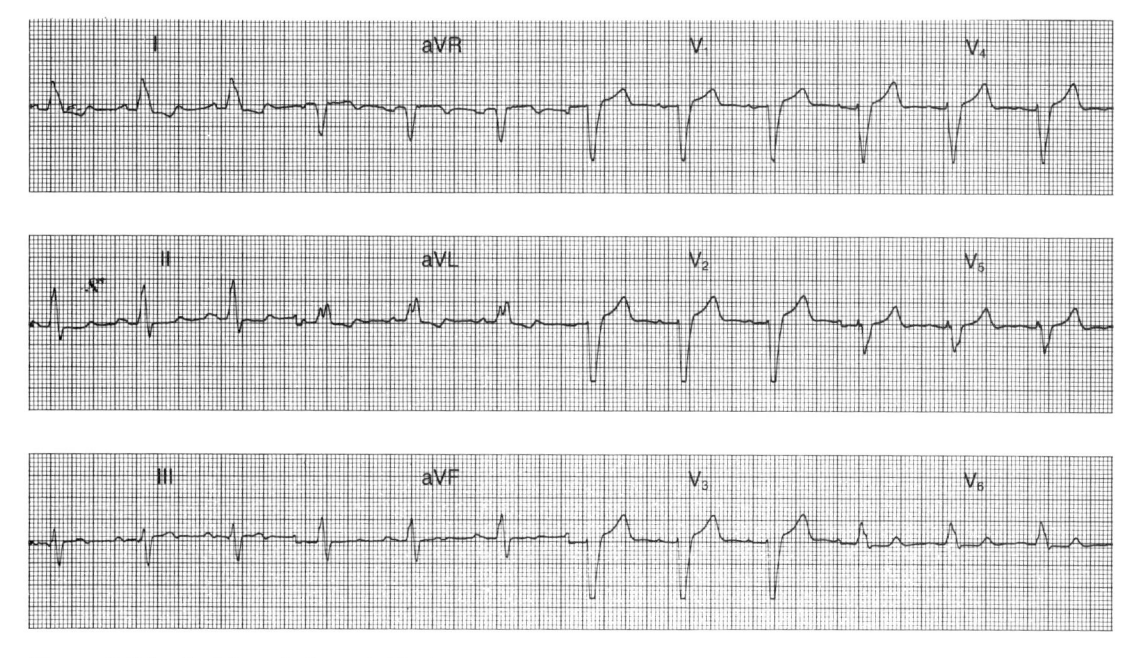

Figure 7-34 Left bundle branch block.

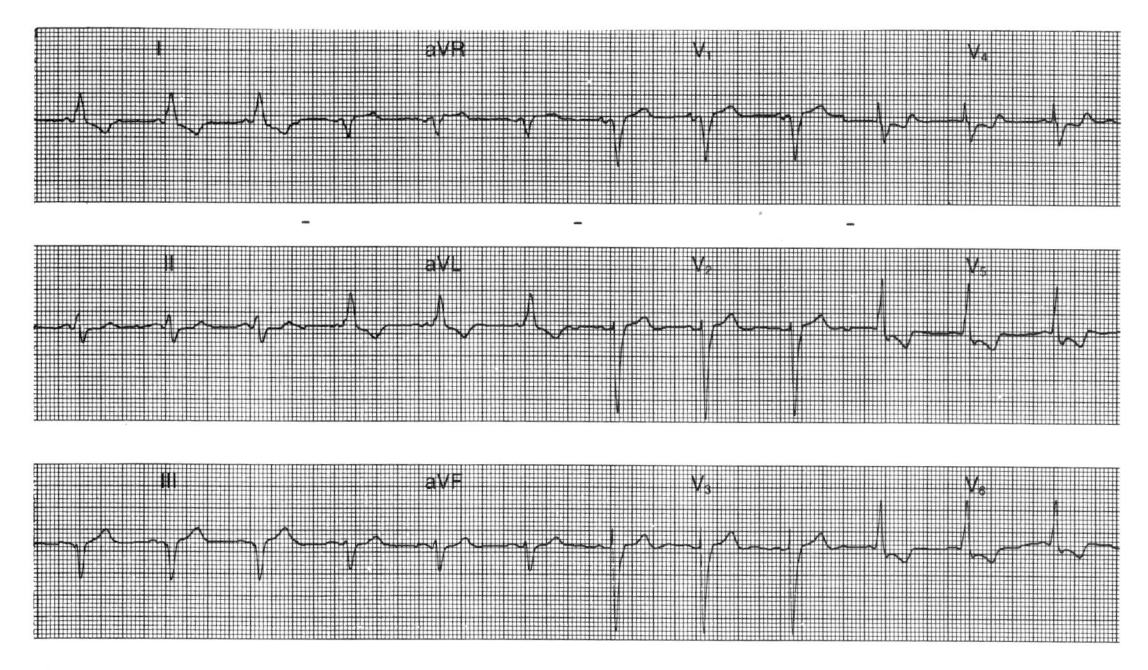

Figure 7-35 Left bundle branch block, left atrial hypertrophy, and left axis deviation.

Left Anterior Fascicular Block: This represents delay or blockage of the anterior fascicle of the left bundle branch. It is sometimes referred to as *left anterior hemiblock.* The electrical impulse travels down the normal conduction pathways to the left bundle branch. Conduction is delayed or blocked at the anterior fascicle so the impulse continues down the posterior fascicle. Through the connection of Purkinje's fibers between the anterior and posterior fascicles, the anterior and superior portion of the left ventricle are depolarized. Because of the change in direction of depolarization in the left ventricle, the QRS axis will become −40° or greater and a small Q wave will be seen in lead I (Figures 7-36 through 7-39).

Left Posterior Fascicular Block: This is a delay or blockage of the posterior fascicle of the left bundle. It is sometimes referred to as left posterior hemiblock. The electrical impulse finds the posterior fascicle blocked, so the impulse proceeds down the anterior fascicle, through the connection of Purkinje's fibers between the two fascicles, and the posterior portion of the left ventricle is depolarized. Because of the change of direction of depolarization in the left ventricle, the QRS axis will shift right to +120° or greater and a small Q wave in lead III will be seen (Figures 7-40 through 7-42).

(Text continues on page 114)

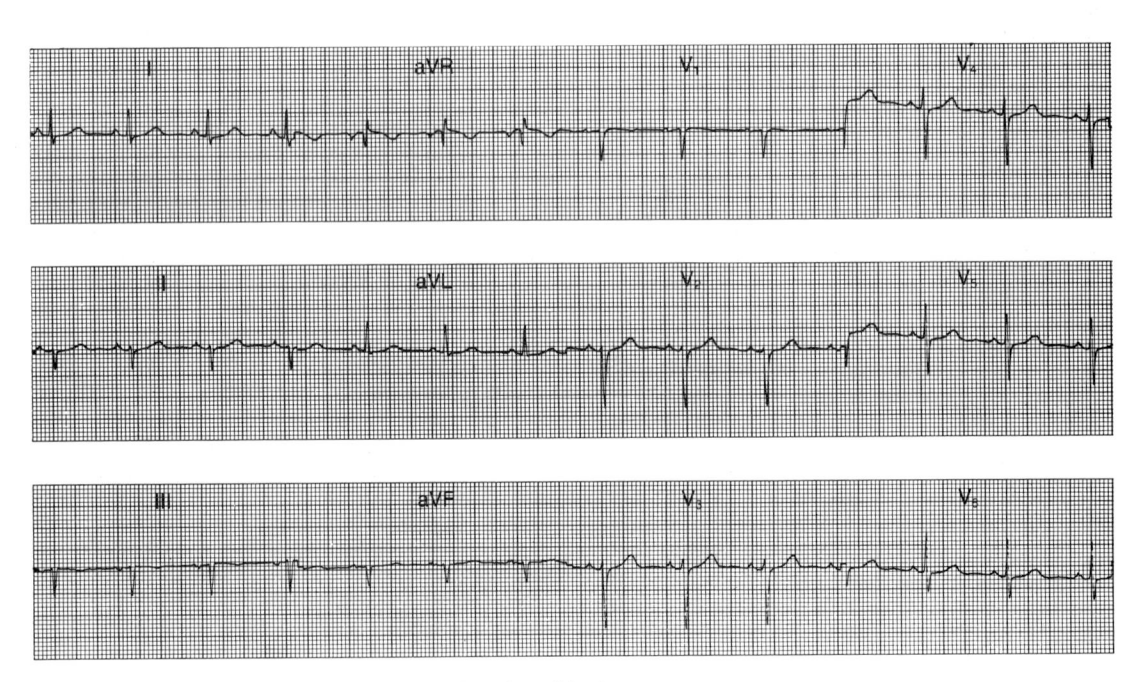

Figure 7-36 Left anterior fascicular block or hemiblock.

ECG Graph Paper and Measurements 111

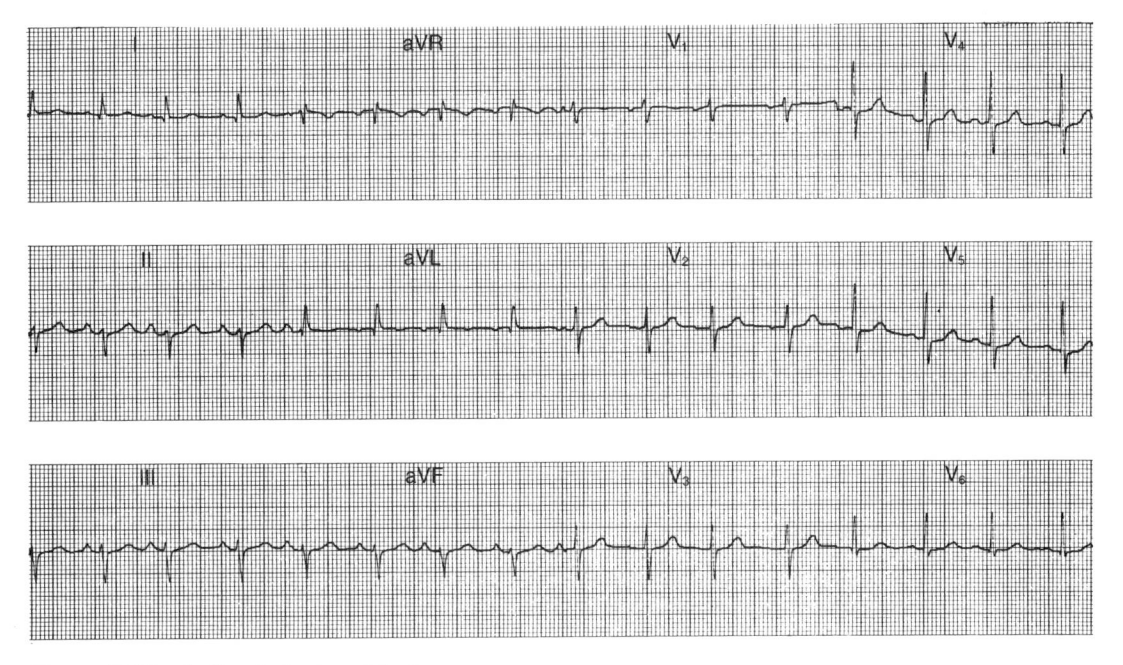

Figure 7-37 Left anterior hemiblock.

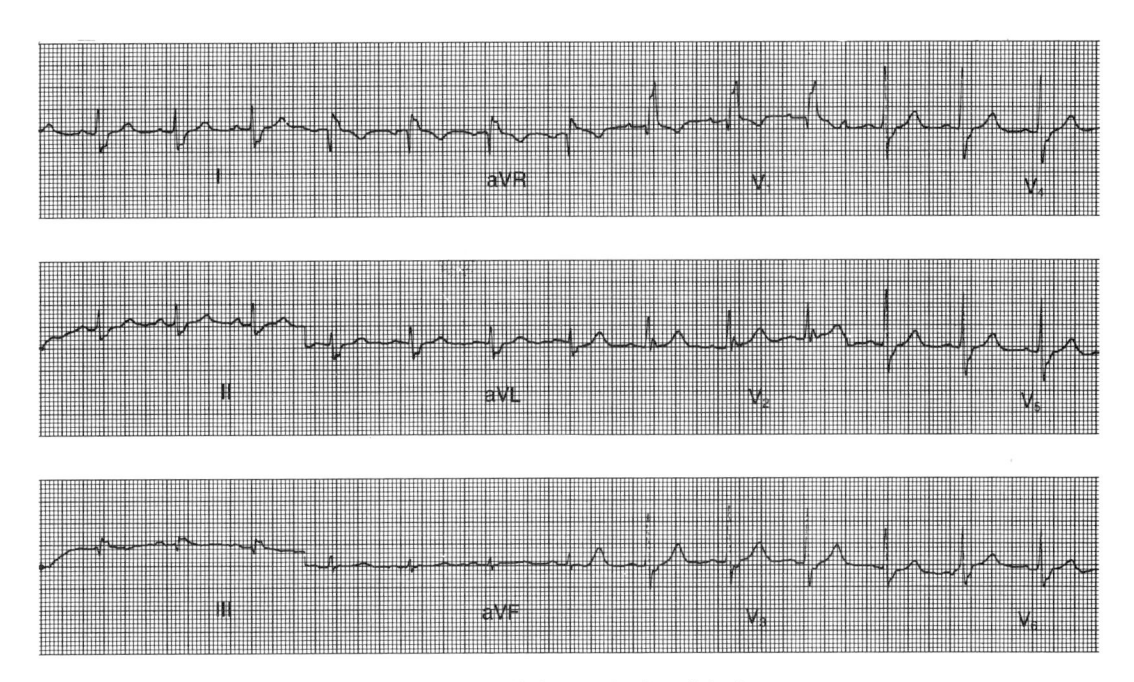

Figure 7-38 Right bundle branch block and left anterior hemiblock.

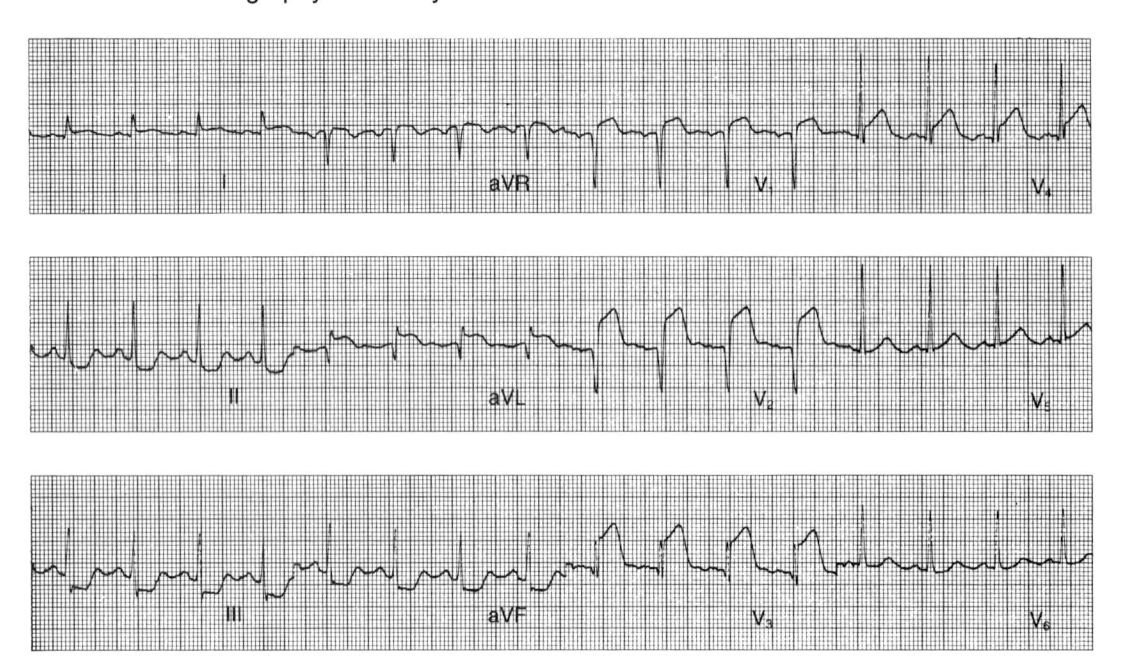

Figure 7-39 Right bundle branch block and left anterior hemiblock.

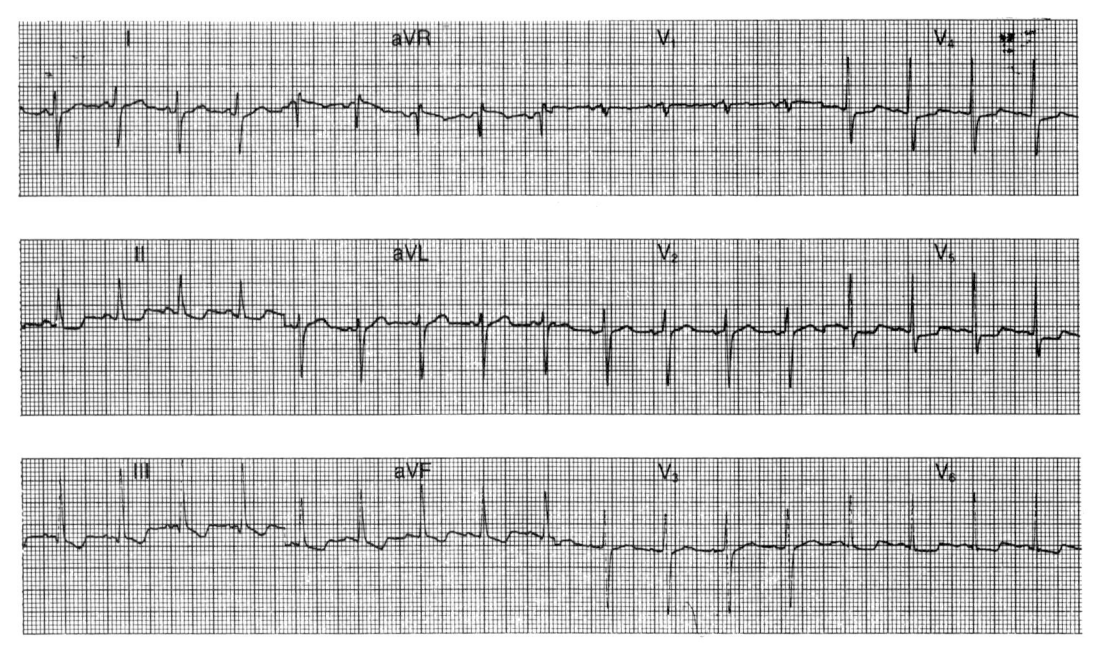

Figure 7-40 Left posterior hemiblock.

ECG Graph Paper and Measurements 113

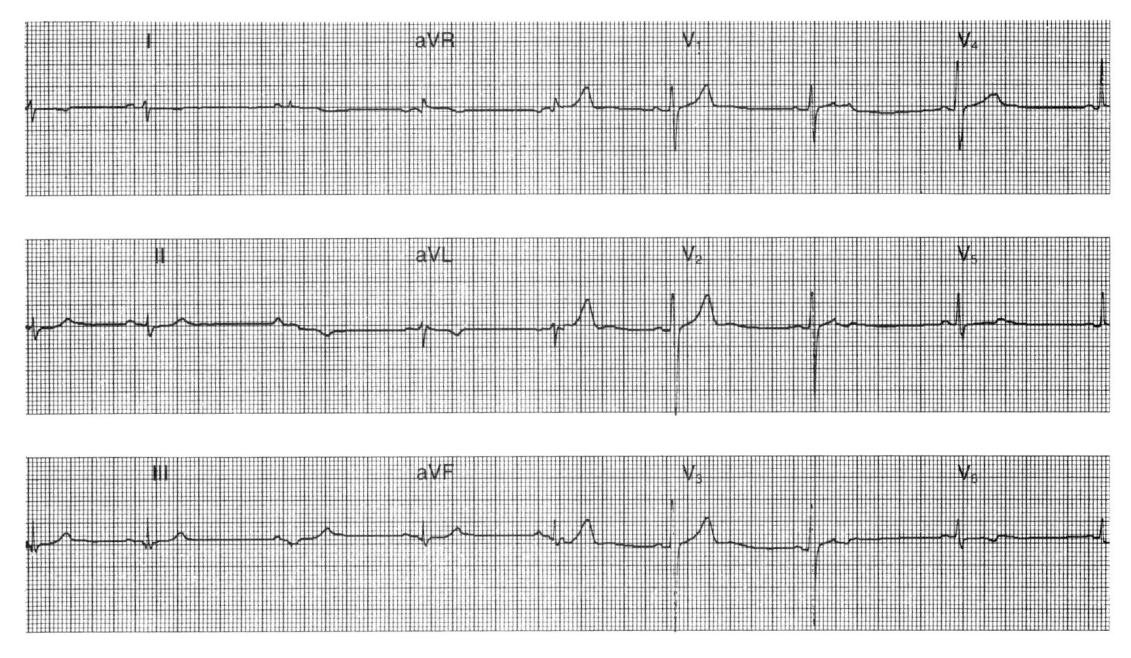

Figure 7-41 Left posterior hemiblock.

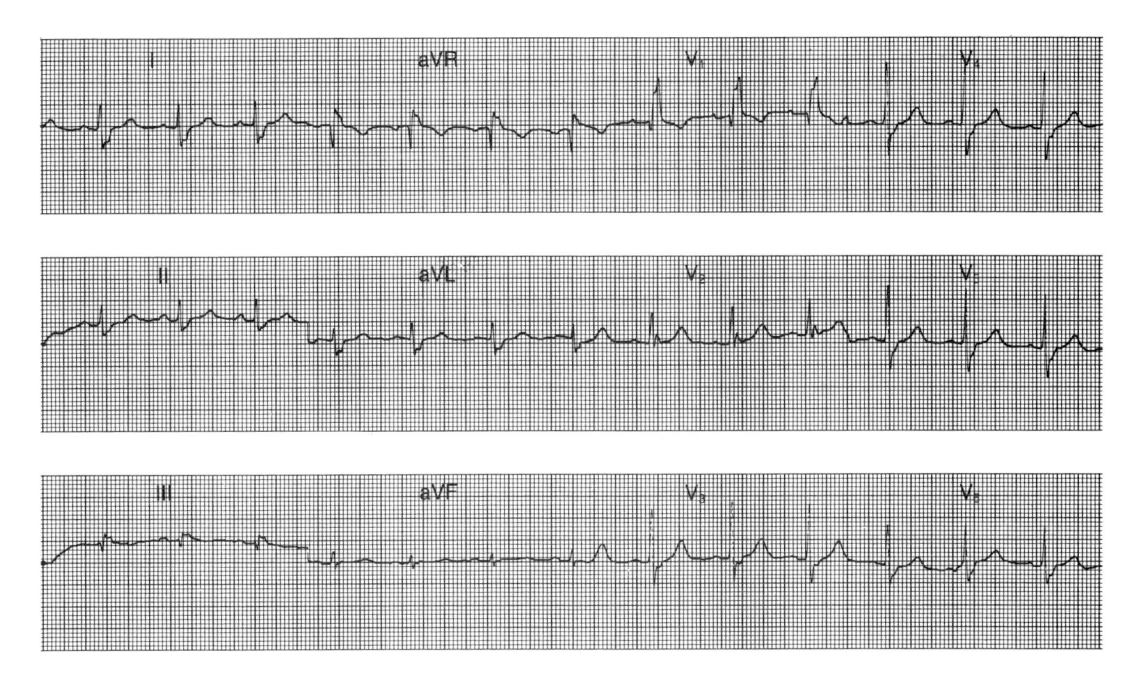

Figure 7-42 Right bundle branch block and left posterior hemiblock.

Ischemia, Injury, Infarction

The heart muscle itself must receive a sufficient supply of blood via its own network of arteries, called the *coronary arteries*. A narrowing of these arteries, often caused by atherosclerosis, results in a diminished blood supply to the heart muscle. Lack of adequate oxygenated blood results in *ischemia*. If the heart remains without adequate oxygenated blood, *injury* to the left heart muscle will occur. And finally, if the blood supply is not returned, death of a portion of the left ventricular muscle will occur and is termed *infarction*.

Ischemia is a lack of sufficient oxygenated blood to the left ventricle, and is manifested on the ECG by symmetrically inverted T waves or ST depression.

Injury is a stage beyond ischemia and is displayed on the ECG by ST elevation. Like ischemia, injury is a reversible process and no permanent damage necessarily occurs.

Infarction is necrosis or death of tissue, usually in a portion of the left ventricular myocardial wall. It follows the stages of ischemia and injury if an adequate blood supply is not returned. Infarction is demonstrated on an ECG by significant Q waves. Q waves are considered significant if they are either one third the height of the R wave or .04 second wide. If neither of these conditions is met, the Q waves are not diagnostic of infarction. Q waves generally appear within 24 hours of the onset of infarction (Figure 7-43).

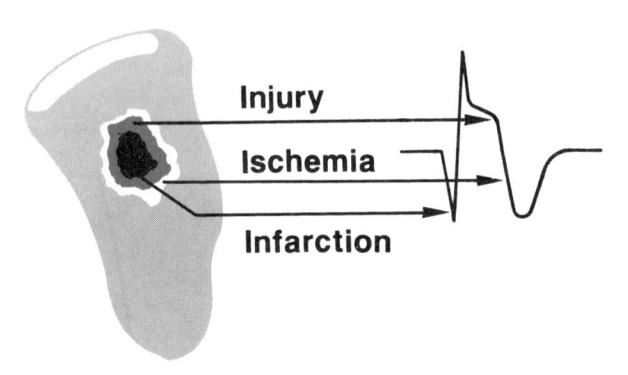

Figure 7-43 Infarction, injury, and ischemia of the left ventricle. (From Davis D: How to Quickly and Accurately Master ECG Interpretation. Philadelphia, JB Lippincott, 1985)

Ischemia, Injury, Infarction

The sequence of stages in the development and evolution of an infarction usually proceeds as follows, although all of the stages are not always recorded on an ECG:

1. An area of left ventricular muscle is injured and ST elevation occurs.
2. Q waves develop in the ECG leads over the infarcted area.
3. T wave inversion occurs in the ECG leads over the infarcted area.
4. ST elevation returns to baseline and T waves remain inverted in the ECG leads over the infarcted area.

The age of an infarction can often be determined by observing the ECG leads over the infarcted area. If the ST segments are elevated, the infarction is probably acute. If the ST segments are at baseline and the T waves are inverted, an infarct is present with an age indeterminate. If the ST segments are at baseline and the T waves are upright, we might conclude that the infarction is old. It is often difficult to make exact determinations from isolated ECGs.

The left ventricle is divided into four main locations: anterior, lateral, inferior, and posterior. Leads V_1, V_2, V_3, and V_4 are located over the anterior portion of the left ventricle. Leads I, aVL, V_5, and V_6 are positioned over the lateral portion of the left ventricle. Leads II, III, and aVF lie over the inferior portion of the left ventricle. No leads are routinely placed over the posterior section of the left ventricle but by observing the opposite or anterior wall and noting the increased R wave voltages in V_1 and V_2, determinations regarding a posterior infarction can often be made.

An infarction can be determined by identifying *significant Q waves* in at least *two* ECG leads for each infarct location or in the case of a posterior infarction, tall R waves in V_1 and V_2.

Anterior infarction	Q waves in V_1, V_2, V_3, V_4
Lateral infarction	Q waves in I, aVL, V_5, V_6
Inferior infarction	Q waves II, III, aVF
Posterior infarction	Tall R wave V_1 and V_2, accompanying an inferior infarction

Various types of infarction are displayed in Figures 7-44 through 7-54.

(Text continues on page 121)

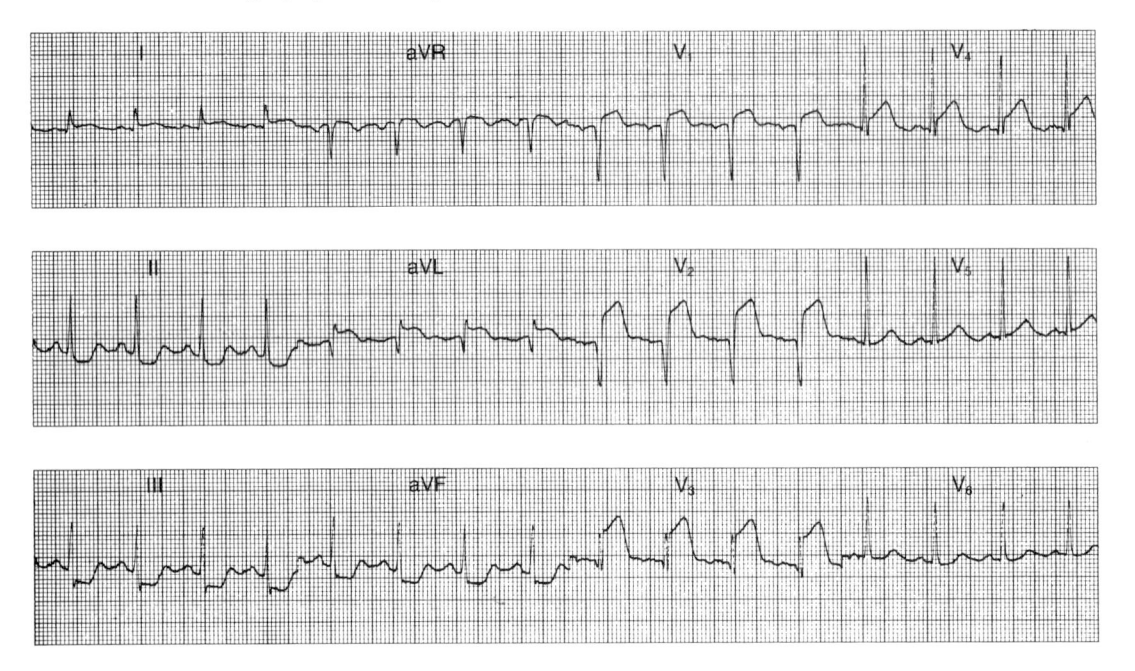

Figure 7-44 Acute anterior infarction.

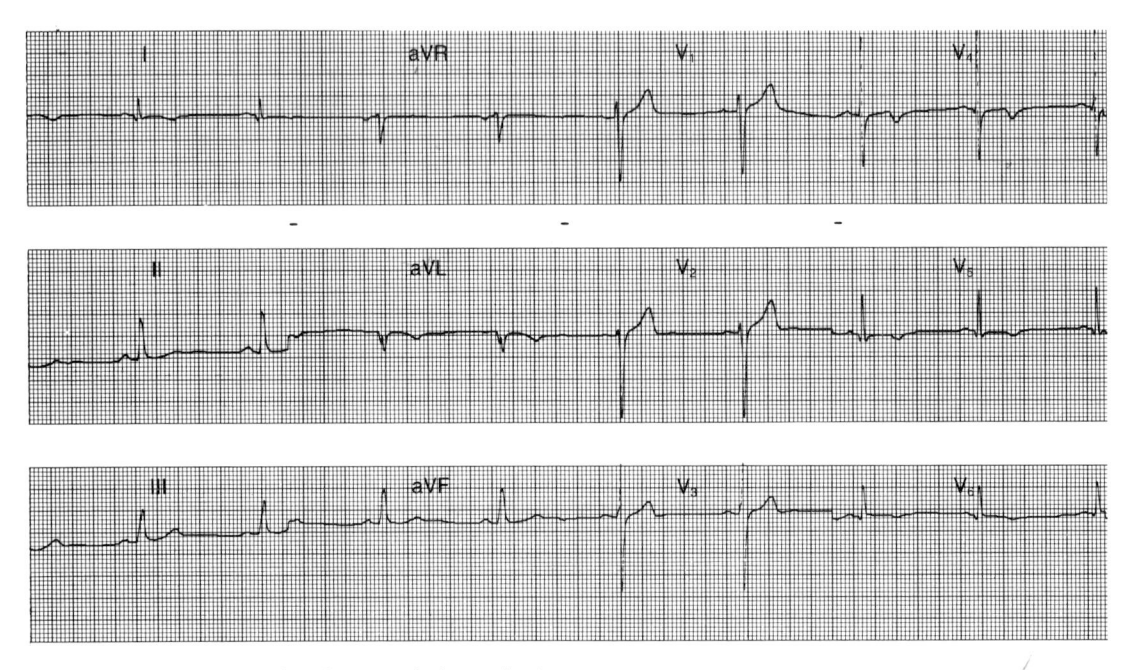

Figure 7-45 Lateral infarction, age indeterminate.

Ischemia, Injury, Infarction   117

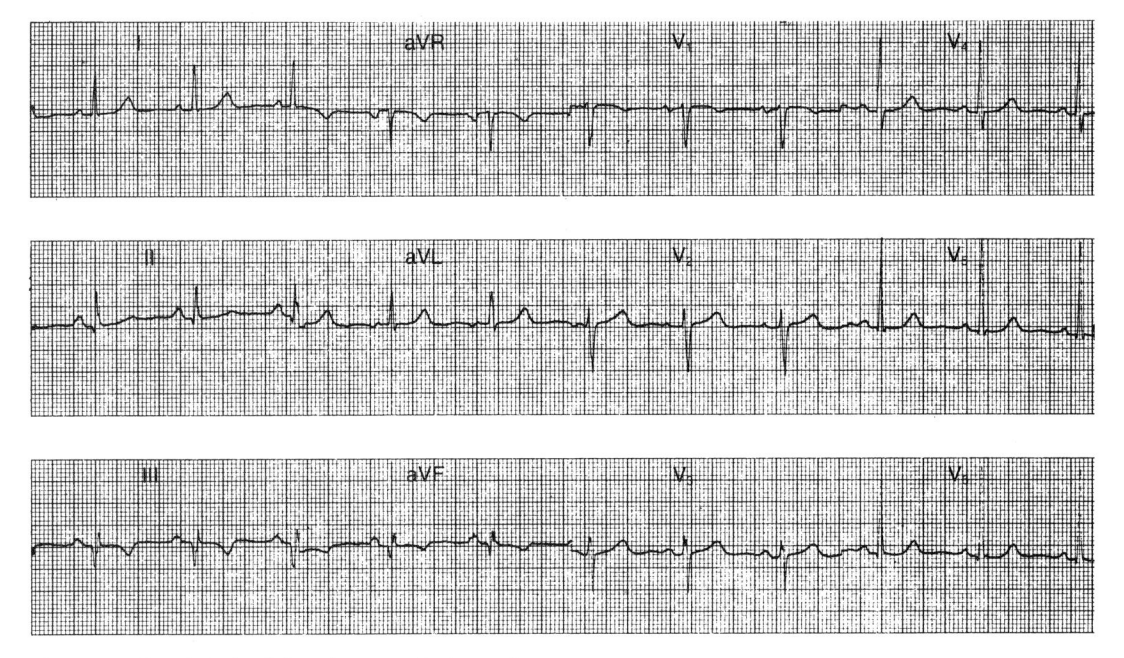

Figure 7-46   Inferior infarction, age indeterminate.

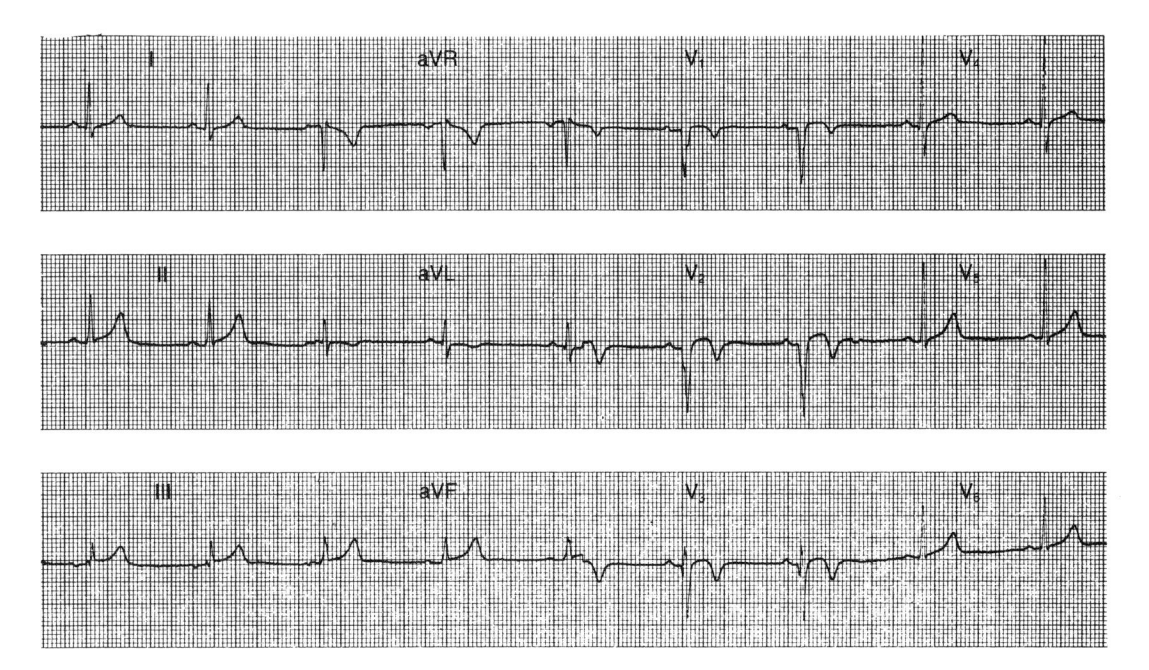

Figure 7-47   Anterior infarction, age indeterminate.

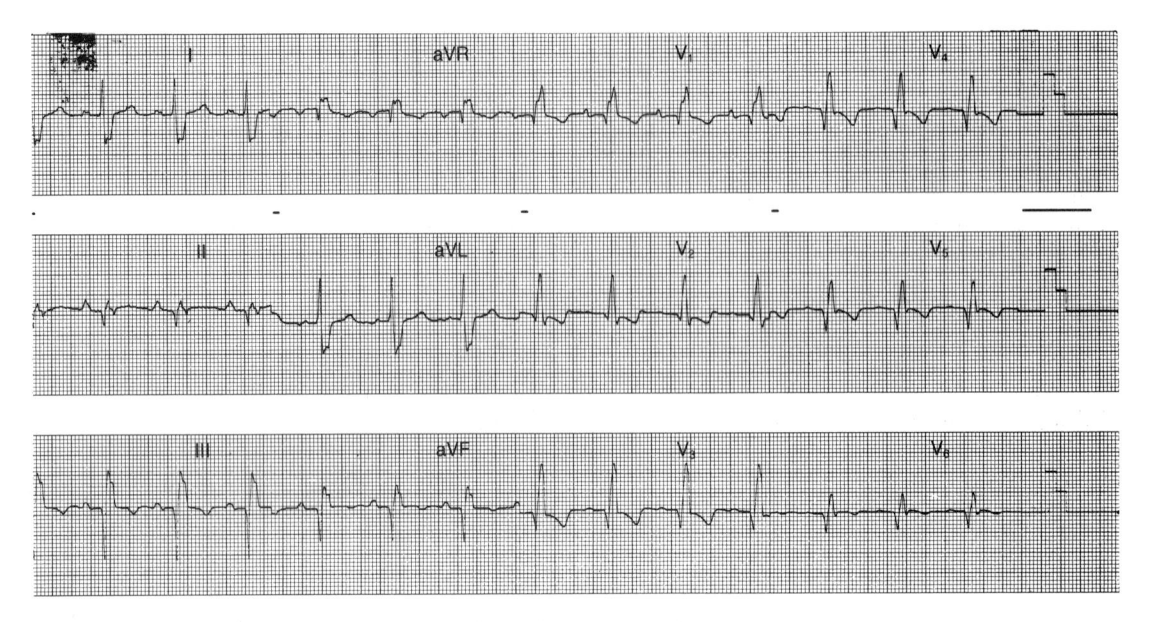

Figure 7-48 Right bundle branch block, first-degree AV block, right atrial hypertrophy, and inferior, anterior, and lateral infarctions, age indeterminate.

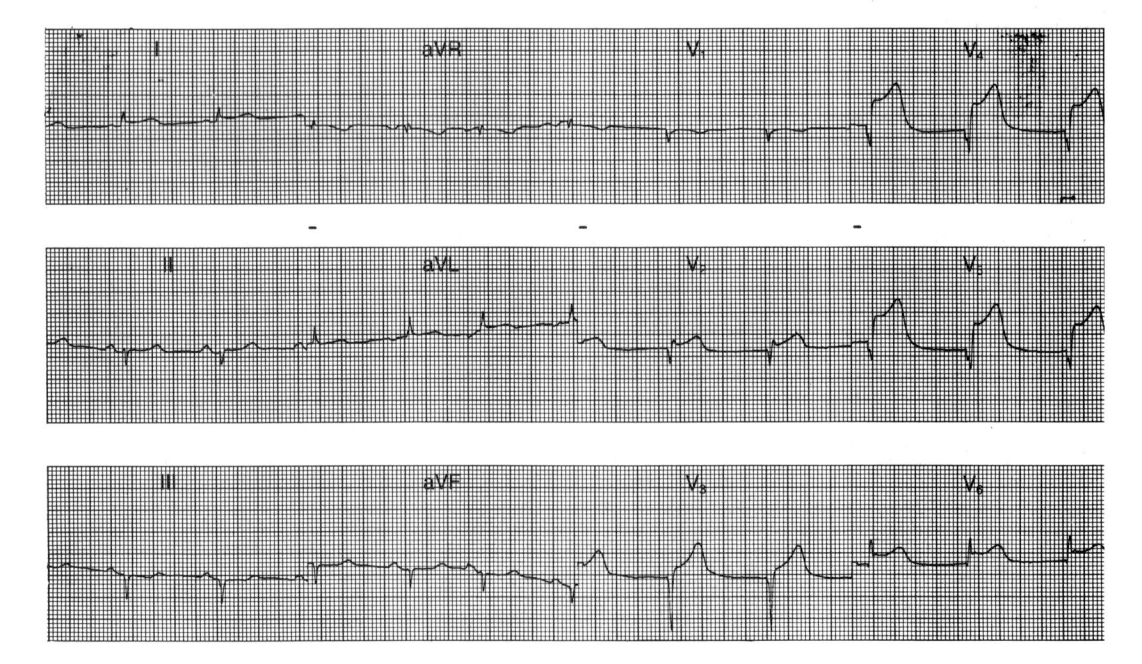

Figure 7-49 Old inferior infarction and acute anterior and lateral infarctions.

Ischemia, Injury, Infarction 119

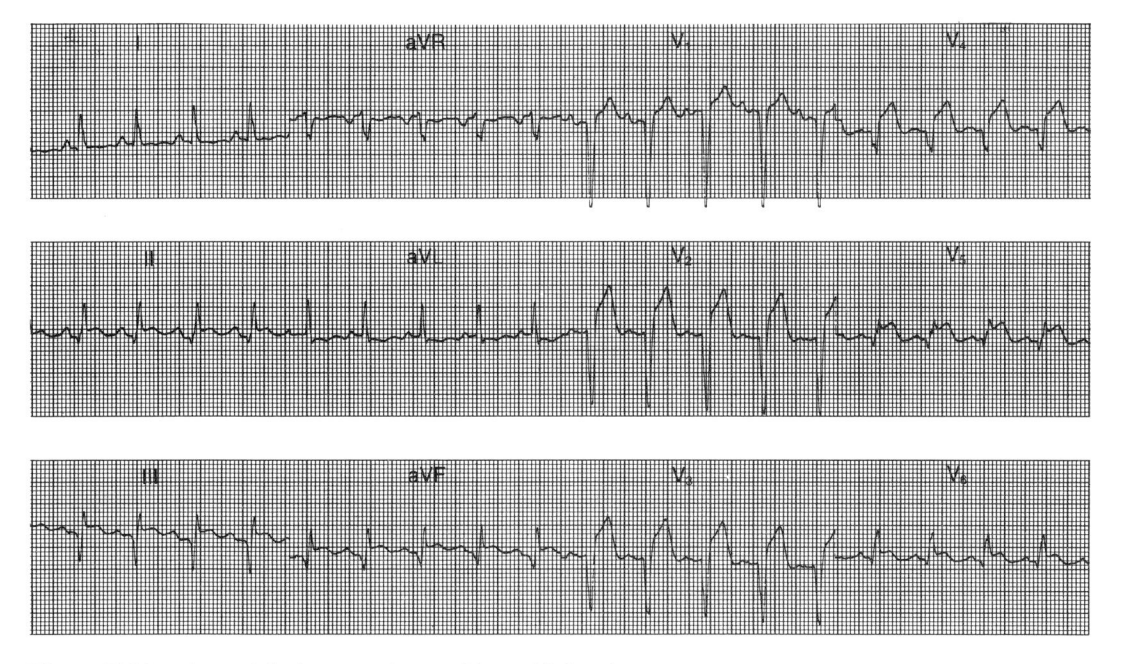

Figure 7-50 Acute inferior, anterior, and lateral infarctions.

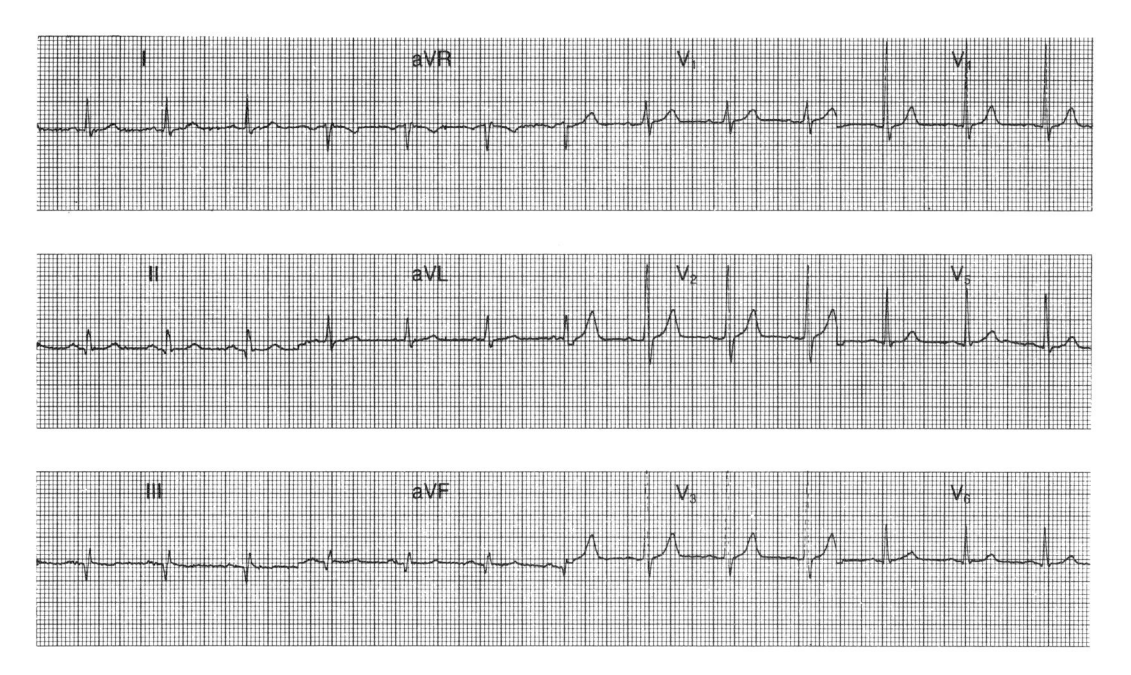

Figure 7-51 Old inferior and posterior infarctions.

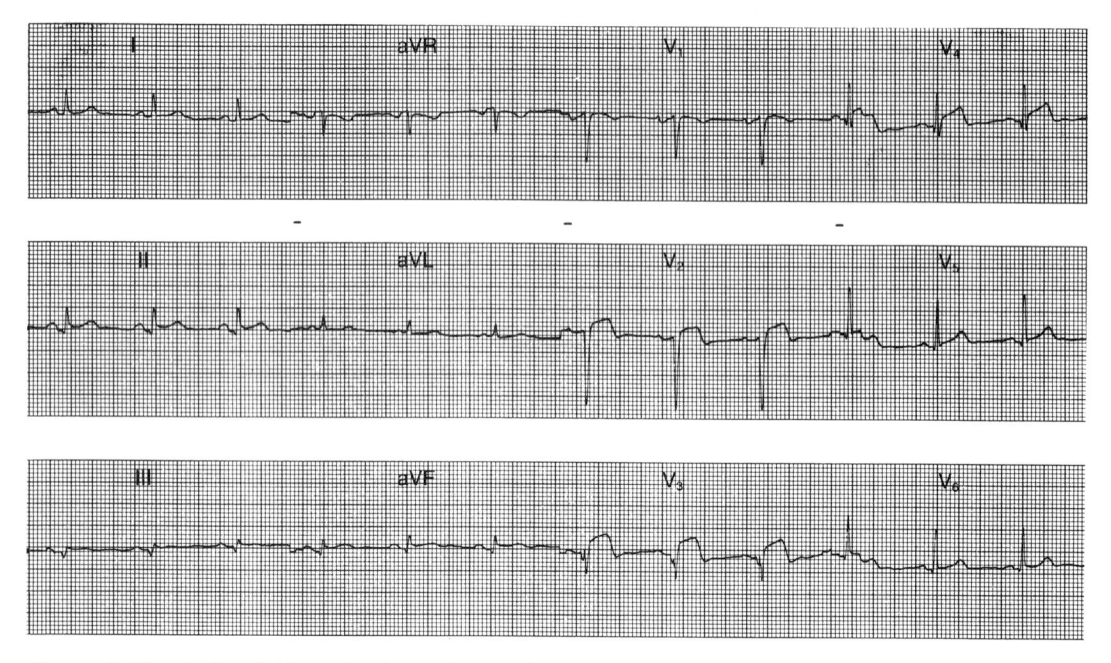

Figure 7-52 Left atrial hypertrophy and acute inferior and anterior infarctions.

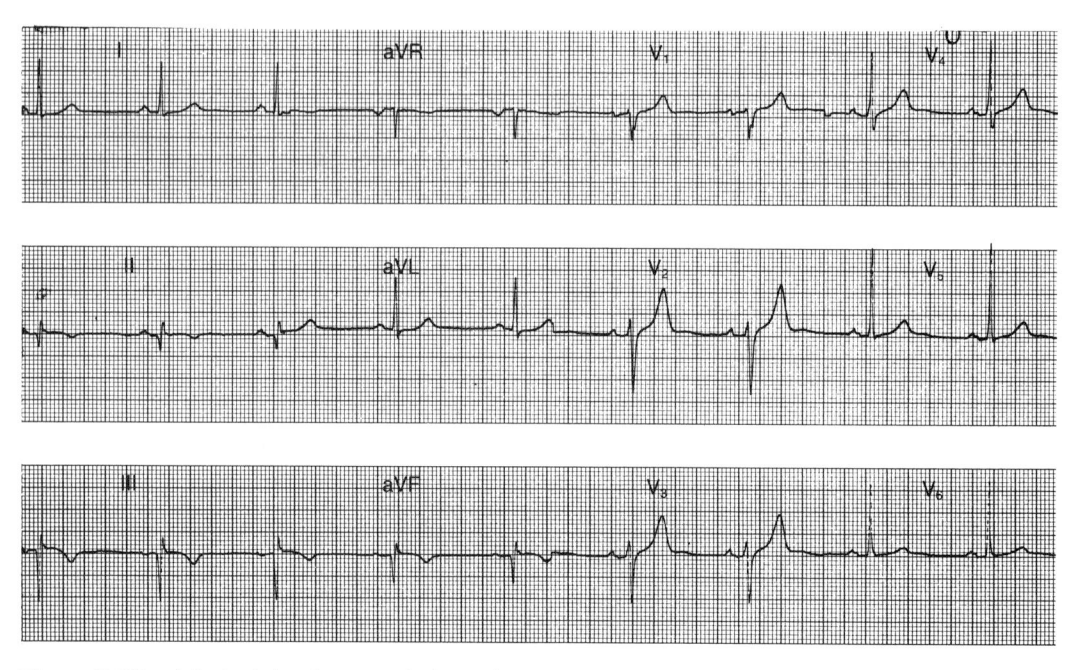

Figure 7-53 Inferior infarction, age indeterminate.

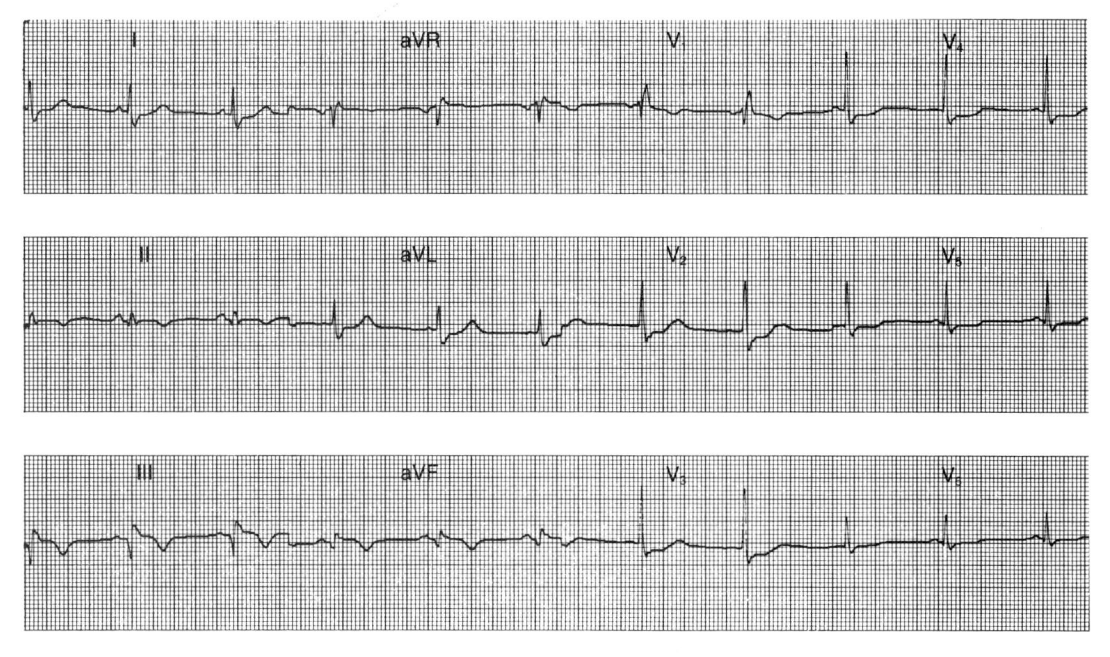

Figure 7-54 Right bundle branch block and inferior infarction, age indeterminate.

Miscellaneous ECG Patterns

Occasionally there are ST-T changes on the ECG that do not fit into any ECG pattern previously discussed. Proper interpretation will depend on a careful clinical evaluation, coupled with the ECG.

Digitalis: The effects of digitalis are characterized on the ECG by shortening, scooping, and downward sloping of the ST segment in leads with tall R waves (Figure 7-55).

Quinidine: A prolonged QT interval and ST-T changes are seen with the use of quinidine (Figure 7-56).

Pericarditis: An inflammation of the pericardial sac encasing the heart is demonstrated on the ECG by concave ST segment elevation throughout the ECG (Figure 7-57).

Early Repolarization: This normal variant is usually seen in young men who demonstrate ST elevation especially in the left chest leads. This ECG pattern is often difficult to differentiate from pericarditis. Serial ECGs will show an evolution of pericarditis by gradually returning ST segments to baseline and subsequent T wave inversion. The early repolarization variant will be unchanged by time (Figure 7-58).

Hypokalemia: A low potassium concentration is suggested on an ECG by the presence of large U waves and flattened T waves (Figure 7-59).

Hyperkalemia: Excess potassium concentration is indicated on an ECG by peaked or tent-shaped T waves (Figure 7-60).

(*Text continues on page 125*)

122 Electrocardiography and Arrhythmias

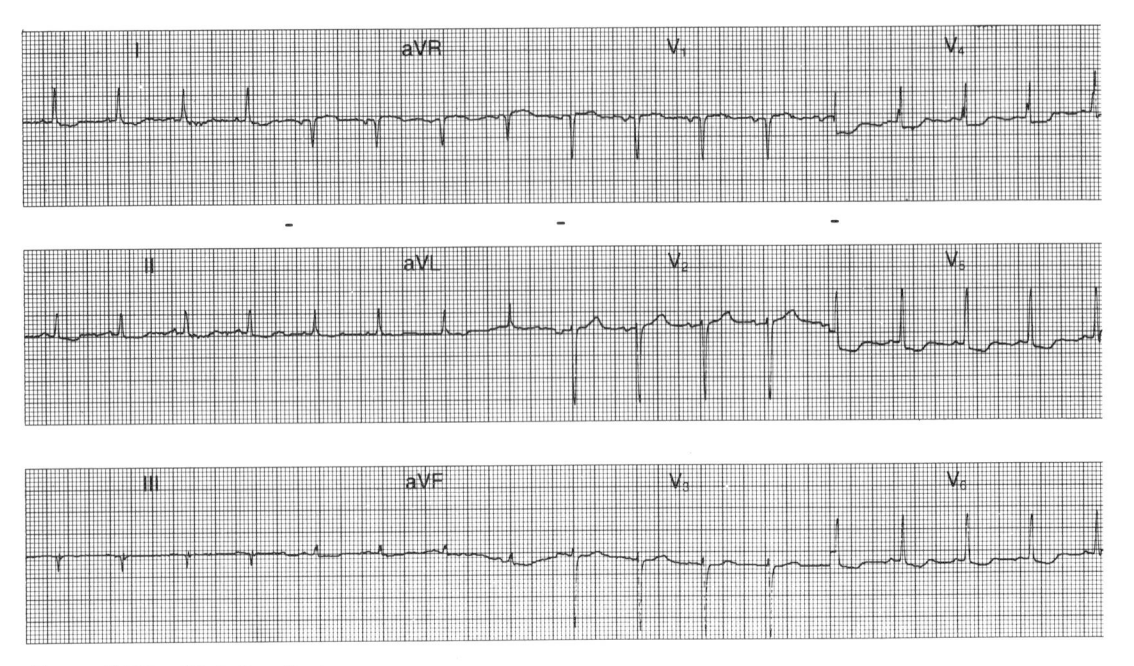

Figure 7-55 Digitalis effect.

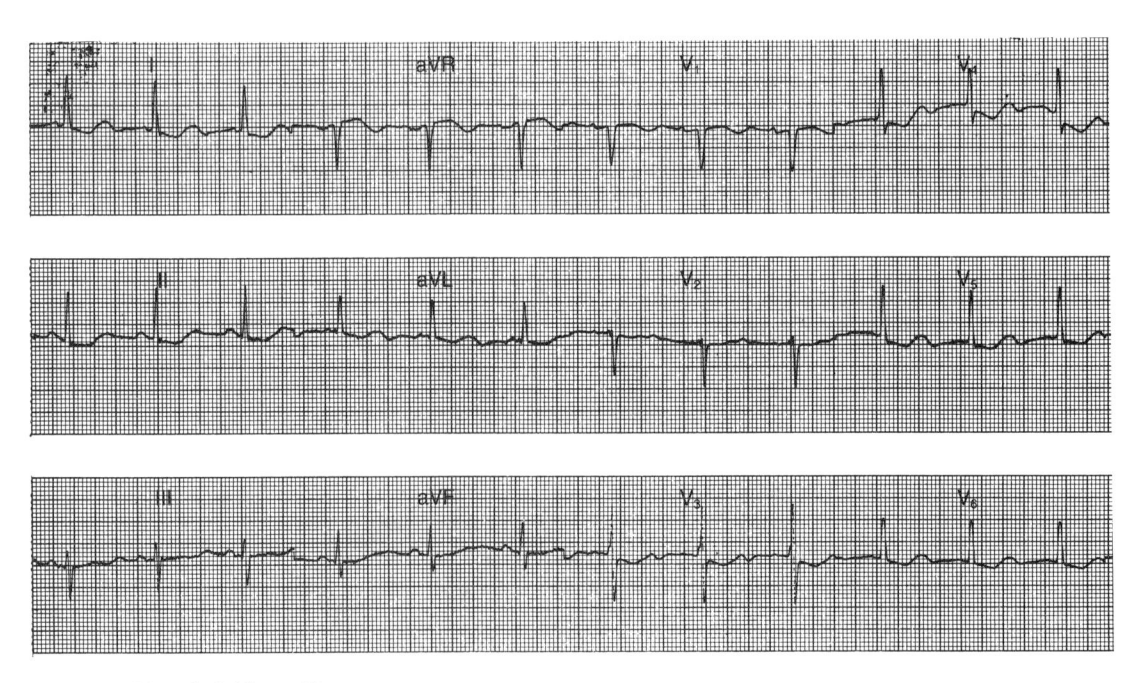

Figure 7-56 Quinidine effect.

Miscellaneous ECG Patterns   123

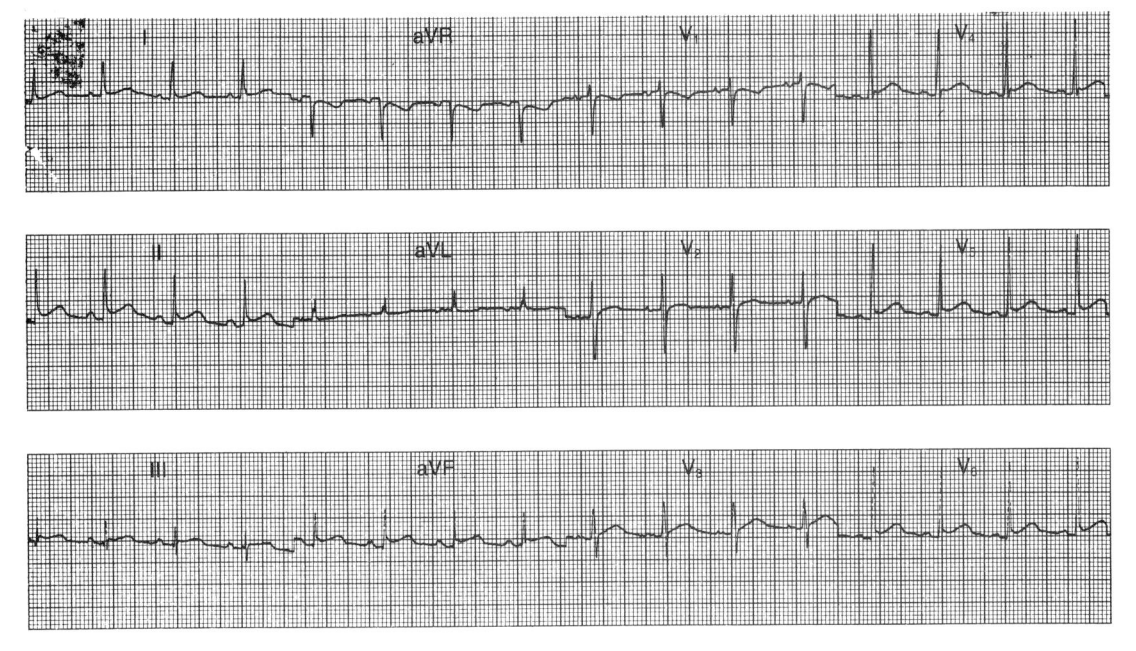

Figure 7-57   Pericarditis.

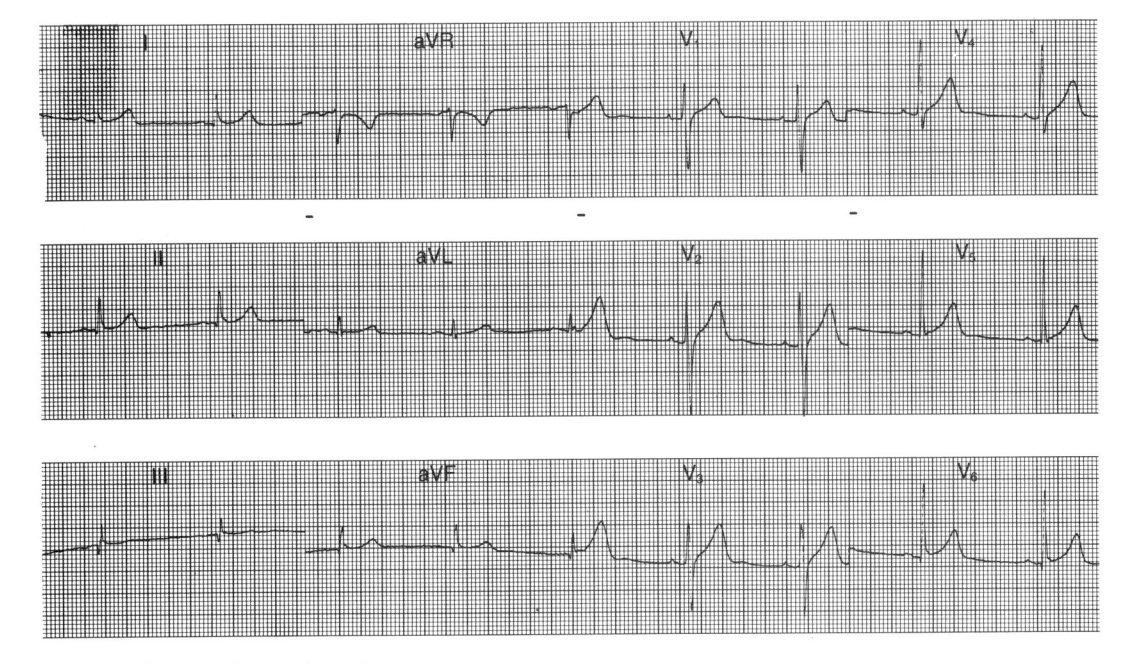

Figure 7-58   Early repolarization.

124 Electrocardiography and Arrhythmias

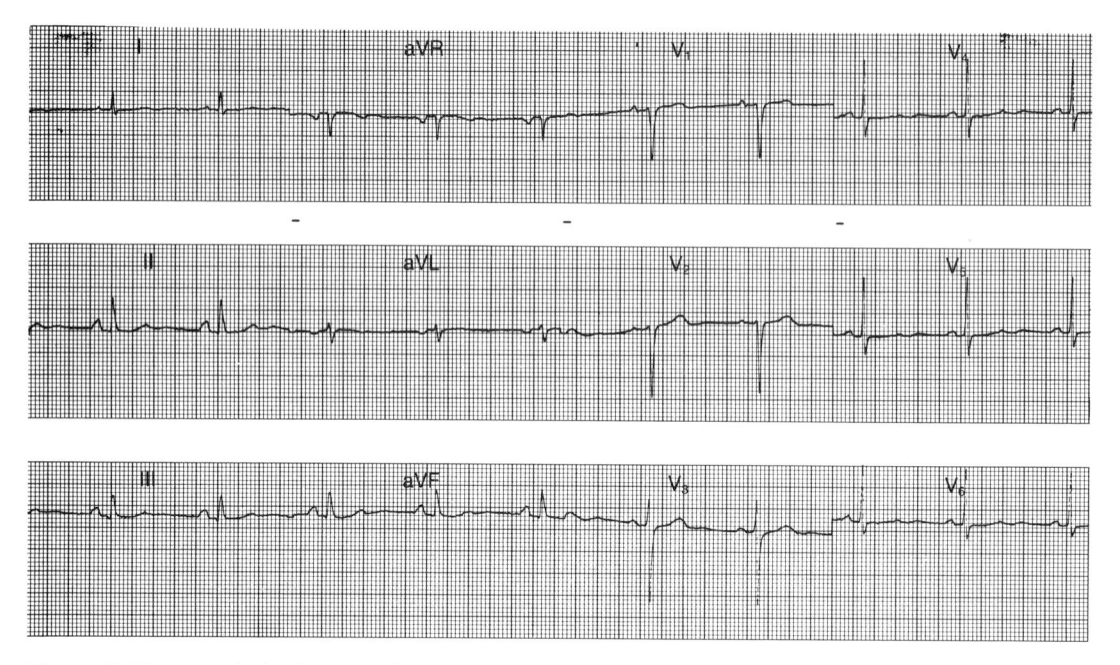

Figure 7-59 Hypokalemia and right atrial hypertrophy.

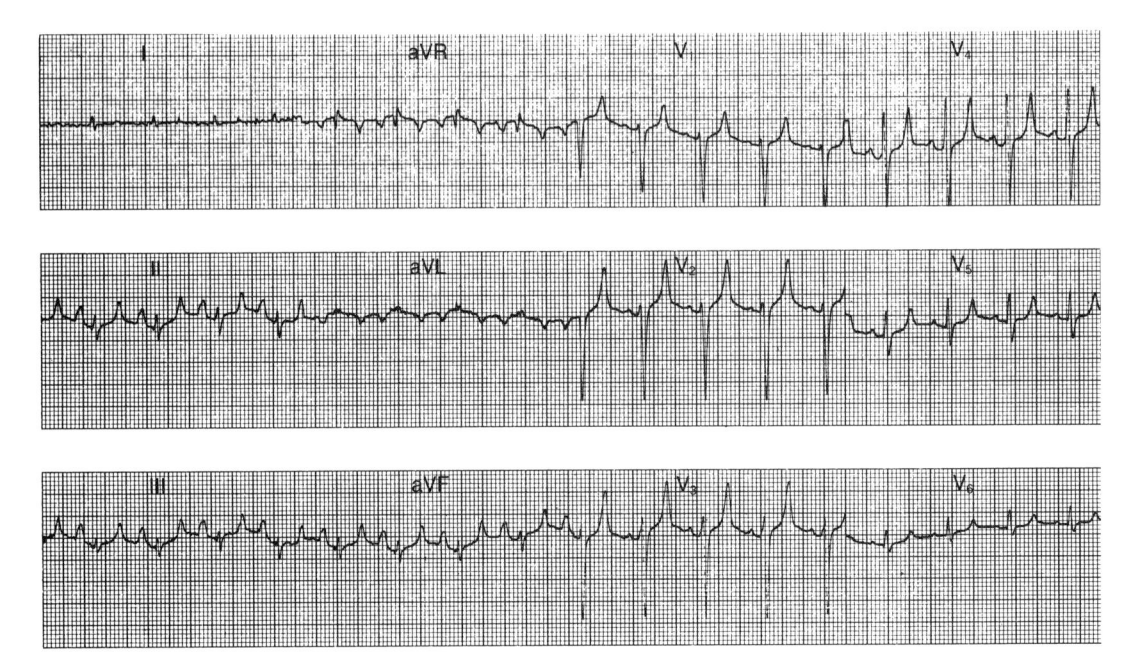

Figure 7-60 Hyperkalemia and right atrial hypertrophy.

Miscellaneous ECG Patterns **125**

Hypocalcemia: A low amount of calcium is suggested by a prolonged ST segment (Figure 7-61).

Hypercalcemia: An overload of calcium may be indicated by a shortened ST segment (Figure 7-62).

Dextrocardia: This is a congenital anomaly in which both the atria and ventricles are transposed to the right side of the chest cavity. Lead I on an ECG will have negative P, QRS and T waves and lead aVR will depict a positive P, QRS, and T wave. The R wave progression in the chest leads will be abnormal. The tallest R wave will be found in V_1 and as the chest leads move away from the transposed heart the R waves will become progressively smaller and then nonexistant (Figure 7-63).

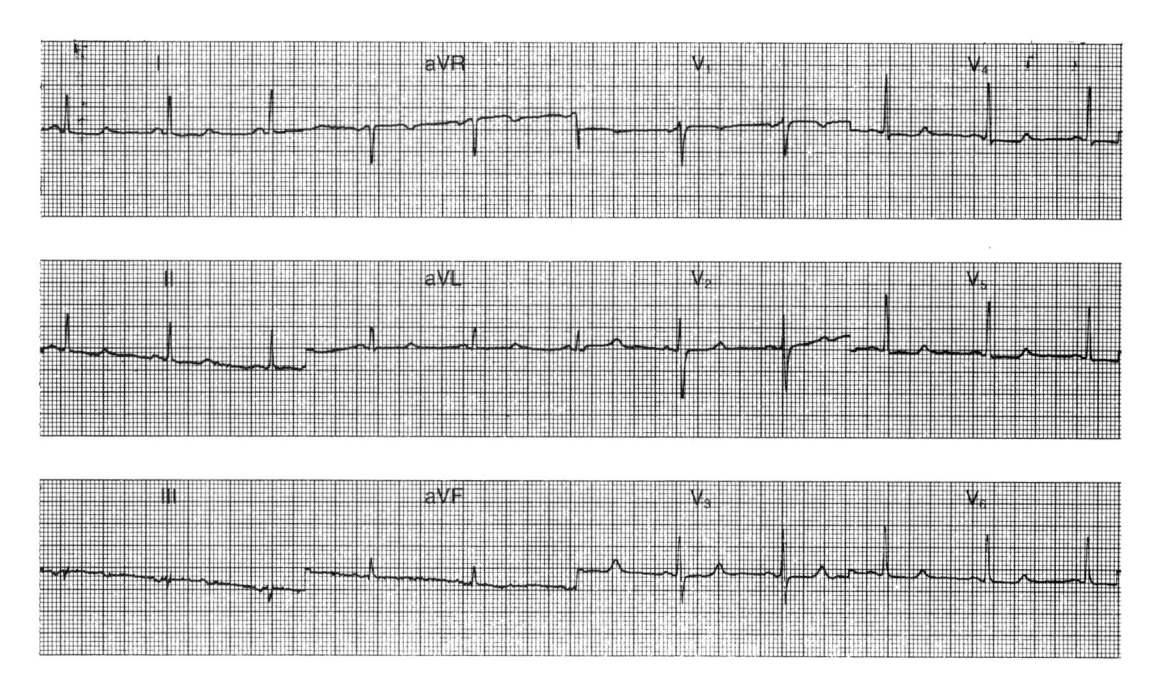

Figure 7-61 Hypocalcemia.

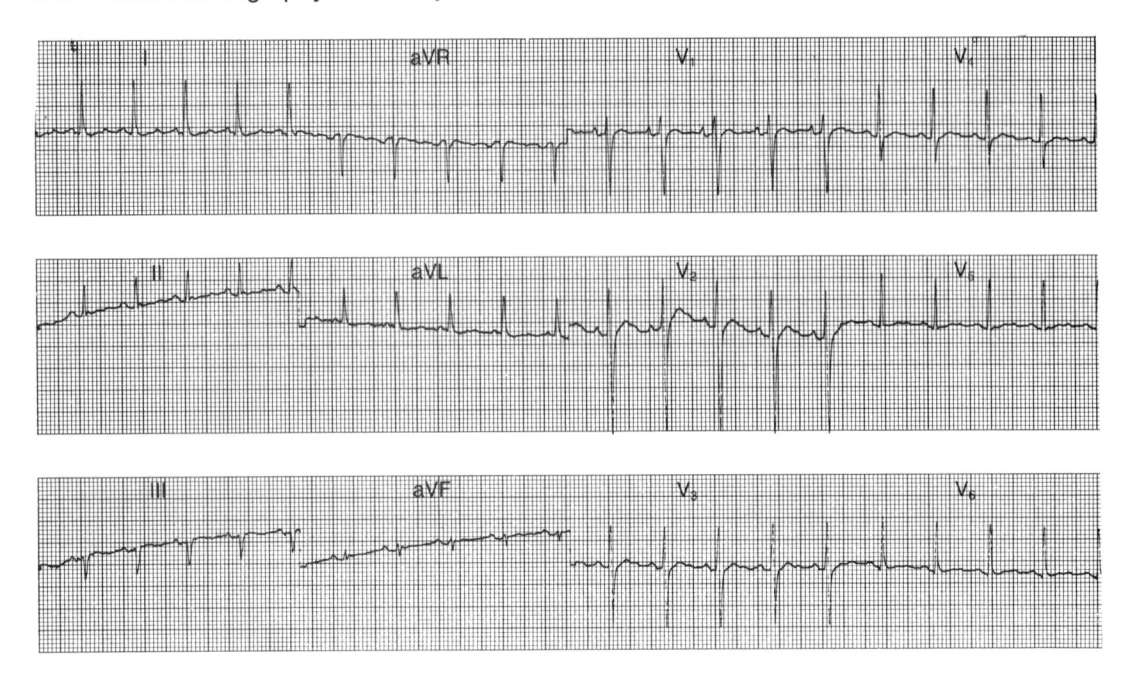

Figure 7-62 Hypercalcemia.

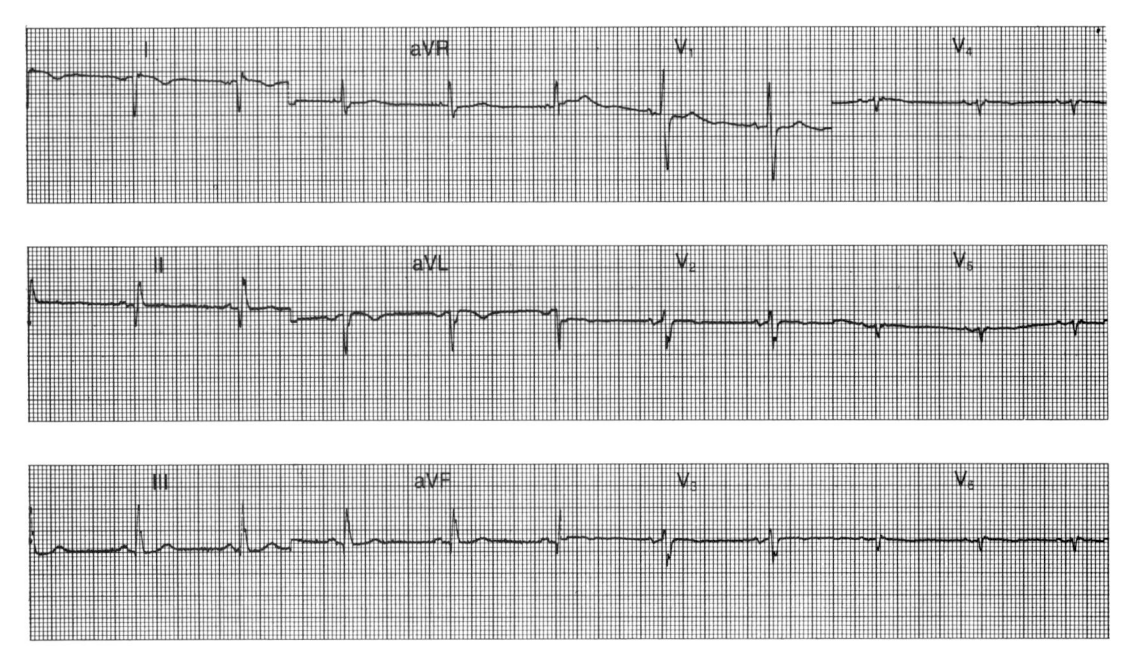

Figure 7-63 Dextrocardia.

Sinus Rhythms

All sinus rhythms begin in the SA node; therefore they are always preceded by a sinus P wave. The PR interval is of constant duration and the atrial and ventricular rates are identical. The sinus rhythms are distinguished from one another by rate or regularity of rhythm. The rhythms may be slightly irregular—the R–R intervals may vary less than .16 second.

Sinus bradycardia—below 60 beats per minute
Sinus rhythm—60–100 beats per minute
Sinus tachycardia—above 100 beats per minute
Sinus arrhythmia—The P–P and R–R cycles vary more than .16 second

(See Figure 7-64 for a depiction of these sinus rhythms.)

What Is an Arrhythmia?

An arrhythmia is a disturbance in normal heart conduction and can take on various configurations. The sinus node is the pacemaker of the heart but there are other potential pacemaker sites in the atria, AV junction, and ventricular tissue.

Extrasystoles

Extrasystoles are extra heart beats that occur prematurely in the cardiac cycle and arise from a pacemaker other than the sinus node in either the atria, AV junction, or ventricles. If the premature beats arise from the exact same area of either the atria, AV junction, or ventricles, then these premature beats are termed *unifocal* (one focus) and will resemble one another. If more than one ectopic focus is firing in either the atria, AV junction, or ventricles, then we call these premature beats *multifocal* (more than one focus) and they then will vary in their configuration (Figure 7-65).

Atrial Premature Contraction (APC). An APC is a premature beat that arises from an area in the atria other than the SA node. The atria are depolarized early, and in a direction that is different than normal atrial depolarization from the sinus node. Therefore, the P wave will look slightly different than the sinus P wave. Conduction then proceeds normally for the remainder of the cardiac cycle, demonstrating a QRS complex that is of the same configuration as the sinus beats. The regularity of the sinus cycle is temporarily disturbed by the APC, causing the SA node to reset its cycle (Figure 7-66).

Nonconducted APC. If an APC occurs extremely early in the cardiac cycle and falls on the T wave of the previous beat, the impulse is often unable to be conducted to the ventricles. It finds a portion of the electrical conduction system beyond the atria refractory from the previous beat and does not allow a QRS complex to be inscribed. An early ectopic P wave with no QRS is recorded and is followed by a pause (Figure 7-67).

(Text continues on page 130)

128 Electrocardiography and Arrhythmias

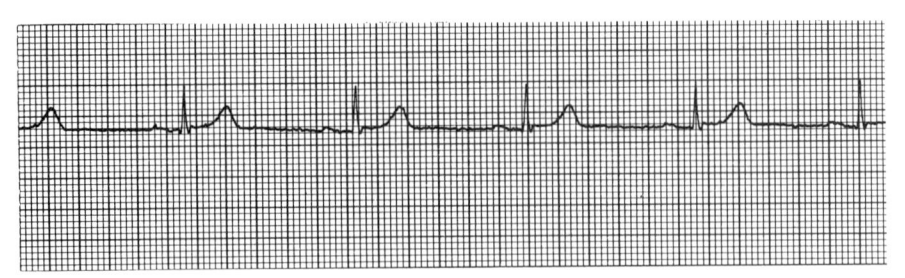

A Sinus bradycardia (56 beats per minute)

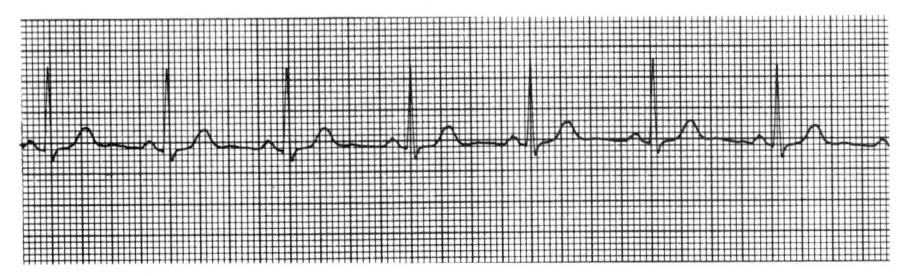

B Sinus rhythm (75 beats per minute)

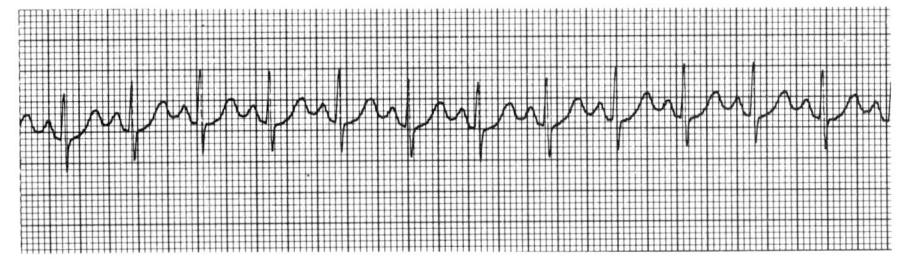

C Sinus tachycardia (131 beats per minute)

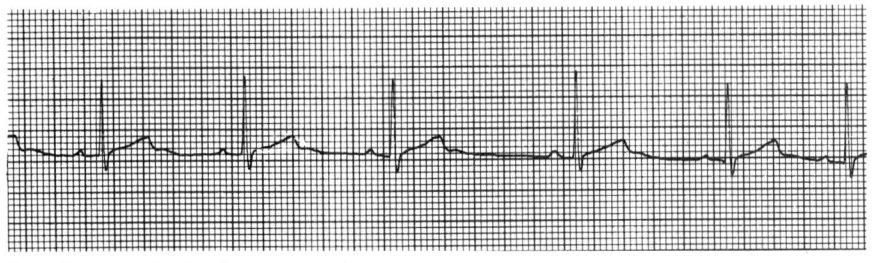

D Sinus arrhythmia

Figure 7-64 Sinus rhythms. (*A*) Sinus bradycardia: 56 beats per minute. (*B*) Sinus rhythm: 75 beats per minute. (*C*) Sinus tachycardia: 131 beats per minute. (*D*) Sinus arrhythmia.

Sinus Rhythms 129

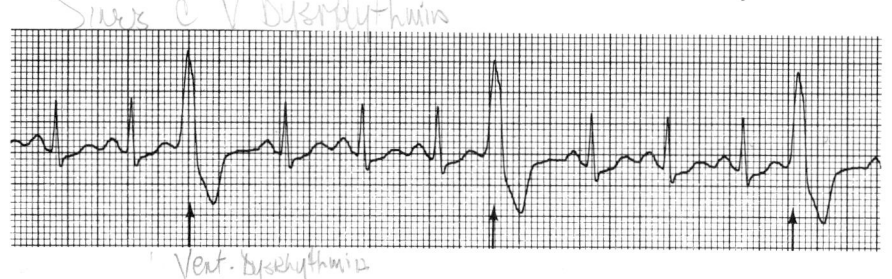

A Unifocal premature beats

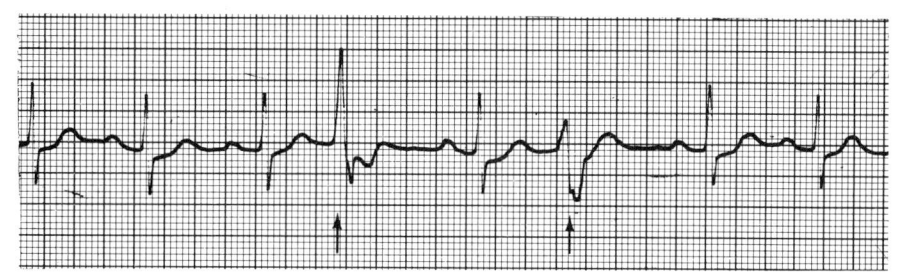

B Multifocal premature beats

Figure 7-65   Extrasystoles.

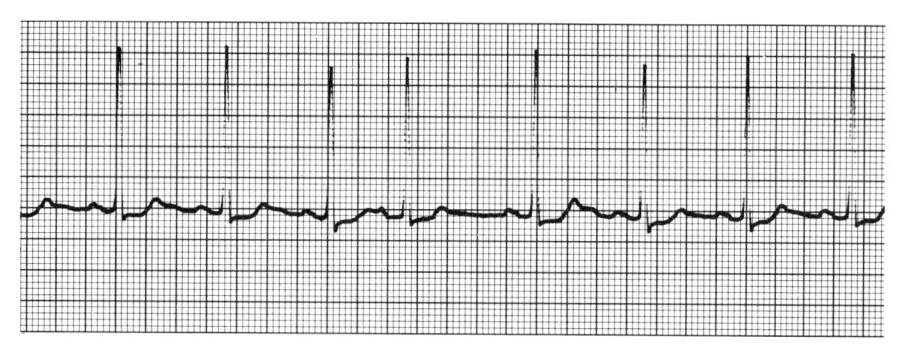

Figure 7-66   Sinus rhythm with one isolated APC.

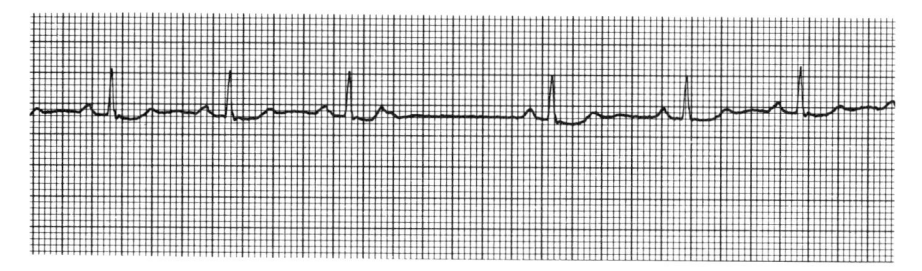

Figure 7-67   Sinus rhythm with one nonconducted APC.

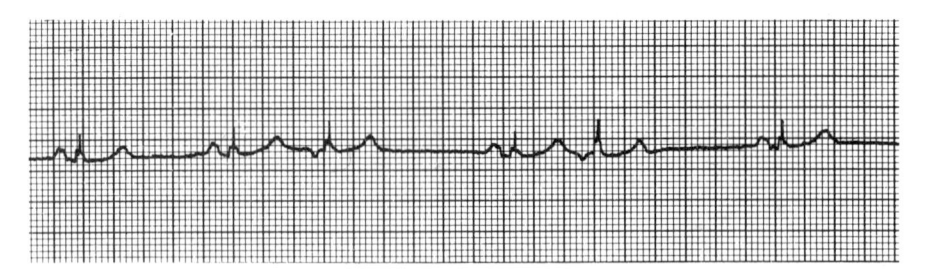

Figure 7-68 Sinus bradycardia with two isolated JPCs.

Junctional Premature Contraction (JPC). A JPC is an early ectopic impulse that begins in the tissue surrounding the AV node and travels forward (antegradely) through the normal conduction pathways, inscribing a QRS that resembles a QRS of the sinus beats. Simultaneously, the impulse travels backward (retrogradely) to depolarize the atria. A negative P wave is inscribed because the atria are depolarized in a backward direction. Depending on whether the antegrade or retrograde conduction is more rapid, the JPC will either have an inverted P wave preceding, buried within, or immediately following the QRS complex. The regularity of the sinus cycle is temporarily disturbed by the JPC, causing the sinus cycle to reset itself (Figure 7-68).

Ventricular Premature Contraction (VPC). A VPC is an early ectopic beat that begins in one of the ventricles and spreads to the other ventricle with some delay because of slow conduction through ventricular myocardium. This delay in conduction produces a widened and different-looking QRS than with the normal sinus beats. The QRS is .12 second or greater in duration. The sinus cycle is not interrupted as with APCs and JPCs and continues on uninterrupted with its regular rhythm.

A malignant VPC is one that falls on the T wave of the previous beat. The T wave is in the relative refractory period of the heart and at a time when the ventricles are quite unstable. A VPC occurring at this time opens the possibility of initiating rapid, repetitive firing of the focus (Figure 7-69).

Escape Beats and Rhythms

Contrary to premature beats, which are always early, escape beats are always late in relation to the cardiac rhythm. When the regular pacemaker does not fire, the escape mechanism fires and rescues the heart from asystole.

AV junctional escape beats fire at an inherent rate of 40 to 60 beats per minute, are always late in relation to the dominant cardiac rhythm, and are preceded by either an inverted P wave, no P wave, an inverted P wave immediately following the QRS, or a sinus P wave with a shorter than normal

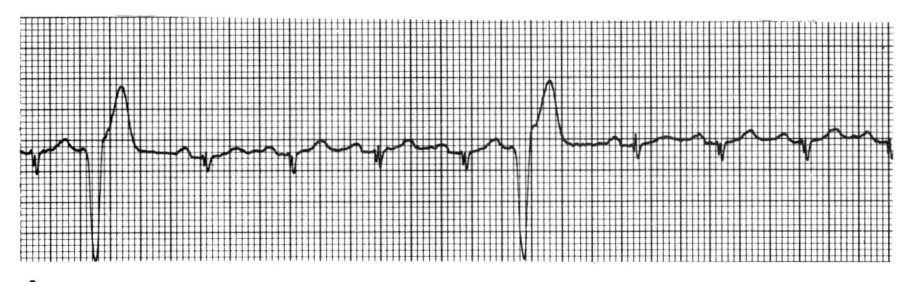

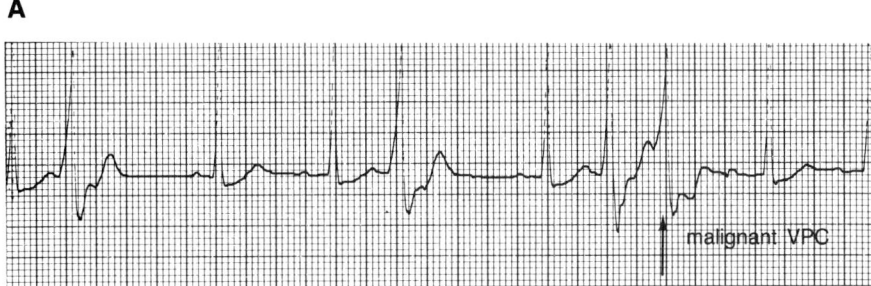

Figure 7-69 (A) Sinus tachycardia with two isolated unifocal VPCs. (B) Sinus rhythm with four unifocal VPCs—one pair and the last VPC malignant.

PR interval. The QRS complex usually resembles the QRS of the dominant rhythm. Six or more junctional escape beats in a row constitute an escape rhythm (Figures 7-70 and 7-71).

Ventricular escape beats fire at an inherent rate below 40 beats per minute, are always late in relation to the dominant cardiac rhythm, and are wide and different in configuration than the beats of the dominant rhythm. Six or more ventricular escape beats in a row constitute a ventricular escape rhythm (Figures 7-72 and 7-73).

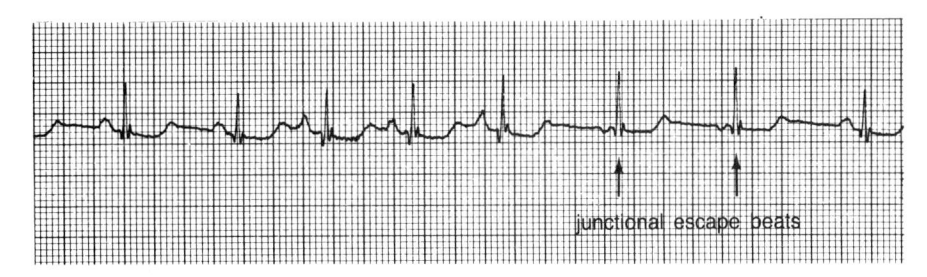

Figure 7-70 Sinus rhythm with three APCs in a row followed by two junctional escape beats.

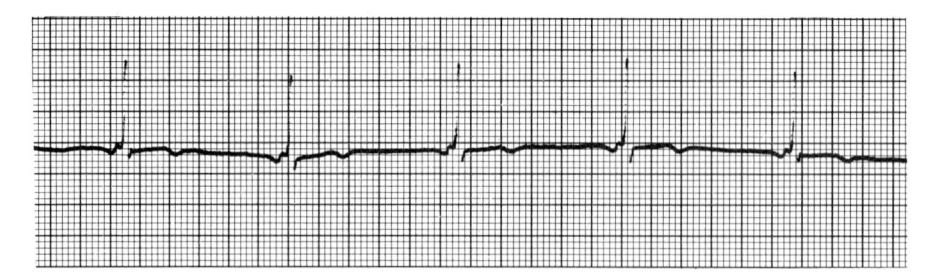

Figure 7-71 Junctional escape rhythm: 54 beats per minute.

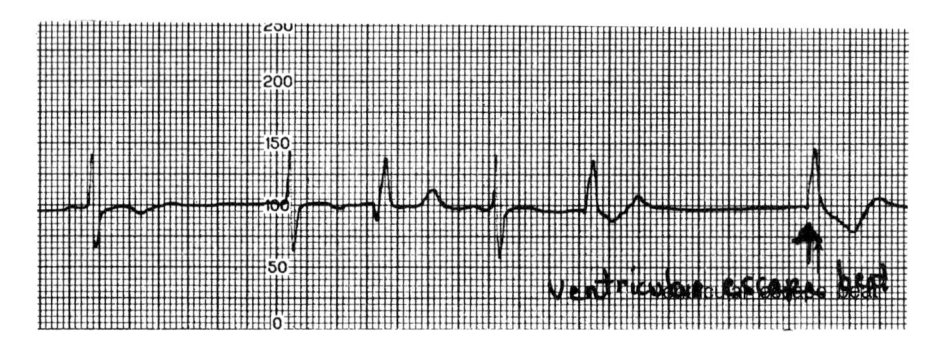

Figure 7-72 Sinus bradycardia with two unifocal VPCs and one ventricular escape beat.

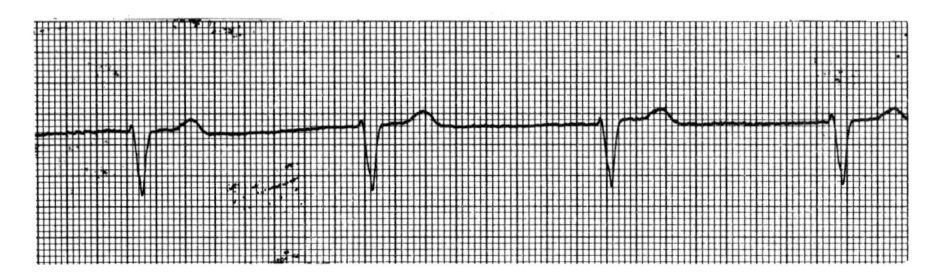

Figure 7-73 Ventricular escape rhythm: 38 beats per minute.

Atrial Ectopic Rhythms

Atrial ectopic rhythms are caused by repetitive and rapid firing of one or more ectopic foci located anywhere in the atria other than the sinus node.

Paroxysmal Atrial Tachycardia (PAT)

PAT is a run of six or more APCs in a row, usually between the rates of 140 to 220 beats per minute. The ectopic P waves are different in configuration from the sinus P waves, the PR interval is of constant duration, and the QRS complexes resemble the QRS complexes of the dominant rhythm (Figure 7-74).

If the atrial tachycardia is slower than 180 beats per minute, probably all of the ectopic atrial impulses will conduct to the ventricles. If the rate is faster, some of the impulses may find the AV node to be refractory, or busy, from the previous beat, and all the ectopic P waves will not be conducted to the ventricles. This is called *PAT with block* (Figure 7-75).

Multifocal Atrial Tachycardia (MAT)

MAT is caused by a repetitive and rapid firing of two or more atrial ectopic foci at a rate between 100 and 200 beats per minute. There are multifocal ectopic P waves with an irregular P–P cycle, the PR interval varies from beat to beat, nonconducted ectopic P waves occur, and the QRS usually resembles the QRS of the dominant rhythm (Figure 7-76).

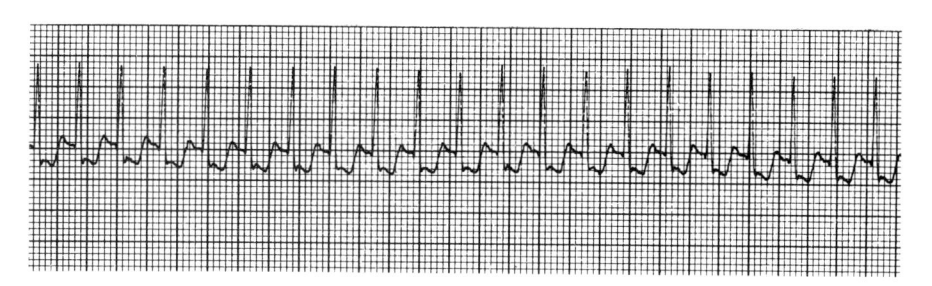

Figure 7-74 Paroxysmal atrial tachycardia.

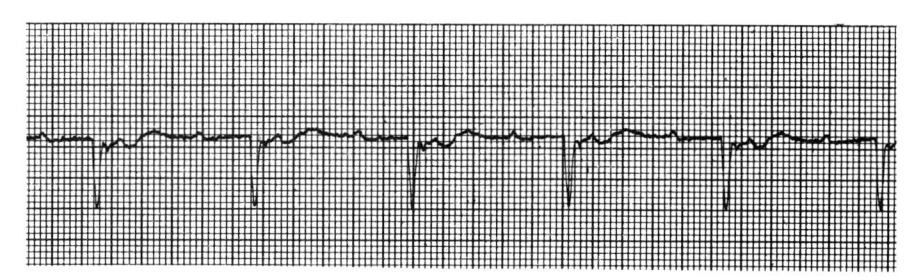

Figure 7-75 Paroxysmal atrial tachycardia: 174 beats per minute with 2:1 block and a ventricular rate of 87 beats per minute.

134 Electrocardiography and Arrhythmias

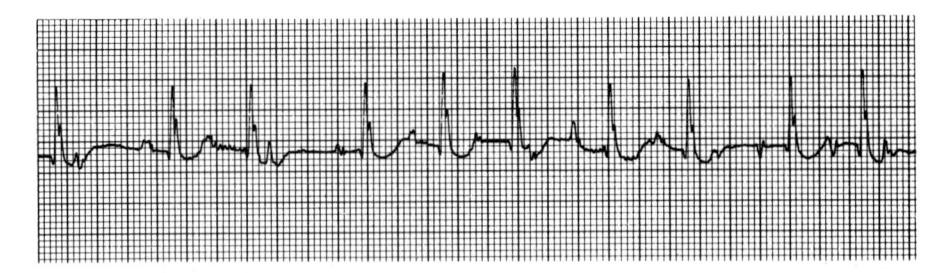

Figure 7-76   Multifocal atrial tachycardia.

Atrial Flutter

One theory of impulse formation in atrial flutter is a rapid and repetitive firing of a unifocal atrial focus at a rate between 220 and 350 beats per minute. Flutter waves (F waves) replace P waves and take on a saw tooth configuration. The rate and regularity of the QRS is variable and depends upon conduction through the AV node of the rapid atrial impulses. The conduction ratio is constant if the R–R cycle is regular, and the conduction ratio is variable if the R–R cycle is irregular (Figures 7-77 and 7-78).

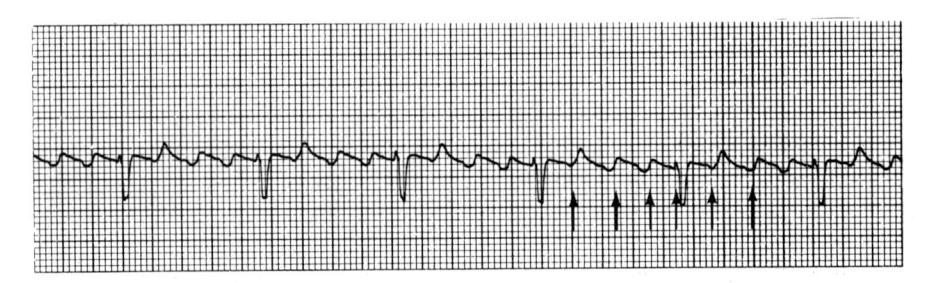

Figure 7-77   Atrial flutter waves.

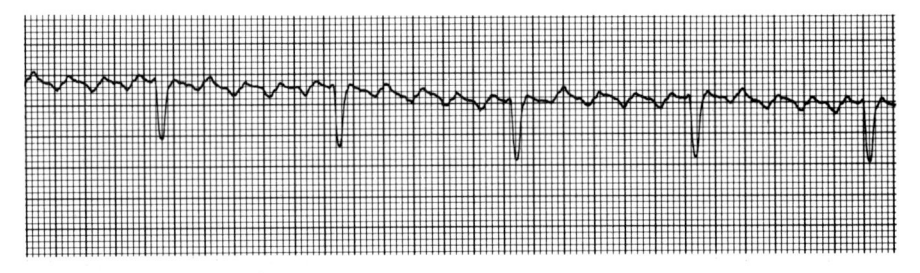

Figure 7-78   Atrial flutter: 275 beats per minute with 4:1 block and ventricular response of 53 beats per minute.

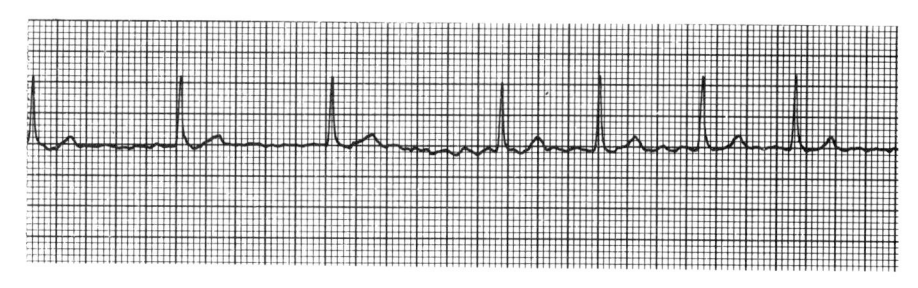

Figure 7-79 Atrial fibrillation with an average ventricular response of 75 beats per minute.

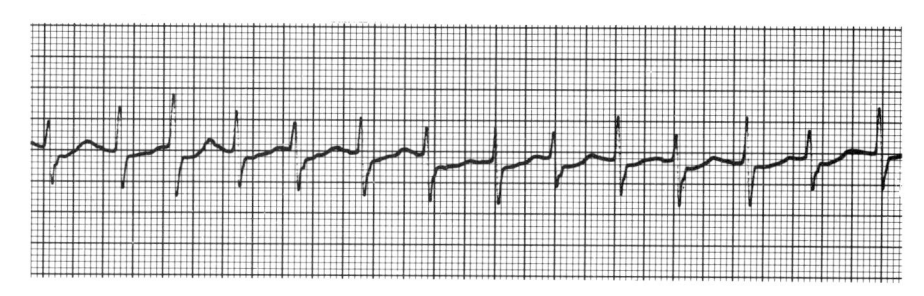

Figure 7-80 Atrial fibrillation with a rapid ventricular response of 145 beats per minute.

Atrial Fibrillation

One theory of impulse formation in atrial fibrillation is that a rapid and repetitive firing of multifocal atrial ectopic foci occurs, at a rate between 350 and 650 beats per minute. These rapidly firing foci produce fibrillatory or f waves that replace P waves and make it difficult to determine the atrial rate. The ventricular rate is irregular because only some of the f waves are able to be conducted intermittently through AV junction to the ventricles (Figures 7-79 and 7-80).

Junctional Rhythms

Accelerated junctional rhythm is a repetitive firing of six or more JPCs at a rate between 60 and 100 beats per minute. The QRS complexes are either preceded by an inverted P wave, no P waves, or immediately followed by inverted P waves. The QRS complexes resemble the QRS complexes of the dominant rhythm (Figure 7-81).

Junctional tachycardia is a rapid and repetitive firing of six or more JPCs at a rate between 100 and 220 beats per minute. The QRS complexes are either preceded by an inverted P wave, no P waves, or immediately followed by inverted P waves. The QRS complexes resemble the QRS complexes of the dominant rhythm (Figure 7-82).

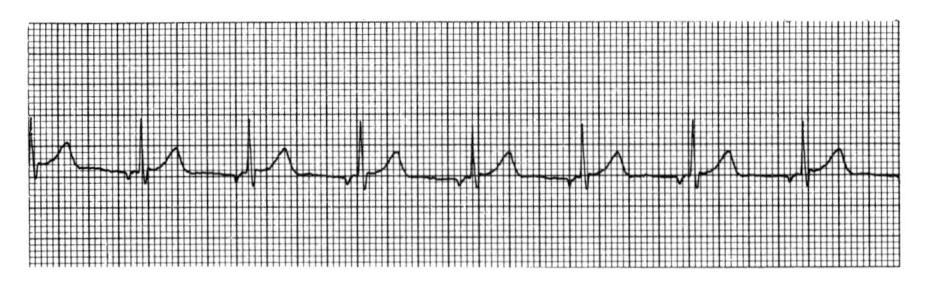

Figure 7-81 Accelerated junctional rhythm: 82 beats per minute.

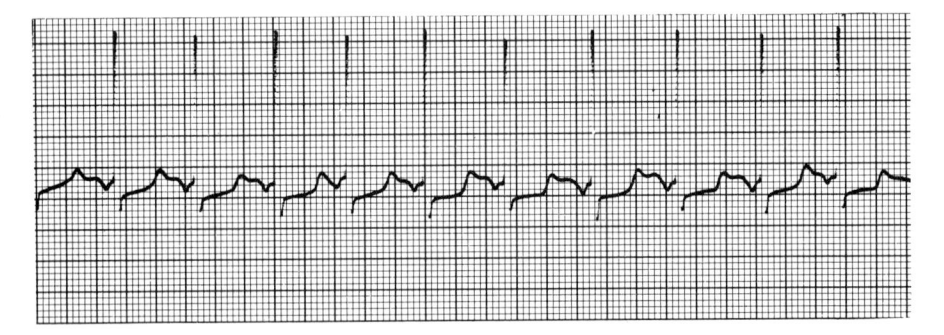

Figure 7-82 Junctional tachycardia: 117 beats per minute.

Ventricular Rhythms

Ventricular rhythms are caused by repetitive firing of an ectopic focus located in the ventricles.

Accelerated Idioventricular Rhythm
Accelerated idioventricular rhythm is a firing of six or more VPCs at a rate of 40 to 100 beats per minute. The QRS complexes are wide and look different than the dominant cardiac rhythm (Figure 7-83).

Ventricular Tachycardia
This is the rapid firing of six or more VPCs in a row at a rate of 100 to 250 beats per minute (Figure 7-84).

Ventricular Flutter
Ventricular flutter is the rapid and repetitive firing of one or more ventricular ectopic foci at a rate of 150 to 300 beats per minute, demonstrating a fairly regular rhythm. The QRS complexes appear to run into one another with no visible ST segments or T waves (Figure 7-85).

Sinus Rhythms

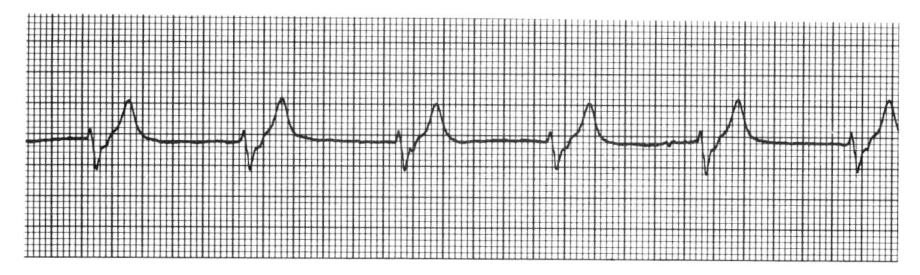

Figure 7-83 Accelerated idioventricular rhythm: 58 beats per minute.

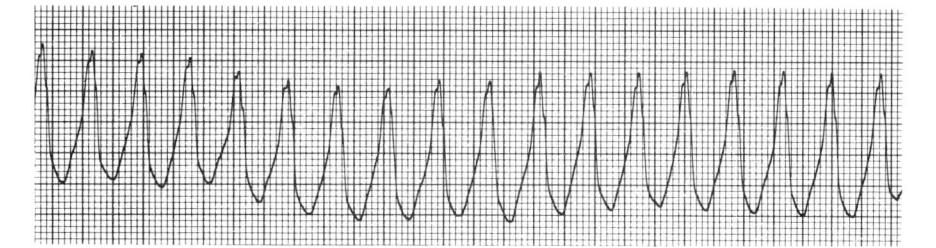

Figure 7-84 Ventricular tachycardia: 180 beats per minute.

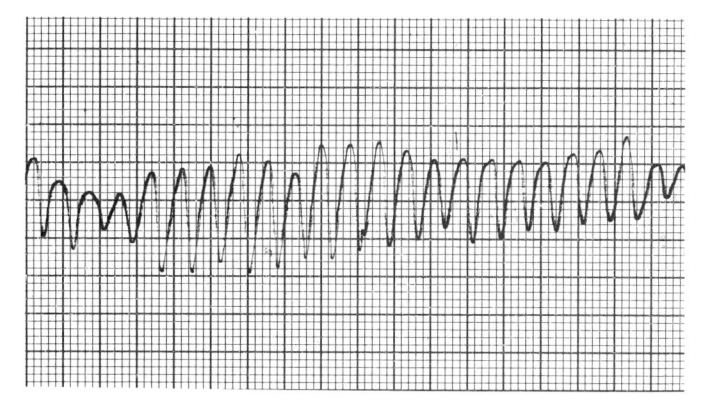

Figure 7-85 Ventricular flutter.

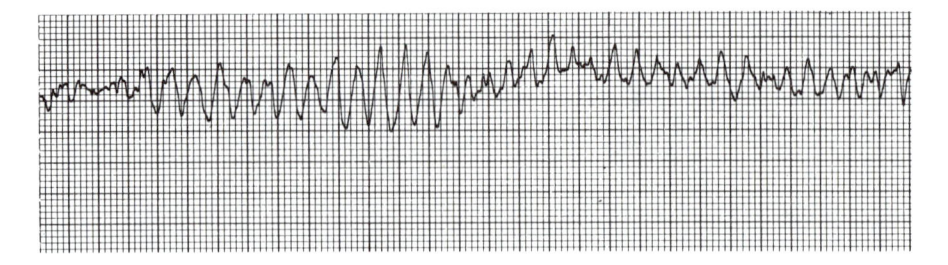

Figure 7-86 Ventricular fibrillation.

Ventricular Fibrillation

Ventricular fibrillation is the firing of multifocal ventricular ectopic foci at a rate of 150 to 500 beats per minute in a highly irregular fashion. No visible QRS complexes can be recognized (Figure 7-86).

AV Dissociation

AV dissociation is a condition in which two rhythms occur in the heart at the same time; the atria and ventricles temporarily beat independently of each other. The sinus node depolarizes the atria and either an ectopic focus in the AV junction or the ventricles depolarize the ventricles. With the atria in sinus rhythm, the P wave floats in and out of the QRS complexes of either the junctional or ventricular focus, but bears no relationship to it (Figure 7-87).

Aberration

Aberration is a variation or change in the QRS complex from its normal configuration; it occurs when a sinus or supraventricular impulse activates the ventricles early and in an abnormal way. The supraventricular impulse finds one of the bundle branches to be refractory from the previous beat, so conduction must take place abnormally from one ventricle first and then to

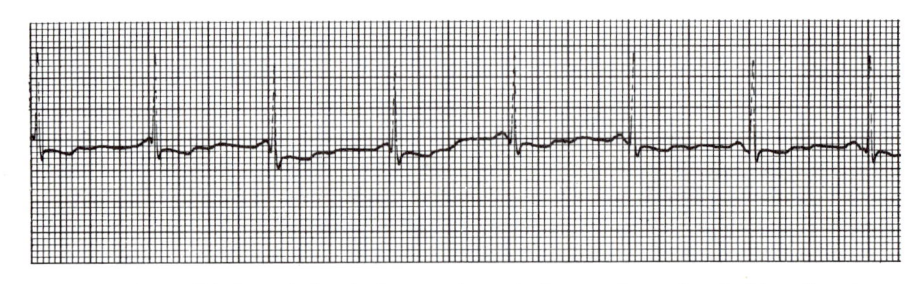

Figure 7-87 AV dissociation between sinus rhythm and accelerated junctional rhythm—75 beats per minute.

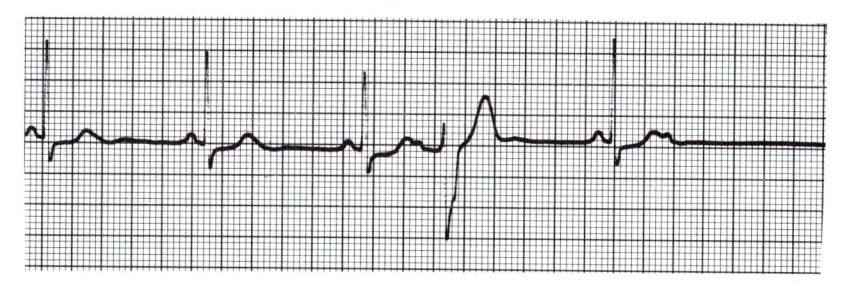

Figure 7-88 Sinus bradycardia showing one APC with aberration and one nonconducted APC.

the other through ventricular myocardium. Because of the delay in conduction a wide and bizarre QRS results. When APCs or JPCs occur very close to the previous beat, usually in the T wave, the QRS complexes of the premature beats are prone to aberration. Also, during irregular ventricular rates, when a long R–R cycle is followed by a short R–R cycle, the beat following the long cycle may be aberrant. This type of aberration is called the *Ashman phenomenon* and is often found in atrial fibrillation.

It is very important to be able to differentiate between supraventricular beats with aberration and VPCs. When trying to differentiate between the two, when sinus rhythm is present, look for the ectopic P waves of the APCs and JPCs hidden in the previous T wave (Figure 7-88).

AV Block

When a supraventricular impulse should be able to be conducted to the ventricles but is not, AV block is considered to be present. When we speak of nonconducted APCs and PAT with block, we are dealing with physiological refractoriness of the conduction system; it is impossible for the heart to conduct when it is still busy from the previous beat. This is considered normal and prevents the heart from beating too rapidly.

First Degree AV Block
This is a delay in conduction of the sinus impulse to the ventricles and is characterized by a PR interval greater than .20 second (Figure 7-89).

Second Degree AV Block Wenckebach
In this condition, the conduction of sinus or supraventricular impulses to the ventricles becomes increasingly more difficult, causing progressively longer PR intervals until a P wave is not conducted. The pause following the dropped P wave enables the AV node to recover and the following P wave is conducted with a normal or slightly shorter PR. The R–R interval becomes progressively shorter until the pause occurs and a junctional or ventricular escape beat may terminate the pause (Figure 7-90).

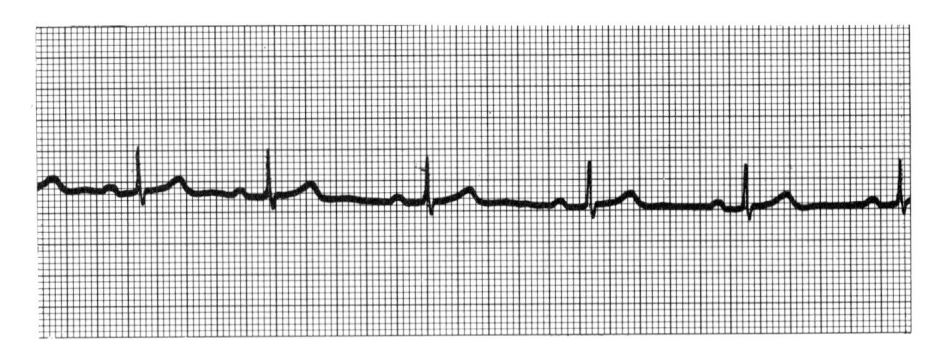

Figure 7-89 Sinus rhythm and first-degree AV block with a PR interval of .24 of a second.

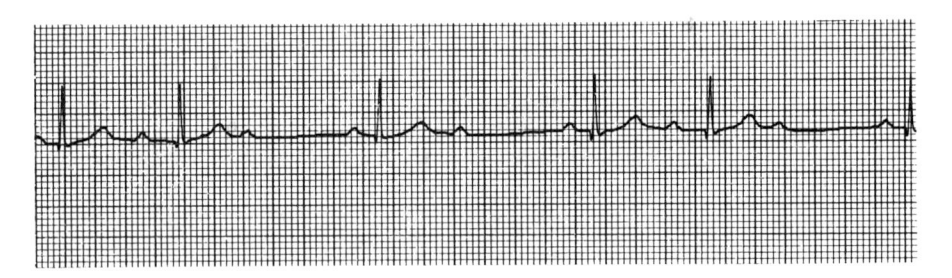

Figure 7-90 Sinus rhythm: 80 beats per minute and second-degree AV block Wenckebach.

Second Degree AV Block Mobitz
Second degree AV block Mobitz is demonstrated by the conduction of sinus or supraventricular impulses to the ventricles with intermittent block of some of the P waves. No more than one P wave in a row is blocked and the PR interval of the conducted beats remains constant (Figure 7-91).

High Grade AV Block
High grade AV block is characterized by the conduction of sinus or supraventricular impulses to the ventricles with intermittent block of more than one P wave in a row and a constant PR interval. In atrial fibrillation or flutter, long ventricular pauses are seen that may be terminated by junctional or ventricular escape beats or rhythms (Figure 7-92).

Complete AV Block
The atria and ventricles beat independently of each other under the control of separate pacemaking foci. There is no relationship between the P waves and the QRS complexes, so the PR interval is always changing. The atria may be under the control of a sinus or supraventricular pacemaker and the

Sinus Rhythms 141

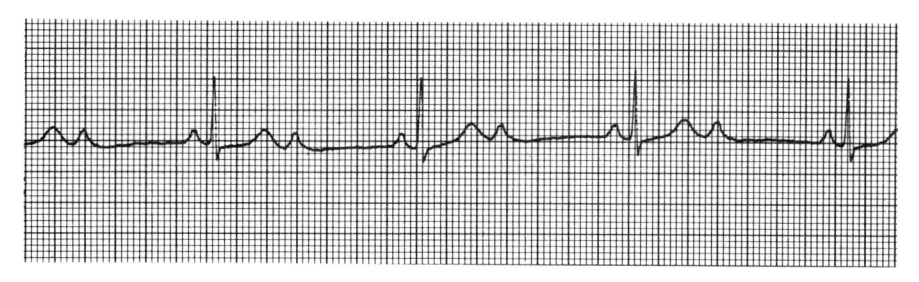

Figure 7-91 Sinus rhythm: 88 beats per minute with second-degree AV block Mobitz and a ventricular rate of 44 beats per minute.

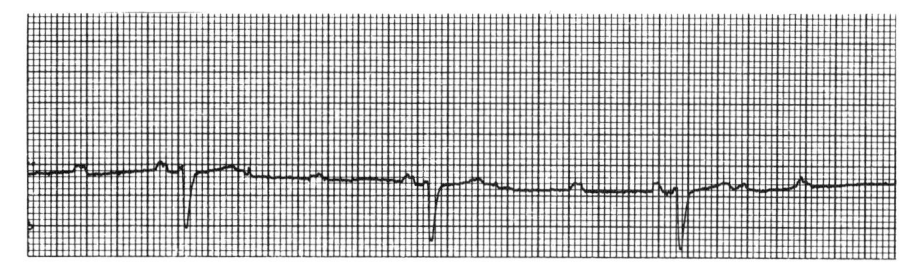

Figure 7-92 Sinus tachycardia: 115 beats per minute with high grade AV block and a ventricular response of 37 beats per minute.

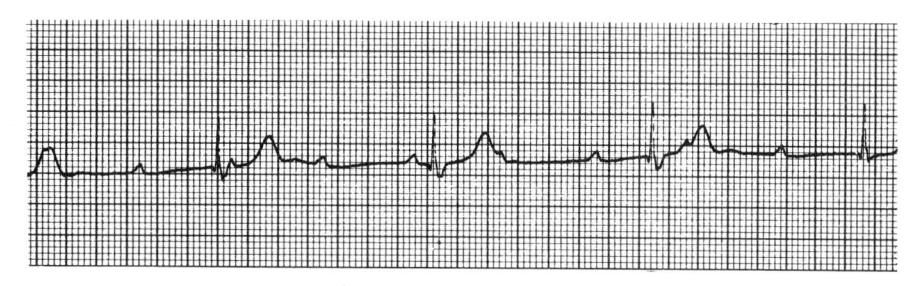

Figure 7-93 Sinus rhythm: 100 beats per minute with complete AV block and an accelerated idioventricular rhythm of 42 beats per minute.

ventricles are rescued either by a junctional escape rhythm when the QRS width is of normal duration, or more likely by a ventricular escape rhythm when the QRS width is wide and of abnormal configuration. The ventricular rate is usually slower than the atrial rate because the escape focus controls the ventricles. In atrial fibrillation with complete AV block, the ventricular rate is unexpectedly regular due to an escape mechanism that rescues the ventricles from asystole (Figure 7-93).

142 Electrocardiography and Arrhythmias

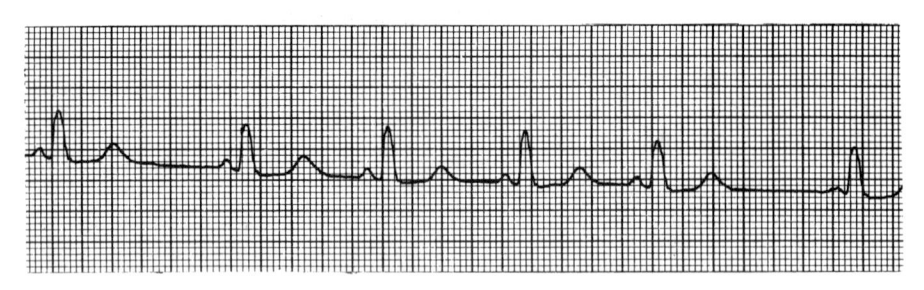

Figure 7-94 Sinus rhythm: 64 beats per minute with second-degree SA block Wenckebach.

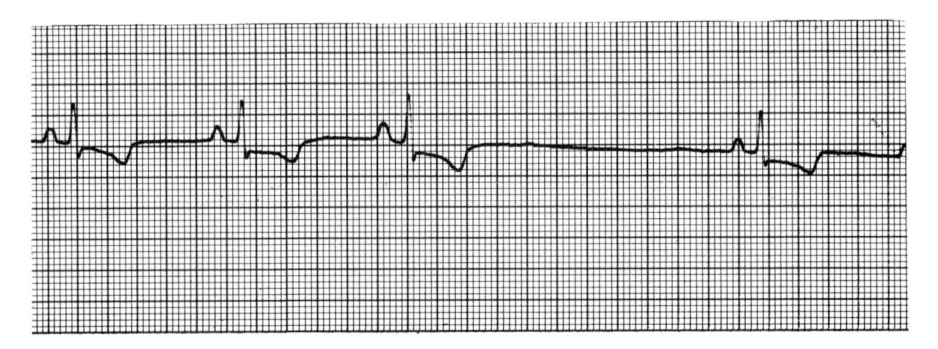

Figure 7-95 Sinus rhythm with second-degree SA block Mobitz.

SA Block

This is a conduction disturbance between the sinus node and the surrounding atrial tissue that can cause a delay or blockage in the conduction of sinus impulses to the atria. With AV block, P waves occur but QRS complexes are absent, while in SA block, both P waves and QRS complexes are absent.

Second Degree SA Block Wenckebach

Second Degree SA Block Wenckebach is characterized by a ventricular pause that measures less than twice the preceding P–P interval and is preceded by progressively shorter P–P intervals before the pause (Figure 7-94).

Second Degree SA Block Mobitz

Second degree SA block Mobitz is characterized by a ventricular pause that measures two, three, or more times the normal P–P interval, and displays a constant P–P cycle before the pause. Junctional or ventricular escape beats may interrupt the long ventricular pauses (Figure 7-95).

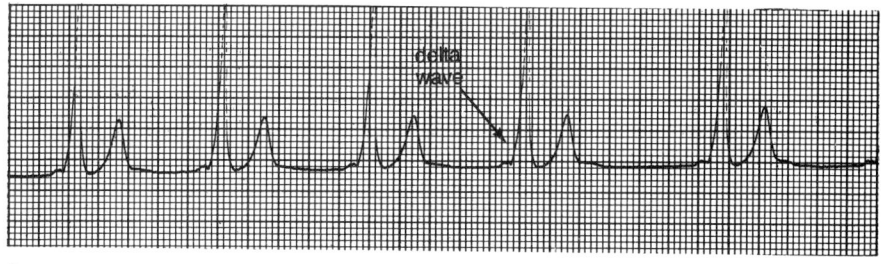

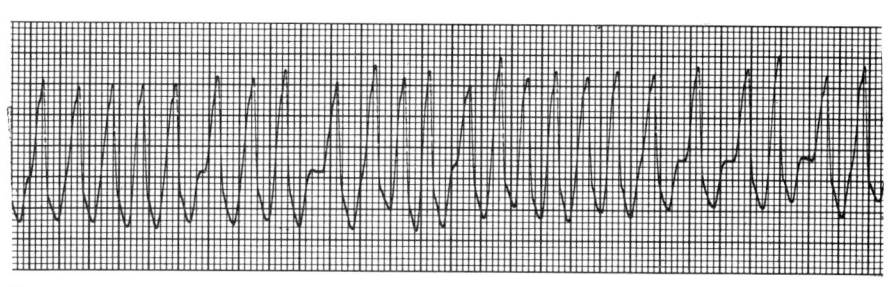

Figure 7-96 (A) WPW: 58 beats per minute. (B) Atrial fibrillation with WPW.

Wolff–Parkinson–White Syndrome (WPW)

In WPW syndrome, an accessory conduction pathway is present between the atria and ventricles. A shortened PR interval is displayed as the impulse conducts rapidly to the ventricles by way of an accessory pathway, a slurring of the initial portion of the QRS (delta wave) occurs and, often, a widened QRS complex will be seen. There will be varying degrees of slurring and widening, depending on both the accessory and normal AV conduction pathways' contribution to ventricular activation. WPW syndrome is associated with intermittent episodes of supraventricular tachycardia that, because of the slurring and width of the QRS in WPW, tend to mimic ventricular tachycardia (Figure 7-96).

Bibliography

Davis D: How To Quickly and Accurately Master ECG Interpretation. Philadelphia, JB Lippincott, 1985

Chapter 8

Graded Exercise Testing (Stress Testing)

Doris Ottoson

It is sometimes difficult to explain a *stress test*, especially to a cardiac patient. They seldom think in terms of exercise, but usually in terms of emotional or mental stress, since this plays a large part in their daily lives and is a major factor of their cardiac conditions. They can understand the test more readily if the difference between a *resting* electrocardiogram and an *exercise* electrocardiogram can be explained.

The basic principle is that, at rest, the heart requires a minimal amount of oxygen-enriched blood to act as a fuel to pump blood throughout the rest of the body. Since that demand is minimal, a normal resting cardiogram is produced. But as the body begins to exercise, the demand on the heart is increased by 8 to 10 times. If the coronary arteries are clogged with cholesterol, the heart obviously cannot meet that demand and thus produces an abnormal electrocardiogram.

During the 1930s and 1940s the abnormal exercise ECG was accepted as a major test in diagnosing coronary artery disease. In the 1950s modern techniques were established. The Master-Step test was one of the major means of testing patients for myocardial ischemia. It was highly effective in producing symptoms of angina and in producing ST–T abnormalities. It was also a very inexpensive test since all that was needed was an ECG machine and a small two-sided staircase. Now it is felt that the treadmill or the bicycle ergometer are more effective and much more reproducible in achieving a maximal exercise test.

The goal of stress testing is to increase the heart rate to a maximal level, which is usually determined by the patient's age and, together with the blood pressure, to levels that normally would not be attained in a person's daily routine. The further the patient is encouraged to exercise will depend on the results seen. A "positive" stress test is determined objectively by changes in the ST–T segment, which must be depressed 1.0 mm or more below the isoelectric line. Subjectively, it is determined by reproducing symptoms of chest pain at a given level of exercise. An abnormal stress test is determined by other factors such as chest pain in the absence of ST–T depression, arrhythmias produced by exercise, severe shortness of breath, or dizziness. Studies indicate that patients showing a positive stress (ST–T depression and chest pain at the early stages of exercise on the treadmill) will have a higher incidence of a myocardial infarction over the next two years.

Basic Exercise Physiology and Normal Responses

Before exercise physiology is discussed, it is important to understand the meaning of the word MET, since METs are used in measuring levels of exercise. A MET is a *metabolic equivalent* and approximates 3.5 ml O_2/kg/min, which is resting oxygen consumption. A healthy individual can be expected to reach a level of exercise, or VO_2 Max, equivalent to approximately 45 ml O_2/kg/min or 13 METs. METs are a convenient and fairly accurate way of measuring oxygen consumption. This can be done more accurately by measuring the volume of expired air per minute and the actual percentage of oxygen extracted during a maximal exercise test. In this process, air is collected in Douglas bags. This involves more equipment and usually is not necessary during a routine stress test.

Basically, the normal cardiovascular system must be able to react normally to increased exercise by delivering more oxygen to harder-working tissues by

1. Increasing the heart rate
2. Increasing blood pressure
3. Increasing stroke volume
4. Increasing oxygen extraction by the capillary beds

Being able to increase the amount of oxygen consumption during exercise depends on

1. The ability to increase respiratory rate (up to 30 to 40 breaths/min in a healthy exercising individual)
2. Ability to increase tidal volume
3. Ability to increase the amount of alveoli ventilated with each breath in order to increase the diffusion of oxygen to a greater area of lung tissue

It is quite normal to see a sudden rise in blood pressure and a greater rise in heart rate during the first minute or two of exercise. This is often due to anxiety, an increased sympathetic tone, and a decrease in vagal tone. As the patient continues to exercise, the heart rate reacts more normally and by the second to third minute the heart rate levels out or reaches a "steady state." This is caused by a balance that has been achieved between oxygen intake and oxygen consumption. The basic formula for determining target heart rates to exercise is the formula 220 minus the patient's age. Studies have shown the heart rate may rise up to 108 beats/min from rest to peak exercise in healthy men. In healthy women the rise is approximately 94 to 109 beats/min from rest to peak exercise. This is known as *chronotropic reserve*. Lesser ranges would be expected in trained athletes.

Normal systolic blood pressure responses to exercise in healthy men may rise up to 60 to 90 mm Hg from rest to peak exercise, with a rise of 40 to 60 mm Hg in healthy women. A normal diastolic blood pressure response would be to decrease slightly, because of the decrease in systemic vascular resistance. Again, it is not abnormal to see a sudden rise in blood pressure during the first three minutes of exercise due to anxiety. As the patient's anxiety decreases and exercise continues, the blood pressure will decrease slightly and then again rise proportionately to increases in exercise. This is known as *inotropic reserve*.

Stroke Volume and Cardiac Output

Depending on the patient's conditioning, cardiac output increases normally with exercise and, as exercise is initiated, the stroke volume increases as increased venous flow takes place. The rise in stroke volume tends to level off just prior to maximal exercise capacity. The normal stroke volume at rest is approximately 50 to 80 ml of blood. To calculate the cardiac output, the formula is stroke volume × heart rate. Therefore, if the stroke volume is 80 ml and the heart rate is 70/min; 80 ml × 70/min = 5,600 ml or 5.6 liters/min, which is an average cardiac output at rest. In a well-conditioned person, the cardiac output may increase up to 30 liters of blood/min.

During exercise, there may be a fall of up to 50% in the systemic vascular resistance caused by the dilatation of the arterial and venous systems and by the opening of large capillary beds in the working muscles. This occurs in order to meet the increase in cardiac output.

Equipment, Patient Preparation, and Lead Systems

In order to assure a functional stress laboratory, accurate and reliable equipment is required. The first choice of methods in exercise testing is a treadmill and second choice would be a bicycle ergometer. Treadmills are easier to use than the bicycle and testing is more reproducible. Sometimes, however, it may be necessary to use a bicycle for patients who may have claudication or back problems or who, for some reason, find it easier to bicycle than to walk on a treadmill. The ECG monitor is the most important piece of equipment. Anything less than a 12 lead ECG system should not even be considered. The treadmill should have capabilities to increase in speed and elevation. Most treadmills are capable of speeds up to 10 or more miles per hour and elevations of up to 25% to 30% grade, although most protocols do not exceed 6 mph or a 25% gradient.

Choice of electrode is very important. Electrodes should have a liquid or gel conductor of silver chloride and should not be very large, in order to avoid overlapping. The patient's skin should be clean and dry, to assure quality tracings. Male patients should be shaven at the site of the electrode, if necessary. The skin should then be cleansed with alcohol to remove excess oils. The area of the site of the electrode should be slightly abraded to remove only the superficial layer of skin. This can be done with a piece of dry gauze or a very fine grained sandpaper. The abrasion needs to be only large enough to match the site of the gel on the electrode. Excessive abrasion should be avoided since this can lead to swelling and edema at the prep site and can cause an increase in the electrical resistance between the electrode and the surface of the skin; it can also cause discomfort to the patient and a chance of infection.

Patients should be semifasting for at least 4 hours prior to testing. It is important to avoid large meals and for the patient to eat only if he feels it necessary. The physician should instruct the patient concerning medications to be taken or to be stopped. Men should wear comfortable pants such as sweatpants or shorts, and sneakers or soft rubber-soled shoes. Women should wear bras and can wear a loose, sleeveless blouse or T-shirt, comfortable slacks, and sneakers. Bras are especially necessary in large-breasted women to avoid excessive artifact.

The more leads that are applied, the greater the degree of sensitivity and specificity of the test results. A full 12 lead ECG demonstrates 89% of abnormal ECG responses. The chest leads are applied in the same manner as for a standard ECG, and the limb leads are applied to the corners of the torso. Some laboratories find it best to apply the limb lead electrodes to the thickest part of the limbs although we have found that causes excessive muscle artifact; it is better if these leads are applied to the boniest area of the limbs where there is less muscle. Monitoring leads, II, aVF and, more importantly V_5, will give the most information since they cover the largest areas of possible myocardial ischemia.

There are other lead systems available, but they add to the need for the application of more electrodes as well as the need for a multichannel recorder that can be a major expense.

Interview

The patient interview may be the most important part of the procedure. It is very important for the technician, for the attending physician, *and* for the patient to determine why the test has been ordered and exactly what they hope to find. It is especially necessary to determine what type of symptoms, if any, the patient has been experiencing. Encouraging the patient to describe his symptoms, whether they are typical or atypical, will provide the technician with definite insight as to what to expect once the patient is on the treadmill. The technician should inquire if the patient has ever experienced exertional chest pain, rest pain, dizziness, palpitation, shortness of breath, or chest pain in cold weather, and exactly where in the chest such pain is located. Questions regarding radiation of the pain, its duration, and what relieves it are also important, as are questions about family history, high blood pressure, smoking habits, any history of diabetes or a heart murmur.

Maintaining an adequate history together with a thorough cardiac exam will make the test easier and safer to conduct. It should be emphasized to the patient that he must alert the technician to anything out of the ordinary the patient may be feeling, such as chest discomforts (typical or atypical), dizziness, undue shortness of breath or fatigue. Good communication with the patient assures a safer test. A patient consent must be obtained and the risks of the test must be explained, including risks of heart attack, stroke, or possible death. After conducting the interview, explaining the test, and obtaining consent, it is now important for the patient to try and relax, something almost impossible to do.

Resting cardiograms while the patient is supine and standing, as well as resting blood pressures must be obtained to use as controls. An ECG with a hyperventilation exercise should be done to rule out labile ST–T wave changes, which are very common and thought to be normal, especially in young women. The physician overseeing the test must conduct a physical exam, auscultating before and after exercise.

Since there are risks involved, the test should never be conducted without an emergency cart and defibrillator. The kit should include syringes, intravenous equipment, and an Ambu-bag. The medications that should be available are fairly standard on most carts, according to hospital protocol. Nitroglycerine preparations should be on hand at all times.

Although all precautionary measures are followed, life-threatening situations may arise. One of the most common (approximately 1 in 5000) is the development of arrhythmias requiring intravenous treatment or possible cardioversions. Myocardial infarction is a rare complication and should be managed by stabilizing the patient and transferring him to the coronary care unit. Average studies have shown overall mortality to be 1 in 10,000. Cerebrovascular accidents have also been reported as a rare complication.

By conducting a thorough interview and physical exam, emphasizing good patient communication at all times, and watching carefully for signs and symptoms, the risk involved is greatly reduced.

Indications for Stress Testing

The main reason for stress testing is to make or remove a diagnosis of coronary artery disease. Other reasons include

1. Risk factors
2. Exercise programs—over the age of 40
3. Arrhythmias (diagnosing or treating)
4. Family history of coronary artery disease
5. Insurance exams—new policies
6. Post bypass serial testing

7. Medical therapy
8. Follow-up to cardiac rehabilitation
9. Postmyocardial infarction

Risk Factors for Coronary Artery Disease

1. *Family History*. This particular factor is one that is difficult to escape since genetic factors involved are ones that are learned, such as patterns of diet, behavior, and activity. Studies show that if the parents have premature evidence of atherosclerosis (fathers under the age of 55, mothers under the age of 65), their children have a sevenfold increase in chances of premature coronary death than if their parents did not display such evidence.

2. *Diabetes Mellitus*. Of patients with overt diabetes, nearly three fourths will die of complications due to atherosclerosis. Vascular disease is evidenced very early in patients with diabetes and in men and women under the age of 45. The chance of coronary death is increased five- to sixfold more than the chance of coronary death in the same age group without diabetes. The main reason may be that hyperlipoproteinemia is present in most diabetics, another major risk.

3. *Smoking*. Individuals who smoke one pack of cigarettes daily have shown moderate to advanced atherosclerosis when compared to non-smokers. Nicotine is known to increase the resting heart rate and myocardial oxygen consumption without proportional increases in coronary blood flow.

4. *Hypertension*. In men and women between the ages of 40 to 59, 15% to 20% have a diagnosis of hypertension. Men in this age group have a threefold increase in coronary artery disease, while women have a sixfold increase. Acceleration of the disease is greatly increased when hypertension is combined with other risk factors.

5. *Hyperlipoproteinemia*. Much of atheromatous plaque is comprised of cholesterol, together with other lipids.

6. *Obesity*. Although obesity has never been proven to be a risk factor by itself, it can be related to diabetes and hypertension as well as atherosclerosis.

Studies of psychosocial patterns, such as studies of individuals with type A behavior, have shown that such individuals have a premature increase of coronary events when any one or more risk factor is present.

Formation of atherosclerotic plaque is a localized disease of the arteries that protrude into the lumen; these lesions are whitish to yellow gray in color and consist of fat lipids, smooth muscle cells, and cellular debris. The plaquing takes place as degeneration of the single layer of endothelial cells of the intima occurs. This degeneration causes an opening that exposes the intimal layer to lipids, smooth muscle cells, and cellular debris.

As these breaks appear, it is normal for the body to heal them by sealing the lesions with platelets and endothelial cells. Smooth muscle cells then cover the endothelial cells. This process normally takes place throughout life, but when it can be observed visibly, these cells are now seen as fatty streaks that become the target for inflammatory reaction. The plaque begins to form as lipids, fibrinogen, collagen, elastin, and smooth muscle cells deposit on the fatty streaks. This structural defect in the arterial wall becomes a permanent site for the deposit of fatty substances that accelerate the formation of atherosclerotic plaque.

Stress testing is done more frequently on patients with suspicious chest pain to rule out angina or coronary artery disease. Patients who present with typical symptoms such as exertional chest pain or pressure, radiating to the jaw, arms, neck, or back, are tested to establish a diagnosis. Fortunately for some patients who present with these symptoms, they are not suffering from angina but possibly from some type of gastrointestinal disorder or muscle pain that can mimic angina; such patients are being tested to help remove a diagnosis of presumed coronary artery disease.

Patients who have symptoms of arrhythmia or proven arrhythmia undergo stress testing to evaluate possible forms of treatment. This is quite helpful in patients with ventricular arrhythmias.

The presence of risk factors, especially in those patients with a positive family history of premature coronary artery disease, indicates the necessity for serial stress tests done as a preventive measure. These patients should be encouraged to eliminate any controllable risk factors.

Conducting a stress test on a patient who has had a myocardial infarction should be done prior to discharge and can be done very safely in as little as 8 to 10 days postmyocardial infarction. Selection of these patients should be done cautiously; only those who have had fairly uncomplicated courses may be stressed and then only to a low level of exercise and heart rate (approximately 5 to 6 METs and 70% target heart rate). The results of exercise subjectively and objectively give the physician a good idea of what the prognosis is and how aggressively the patient should be treated. It also gives the patient encouragement to go home, partake in minimal household activities, and begin a limited walking program. The patient no longer feels like an invalid and it gives him and his family a sense of security.

In those patients who have had coronary artery bypass grafting, stress testing can be done 4 to 6 weeks after surgery to help access patency of the grafts by ECG and to evaluate the patient for any symptoms. It may also be used as a baseline for the patient who chooses to join a cardiac rehabilitation program. Serial stress testing is then done periodically to evaluate progress.

For the cardiac patient who is receiving medical therapy, stress testing is performed periodically as a follow-up to make sure that his condition is not deteriorating, and that his medications and dosages are at appropriate levels.

Cardiac rehabilitation patients undergo stress testing as often as necessary to reevaluate progress and update exercise prescriptions.

Before discussing the actual methodology of stress testing it is important to understand that this particular noninvasive test is not 100% foolproof. There are various underlying conditions other than coronary artery disease that may cause a positive or abnormal stress test. It has been estimated that a patient generally must have a 50% to 75% narrowing in at least one coronary artery before diagnostic ECG abnormalities will occur. To better understand the reliability of the results the terms *sensitivity* and *specificity* should be defined.

Sensitivity represents the number of patients who have angiographically-proven coronary disease and a positive stress test.

Specificity represents the number of patients with angiographically-proven normal coronaries who have negative or normal stress tests.

True positive is a term applied to those individuals who have positive or abnormal tests and proven coronary artery disease.
False positive represents the positive or abnormal stress test in those with proven normal coronaries. These two terms define sensitivity.
True negatives are patients with normal angiograms and normal stress tests.
False negative represents those who have abnormal angiograms and normal stress tests.

So the term positive refers to the sensitivity of the test and the term negative refers to its specificity.

In diagnosing the results of the stress test, all factors must be taken into account, such as level of exercise achieved, heart rate response, blood pressure response, symptoms if any, previous medical history, risk factors and, most important, any changes in the ST segment that may occur with exercise.

Maximal and Submaximal Testing

Stress tests may be divided into two major categories: maximal and submaximal. The maximal stress test is achieved by encouraging the patient to exercise to the ultimate point possible, in order to obtain the most reliable results. This is especially important in those patients who are undertaking a stress test to make or remove a diagnosis or to evaluate therapy. It is best when these tests are symptom-limited by fatigue, shortness of breath or leg fatigue. Then the technician knows that the patient has probably reached his VO_2 max and that the test is fairly reliable. In order to make *any* conclusions, the patient must achieve a heart rate of at least 85% of the predicted maximal target heart rate. Submaximal testing on postmyocardial infarction patients is usually terminated when a predicted submaximal heart rate is achieved, usually 70%. That is assuming the ECG remains unchanged and the patient is asymptomatic. Medications, especially beta-blockers, can also alter the effect of the ECG and the patient's performance.

Protocols

The protocols can usually be modified according to the patient's capabilities. The speeds and elevation of the treadmill can always be decreased or increased. The most common protocol used is the Bruce protocol. The treadmill starts out slowly enough to give the patient time to warm up and builds speed every three minutes. During all protocols the ECG is monitored and recorded just prior to an increase, as is the blood pressure. The Bruce protocol can be used for all maximal tests. For submaximal tests, a Naughton protocol may be used. The Naughton is a slow-moving 2-minute-stage protocol. Again the ECG and blood pressure are recorded before moving to the next stage. The MET level should not show more than two increases per stage. Logically the higher the MET achieved the better. The ECG and blood pressure should be monitored during the recovery period until the patient is baseline, usually 6 to 8 minutes after completion of the test.

The chart in Figure 8-1 shows how oxygen requirements increase with work loads in various exercise tests.

The MET reached also helps to classify the healthy individual as well as the patient with coronary disease by functional class. The American Heart Association has established such a classification.

FUNCTIONAL CLASS	METS	O₂ REQUIREMENTS ml O₂/kg/min	STEP TEST NAGLE BALKE NAUGHTON* 2 min stages 30 steps/min	TREADMILL TESTS BRUCE† 3-min stages	KATTUS‡ 3-min stages	BALKE** % grade at 3.4 mph	BALKE** % grade at 3 mph	BICYCLE ERGOMETER**
NORMAL AND I	16	56.0	(Step height increased 4 cm q 2 min) Height (cm)		mph % gr 4 22	26		For 70 kg body weight kgm/min 1500
	15	52.5		mph % gr 4.2 16		24		
	14	49.0				22		
	13	45.5				20		
	12	42.0	40		4 18	18	22.5	1350
	11	38.5	36			16	20.0	1200
	10	35.0	32	3.4 14	4 14	14	17.5	1050
	9	31.5	28			12	15.0	900
	8	28.0	24		4 10	10	12.5	750
	7	24.5	20	2.5 12	3 10	8	10.0	
II	6	21.0	16			6	7.5	600
	5	17.5	12	1.7 10	2 10	4	5.0	450
	4	14.0	8			2	2.5	300
III	3	10.5	4				0.0	
	2	7.0						150
IV	1	3.5						

  *Nagle FS, Balke B, Naughton JP: Gradational step tests for assessing work capacity. *J Appl Physiol* 20:745–748, 1965.
  †Bruce RA: Multi-stage treadmill test of submaximal and maximal exercise.
  ‡Kattus AA, Jorgensen CR, Worden RE, Alvaro AB: ST segment depression with near-maximal exercise in detection of preclinical coronary heart disease. *Circulation* 41:585–595, 1971.
  **Fox SM, Naughton JP, Haskell WL: Physical activity and the prevention of coronary heart disease. *Am Clin Res* 3:404, 1971.

Figure 8-1 Oxygen requirements increase with work loads from bottom of chart to top in various exercise tests of the step, treadmill, and bicycle ergometer types. (By permission of American Heart Association, Inc.)

Physiological Classes	Functional Classes
I: No angina at maximal activity	I: 9 METs or higher
II: Angina at maximal activity	II: 5–7 METs
III: Angina at minimal activity	III: 3–5 METs
IV: Angina at rest	IV: Below 3 METs

The above work capacities described in METs are good indicators of capable work loads.

Patient Selection

The types of patients who should undergo stress testing have already been discussed. Again, these patients should be evaluated very carefully. There are patients who should not be considered for this test because of the danger and risk involved. Below are absolute contraindications to stress testing—absolute meaning *under no circumstances* should they be evaluated.

1. Acute infarction. If the patient is suspected of having an infarction, all test results should be reviewed, including cardiac isoenzyme tests and serial ECGs. The complete set of cardiac isoenzyme tests must be negative before considering stress testing. Even if the first two sets are negative and the ECGs remain unchanged, the third set can always return positive for infarction. If the patient is exercised, an extension of infarction or worse could occur.
2. Unstable angina or angina at rest. This usually means the patient is on the verge of an impending infarction and exercising the patient before he is stabilized on the proper medications could cause infarction. When stable, a submaximal stress test should be done. A full or maximal test can always be done if the patient remains stable.
3. Ventricular tachycardia or other multifocal ventricular ectopic rhythms. Without the proper control, this could obviously lead to ventricular fibrillation.
4. Severe aortic stenosis. Patients with severe aortic stenosis have a much lower cardiac output and lower blood pressure. Exercising these patients poses great risk, because of failure of the cardiac output and the blood pressure to rise. If anything, they would drop.
5. Recent embolism. Exercise could cause sudden death by displacing an embolus, whether systemic or pulmonary, into the blood stream.
6. Known or suspected thrombophlebitis. Exercise could cause an embolism.
7. Active myocarditis. Usual treatment for such diseases is bedrest, and overexertion could cause sudden death.
8. Congestive heart failure. Pulmonary edema could result.
9. Dissecting aneurysm. Sudden death.
10. Acute infectious diseases. Fever.
11. Excessive medications. Psychotropics, digitalis.

12. Patients with second or third degree heart blocks.
13. Patients with left main disease or its equivalent.

The following relative contraindications in patients may be evaluated due to the fact that the benefits of exercise testing often outweigh the risks involved. Precautions should be taken and the patient should be watched very closely.

1. Uncontrolled high rate supraventricular arrhythmias
2. Frequent ventricular ectopy
3. Ventricular aneurysm
4. Mild to moderate aortic stenosis
5. Myocardial obstructions (subvalvular, *i.e.* IHSS or cardiomyopathies)
6. Untreated pulmonary or systemic hypertension
7. Uncontrolled metabolic disease (diabetes)
8. Marked cardiac enlargement

Reasons for Termination

1. Ventricular tachycardia. Also, patients developing an increase in ventricular couplets or multifocal PVCs should be considered for stress test termination, based on symptoms and ECG abnormalities.
2. Bradycardia. Failure of heart rate to rise with increasing exercise could be a sign of advanced coronary disease.
3. Failure of blood pressure to rise or a fall in systolic blood pressure represents a very limited cardiac output.
4. Acute myocardial injury—seen by sudden or progressive elevation of ST segments.
5. Angina pectoris.
6. Development of second or third degree AV blocks.
7. Excessive fatigue or dyspnea. Dyspnea may be an anginal equivalent and fatigue usually means the patient has reached his maximum.
8. Failure of monitoring systems.

It is very important to maintain continuous communication with the patient. Occasionally a patient may say he "just doesn't feel right" or he "feels strange." If the patient did not seem overly anxious prior to exercise, it's best to believe him and terminate the test, even in the absence of any of the above reasons. The patient knows his body best and continuing exercise may lead to complications.

Medications

There are several drugs that may alter the effect of an exercise test. They may affect the ECG interpretation, the patient's ability to exercise, or various symptoms. The technician should be familiar with all cardiac drugs.

Below are the major drugs and their possible effects.

1. Antianginal Drugs:
   a. Nitroglycerine compounds. May affect the patient physically (if taken just prior to exercise) by lowering the blood pressure. Nitroglycerine will also allow the patient to exercise longer with less ST–T depression.
   b. Beta-blockers (Inderal, Lopressor, Minipress, Corgard, Tenormin).
   c. Calcium antagonists (Diltiazem).

These drugs may alter overall interpretation by raising the question of a false negative test, especially when attempting to rule out coronary artery disease. A false negative test could be considered if the test were maximal, and there were no abnormalities in the way of symptoms or ECG changes. Does this result occur because the patient is actually normal or in fact does the patient have coronary disease, with the medications controlling symptoms and maximizing coronary circulation, thus preventing ischemia?

2. Antihypertensive Drugs:
   a. Diuretics. If potassium levels have not been checked recently, hypokalemia may be present, causing ST–T wave abnormalities frequently seen in the resting ECG.
   b. Vasodilators
3. Digitalis Preparations. These are well known to produce significant ST segment depression. In patients with ischemia, their depressions will be accentuated and in those with normal coronaries the ST segment may also drop significantly. It would be convenient if the digitalis could be stopped a few days before, but this usually is not possible.

It is best to set up criteria for interpretations and termination since increasing exercise in the presence of significant ST depression in the absence of symptoms is definitely risky. Two or three millimeters of ST depression is definitely suspicious, 4 to 5 millimeters should be considered ischemic, and the patient should be watched very closely if exercise is to continue (Figure 8-2).

4. Quinidine. Prolongs the QT interval and decreases QRS voltage.
5. Antiarrhythmic Drugs. Medications that prolong the QT interval are Norpace, Procainamide, and Amiodarone. The QRS widens with Norpace, Procainamide, Amiodarone, and Flecainide. Beta-blockers Verapamil and Diltiazem will prolong the P–R interval.
6. Psychotropic Drugs. Usually, the heart rate is increased, the T waves are lowered, and the presence of ST depression is common. These drugs have a suppressive effect on left ventricular function causing hypotension. It also prolongs the P–R interval, frequently causing various degrees of AV block.

156 Graded Exercise Testing (Stress Testing)

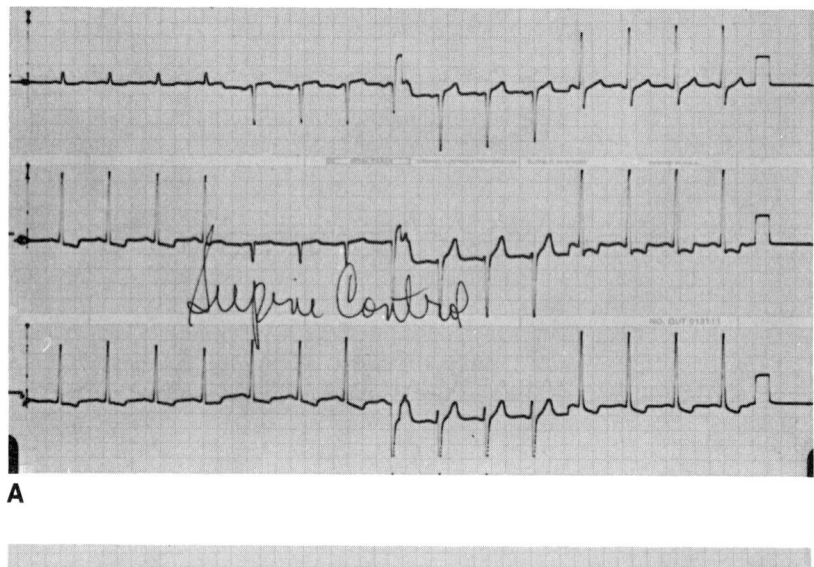

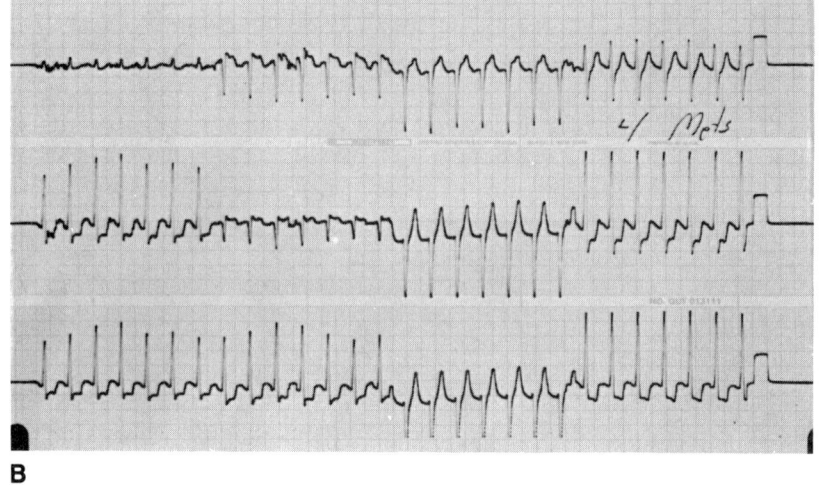

Figure 8-2 (*A*) Digitalis effect: Resting ECG. (*B*) Digitalis effect: Exercise ECG.

Interpretation of the Exercise ECG

Figure 8-3 shows a normal resting ECG and a normal exercise ECG. When interpreting the exercise ECG, there are a few major points to remember:

1. The P–R interval usually becomes shorter.
2. The P wave becomes taller.
3. The total amplitude of the QRS usually decreases, along with the T wave.
4. The normal ST segment will upslope steeply and appear slightly convex, so that within .04 to .06 second after the J point, it will return to baseline.

Interpretation of the Exercise ECG   157

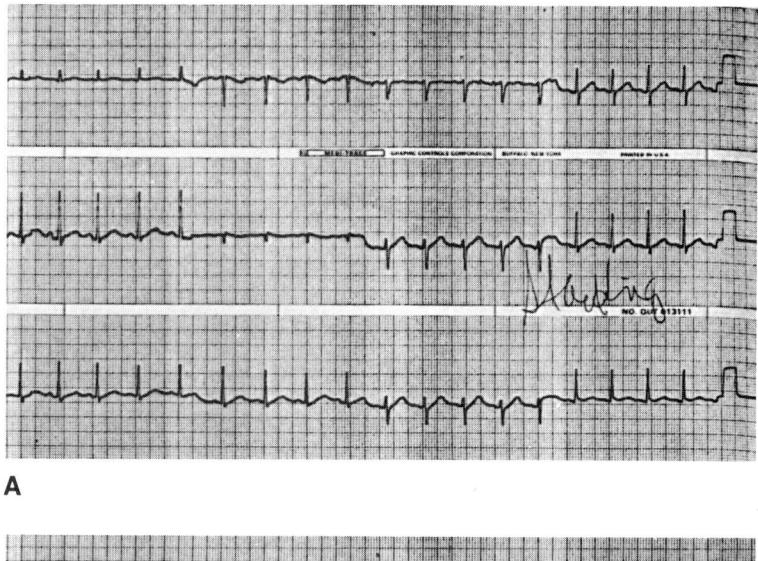

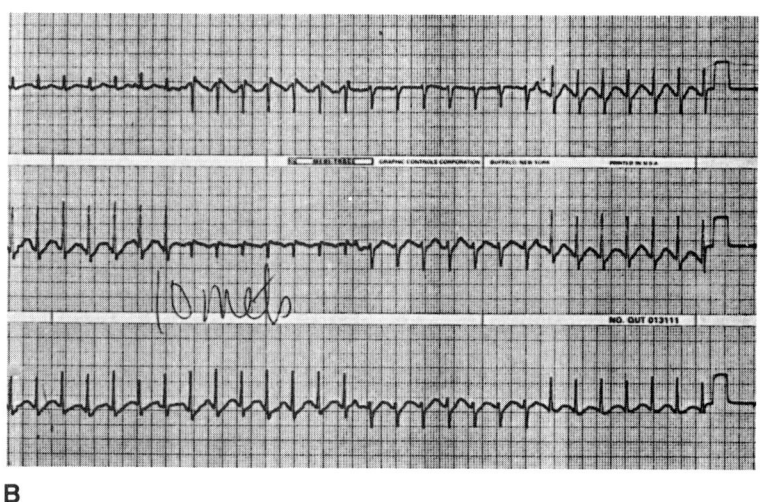

Figure 8-3 (A) Normal resting ECG. (B) Normal exercise ECG.

5. When looking for ischemia, the P–Q segment should be used as the isoelectric line as your point of measurement.

In the presence of ST segment depression, ischemia should be considered first as the cause. The more severe the ST depression, the greater the likelihood of ischemia. The degree of ST depression usually corresponds with the degree of disease. Studies show a major branch must be narrowed by 50% to 75% in order to display ECG abnormalities.

Figure 8-4 shows a resting ECG, for comparison with an ECG showing severe depression.

158 Graded Exercise Testing (Stress Testing)

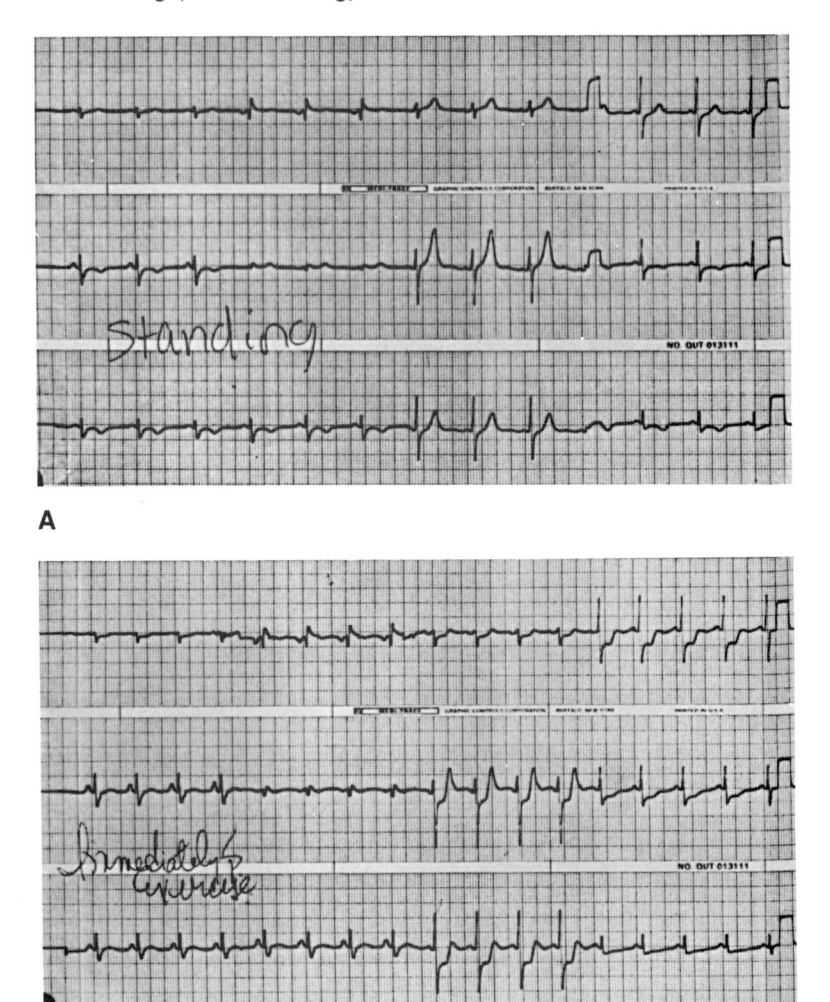

Figure 8-4 (*A*) Resting ECG. (*B*) Severe ST depression.

When ECG abnormalities exist on the resting tracings it may be wiser to choose an alternative form of testing, such as thallium stress testing. Several conditions often display these resting ST abnormalities:

1. Left bundle branch block
2. Left ventricular hypertrophy (hypertension and aortic stenosis)
3. Wolff-Parkinson-White syndrome
4. Digitalis
5. Hypokalemia

Interpretation of the Exercise ECG 159

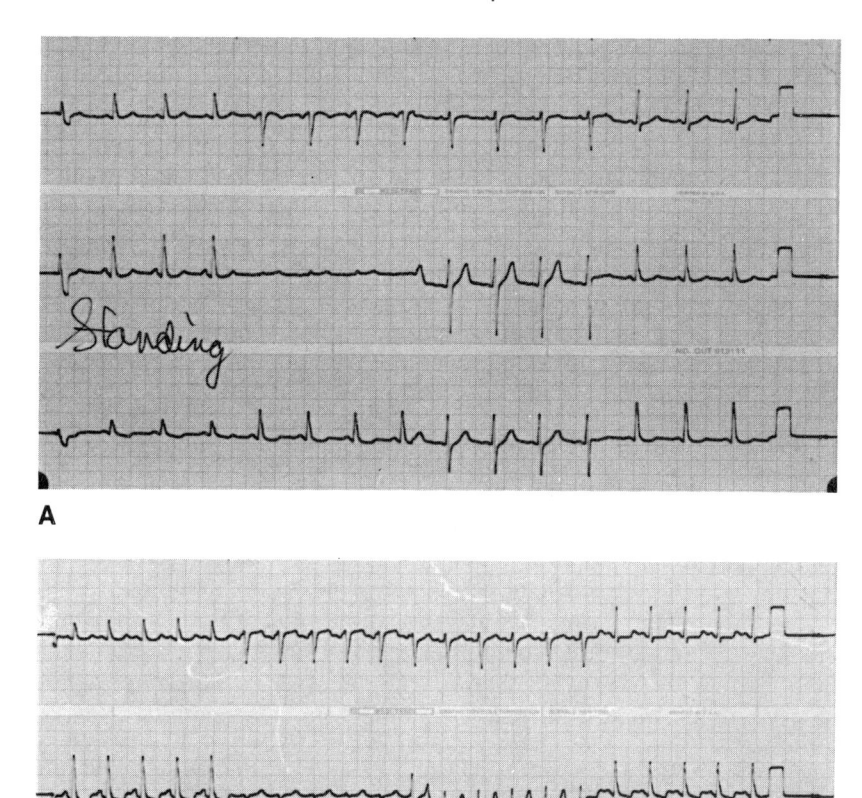

Figure 8-5 (*A*) Resting ECG. (*B*) ECG showing results of hyperventilation procedure.

Postural changes and hyperventilation may often produce diffuse ECG changes in all leads (see Figure 8-5). It usually is not necessary to order a thallium stress test in such cases. More frequently than not, these changes will normalize with increase in exercise.

Hyperventilation routinely done at rest, especially in the younger patient, will very often produce abnormalities of the ST–T segment that are thought to be normal (Figure 8-5). These changes, seen with standing and with hyperventilation, may be due to vasoregulatory asthenia, a syndrome found in young to middle-aged women who are hyperactive emotionally and usually sedentary. They are found to have higher than normal resting heart rates, increased cardiac output, and decreased blood volume.

The hyperventilation procedure should be done with the patient standing. The procedure consists of having the patient breathe, almost pant, very deeply and quickly for approximately 20 seconds or until the ECG displays abnormalities, usually around a heart rate of 100 beats per minute. It is important that this procedure be done since the changes produced are strong evidence against the patient having significant pathology. Because of these particular findings, women have a much higher incidence of false positive results.

J-Point Depression

It is felt by some researchers that it is totally normal for the J-point, the junction between the S wave and the ST segment, to depress (Figure 8-6). Not only is it considered normal, but it is felt that these patients have a better survival rate than those with completely normal ST segments. In most cases this may be true although it is more common than not to see significant J-point depression change to horizontal or downsloping ST segment depression in the recovery period. Therefore, it must be concluded that J-point is only the beginning sign of ischemia in these patients. The criteria for J-point depression to be considered normal is that it must return to the baseline within .08 second.

Upsloping ST Segments

It is recognized that upsloping ST segments are seen and do not return to the baseline as quickly as the J-point depression; they are associated with ishcemia. The slow upsloping ST segment does not return to the baseline within .08 second after the J-point and consist of 1.5 mm depression below the baseline (Figure 8-7). This type is considered to be least specific of ST depression but certainly indicative of ischemia.

Horizontal ST Depression

With the two other types of depression described as being the least specific, the horizontal type is certainly more conclusive of ischemia; only 1.0 mm of ST depression is needed for criteria (Figure 8-8). Most researchers have agreed the 1.0 mm ST depression is a definite criterion for ischemia.

Downsloping ST Depression

In those patients with ischemia and horizontal ST depression, a pattern of downsloping ST and deeply inverted T waves will frequently occur in the

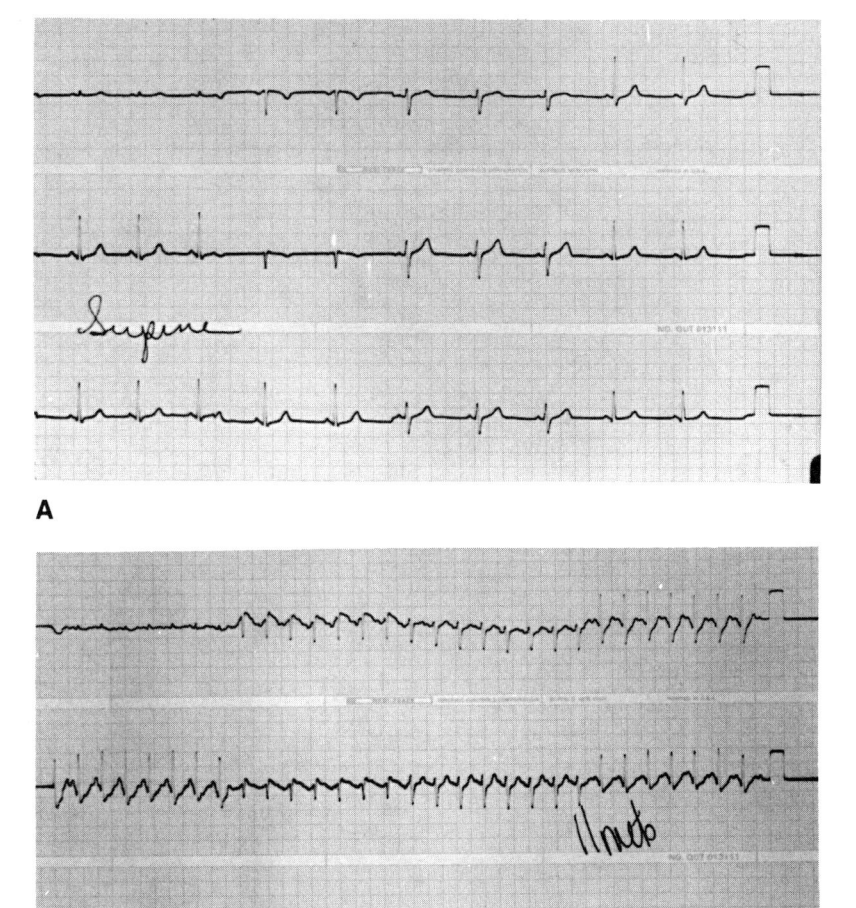

Figure 8-6 (A) Normal resting ECG. (B) J-junctional depression.

recovery period. This is the most specific type of depression and is often associated with significant disease (Figure 8-9).

ST depression that resolves quickly either during the cool-down phase of exercise or early in the recovery is probably not due to ischemia, while the type that persists or worsens has definite coronary pathology. Various factors must be considered when interpreting the exercise ECG, such as the resting tracings, blood pressure response, medications and, most important, the presence of any symptoms.

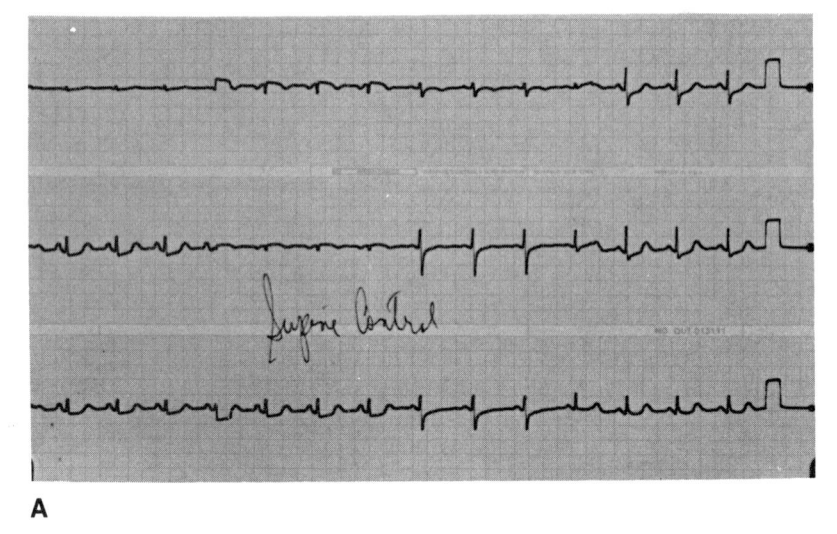

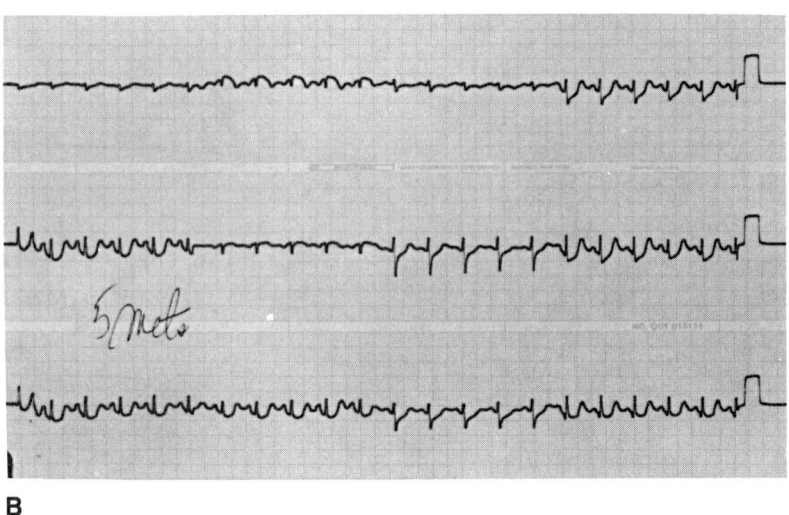

Figure 8-7 (*A*) Resting ECG. (*B*) Slow upsloping ST depression.

Factors Causing False Positive ST Depression in Women

It has been thought that, since women have a higher incidence of false positive results, the criterion should be changed from 1.0 mm of ST depression to 2.0 mm of ST depression, but as yet a definite criterion has not been established other than 1.0 mm.

Interpretation of the Exercise ECG 163

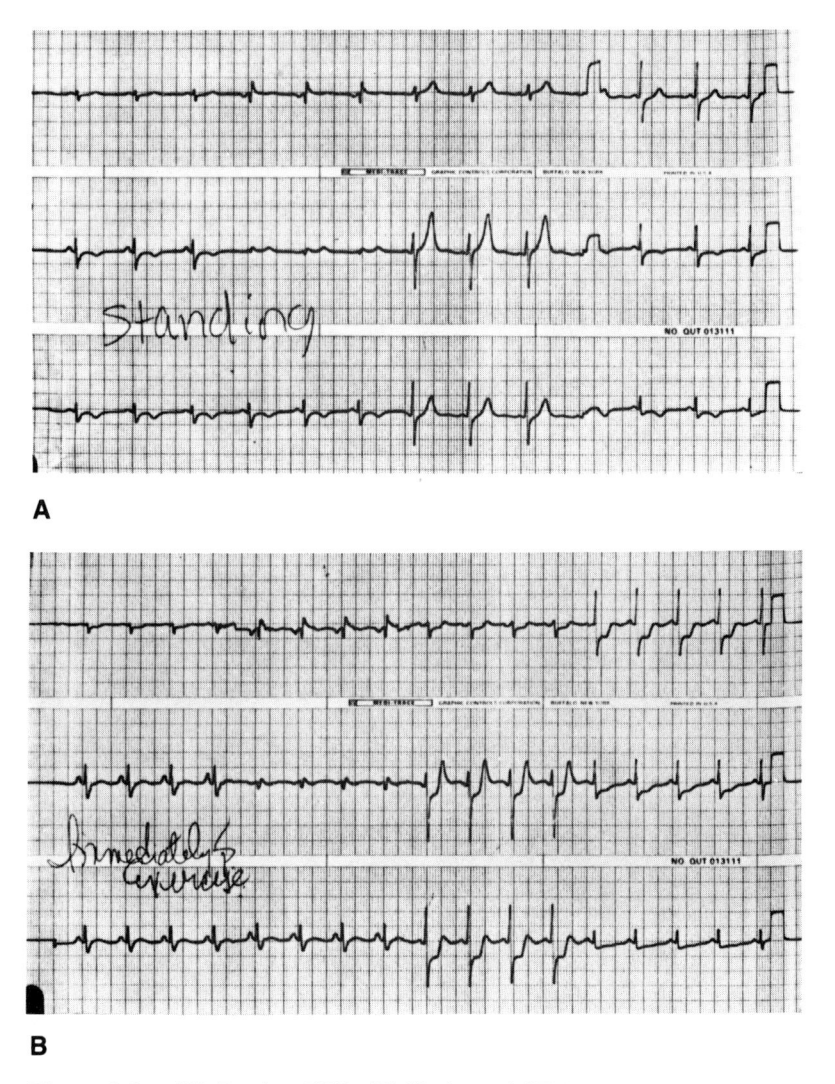

Figure 8-8 (*A*) Resting ECG. (*B*) Horizontal ST depression.

Vasoregulatory Asthenia

Vasoregulatory asthenia frequently occurs in young women. These women usually complain of chest pain with sinus tachycardia and show abnormal resting cardiograms demonstrating ST–T wave abnormalities. These changes are usually emphasized with standing and hyperventilation. As exercise begins, the cardiogram may worsen, but as exercise becomes more

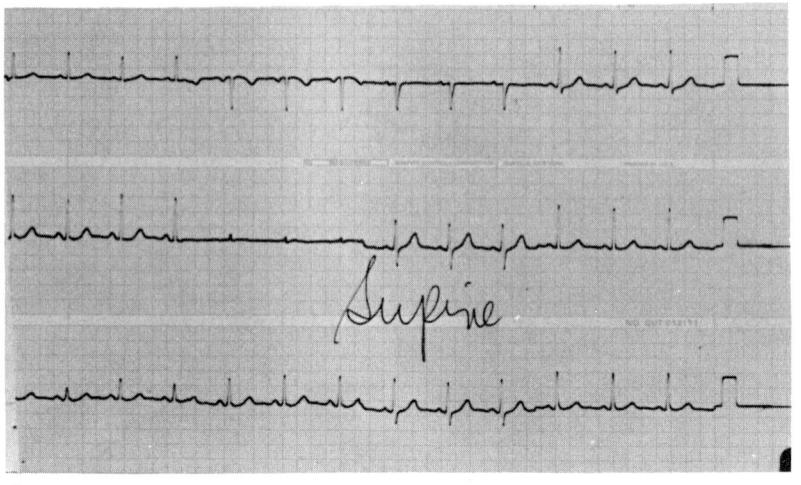

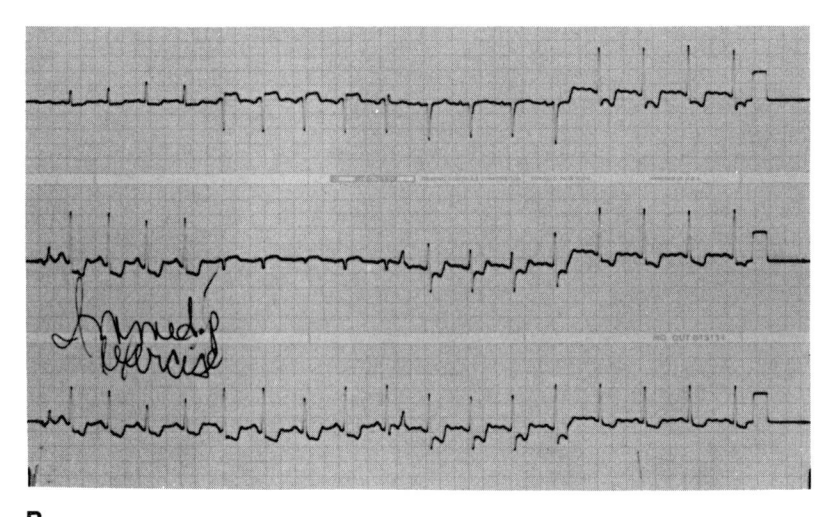

Figure 8-9 (*A*) Normal resting ECG. (*B*) ST depression downsloping.

strenuous the ECG usually improves, demonstrating junctional changes. In the recovery period, the ECG commonly demonstrates horizontal ST segments throughout all leads as seen at rest.

Reynolds' Syndrome
Increased sympathetic tone in patients frequently demonstrates ST abnormalities or T wave inversion during exercise. These changes may sometimes be eliminated on retesting in patients who have been through an exercise program.

Syndrome X

(Angina and normal coronaries). These patients have typical anginal pain with abnormal exercise ECGs, although angiography demonstrates normal coronary anatomy. Abnormalities demonstrated are those of contractility and elevated left ventricular end-diastolic pressure. Evidence shows these patients may be showing the signs of early cardiomyopathies.

ST Depression With Respiration

This abnormality may occur in the healthy individual as well as the patient with significant coronary disease. In the normal subject, it may be due to a sedentary lifestyle and the loss of left ventricular compliance. The abnormality is seen intermittently in a few consecutive beats on the exercise ECG and usually does not demonstrate worsening in the recovery period. Those with disease usually show typical ischemic changes that progress with serial testing. The reason it is only seen in a few beats is that left ventricular filling is influenced by inspiration and expiration. There is an increase in end-diastolic pressure caused by a loss of left ventricular compliance and increased rates of filling, which then produce the ST depression.

Various ST Abnormalities

ST Elevation

In a normal resting cardiogram, ST elevation with exercise is more often than not associated with significant coronary disease. It usually reflects transmural ischemia. ST elevation will be seen very rarely in one lead unless it occurs over the area of previous infarction. This usually represents dyskinesia in that area. When seen in multiple leads such as II, III, aVF, it usually correlates with total or near total occlusion of the artery that supplies that area (Figure 8-10). Continuing exercise in these patients may lead to an infarction. Ventricular ectopy will often accompany the ST elevation, which poses even greater risk. Exercise should be promptly terminated and the patient watched closely.

Patients with previous infarctions may demonstrate ST elevation due to ventricular aneurysms. If an aneurysm is not present, the damaged myocardium may become increasingly akinetic and respond electrically, as with an aneurysm.

Right Bundle Branch Block

Since a right bundle branch block has never been proved to be caused by coronary artery disease, the ST changes seen with exercise are of questionable significance (Figure 8-11). ST depression is commonly seen due to repolarization changes. In order for them to be diagnostic, ST depression must be demonstrated in the lateral precordial leads.

(Text continues on page 168)

166 Graded Exercise Testing (Stress Testing)

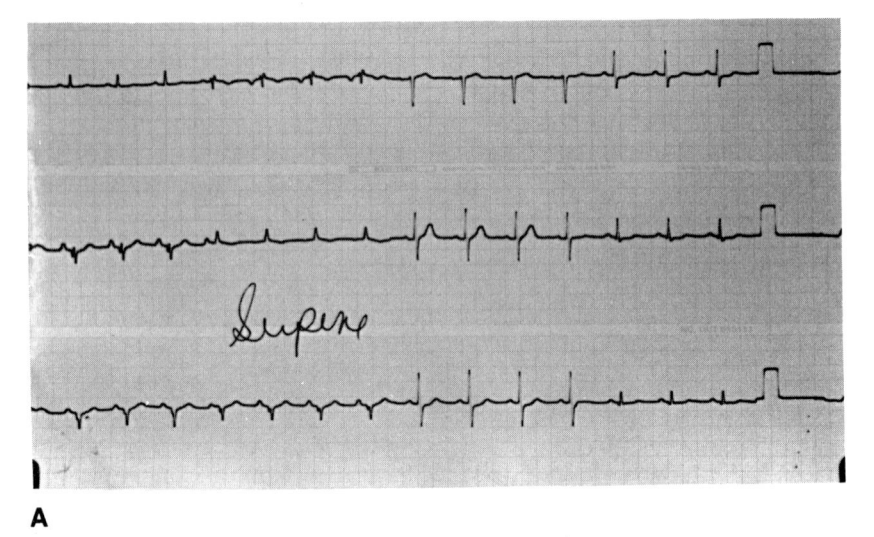

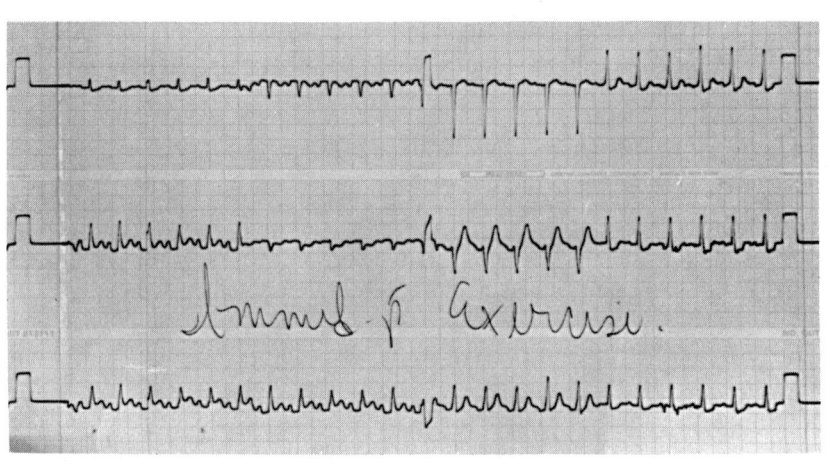

Figure 8-10 (*A*) Resting ECG. (*B*) ST elevation in inferior and anterior leads.

Interpretation of the Exercise ECG 167

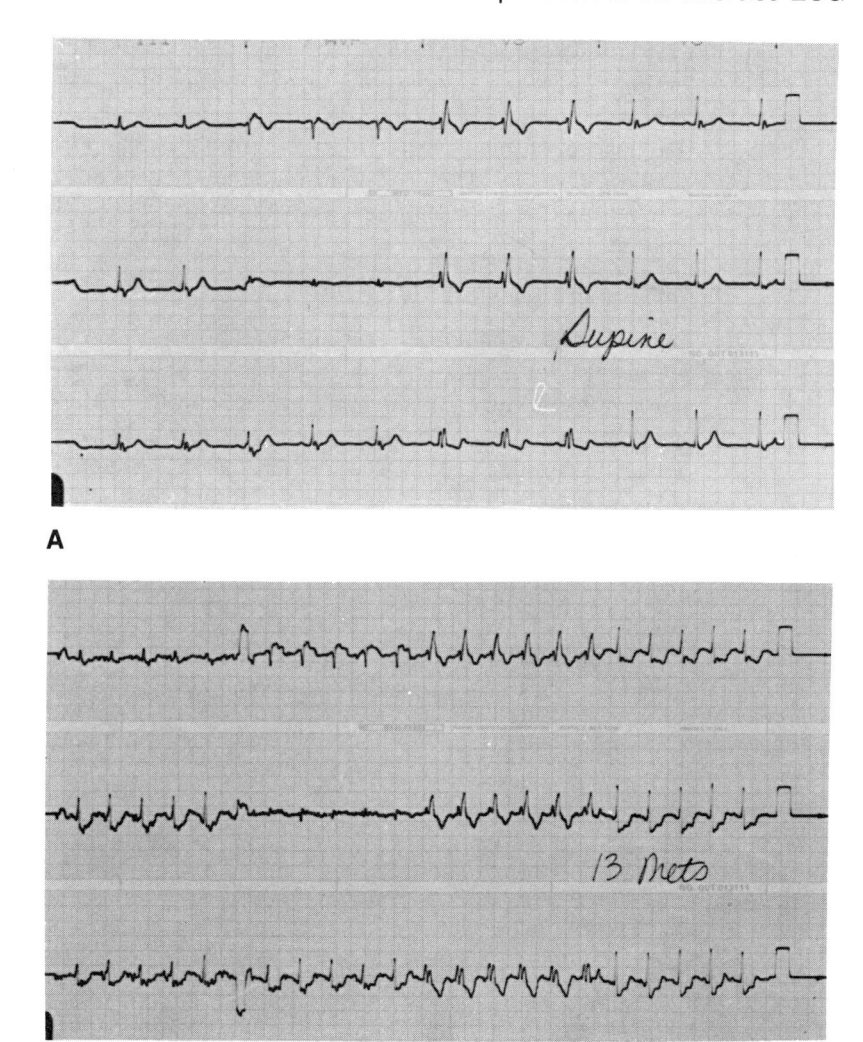

Figure 8-11 (A) Resting ECG. (B) Right bundle branch block changes.

Left Bundle Branch Block

Patients with left bundle branch block often demonstrate widespread ST abnormalities on the resting ECG. For this reason, when trying to make a diagnosis of coronary artery disease, it may be beneficial to proceed with a thallium stress test, since the changes produced with exercise will usually prove to be nondiagnostic or inconclusive.

Wolff-Parkinson-White Syndrome

In the patient who has a history of W-P-W syndrome, exercise may produce a delta wave that may not be seen otherwise. Exercise may also cause the delta wave to disappear in the patient who begins with W-P-W and, frequently, to return in the recovery period. In either case, ST segment of at least 1.0 mm depression is usually present. Evidence shows that in most cases, coronary disease is not present. Again, for this reason, thallium stress testing may be indicated to avoid a false positive result.

T Wave Inversion

It was once thought T wave inversion was a good indicator of myocardial ischemia. This is no longer true, although patients with coronary disease often demonstrate T wave abnormalities. T wave inversion alone must not be considered diagnostic. As previously discussed, this abnormality may be demonstrated by various factors such as postural or hyperventilation changes, vasoregulatory asthenia or, possibly, medications. However, in the presence of angina, these changes should be considered as significant.

U Waves

Studies now show that the presence of a "U" wave produced by exercise and seen during recovery may be indicative of ischemia, especially if the U wave were not present at rest. Inverted "U" waves are more significant. The ECG that demonstrates a "U" wave is fairly reliable and indicative of some degree of left ventricular dysfunction.

Exercise-Induced Arrhythmias

Paroxysmal atrial tachycardia. Sustained P.A.T. initiated by exercise is not that common. If it is produced, and is associated with ST depression this may be considered a good indicator of ischemia.

Ventricular arrhythmias. It is quite common to see PVCs at rest that decrease with exercise and return in the recovery phase. This is especially common in young, healthy individuals. It is also common to see PVCs produced at maximum levels of exercise. Patients developing ventricular arrhythmias at low levels of exercise that do not subside with increased exercise may have a high incidence of coronary disease.

Ventricular tachycardia. Produced by exercise, this arrhythmia has a significant correlation to myocardial ischemia, although it may be seen in young adults and may be considered benign. In the older patient, ischemia should be considered as the underlying cause. Patients with cardiomyopathies also demonstrate an increase in ventricular irritability.

Thallium Stress Testing

In those patients for whom standard stress testing is not going to supply useful information a thallium stress test may be indicated.

These patients include those with

1. Resting ECG abnormalities without chest pain
2. Left bundle branch block
3. Patients on digitalis or diuretics
4. Left ventricular hypertrophy
5. Young women with ST abnormalities

Thallium, a radioactive tracer, is given to the patient intravenously. It first passes through the right side of the heart where it enters the lungs. It then goes into the left heart and through coronary circulation to the myocardium. Thallium is picked up easily because it acts much like potassium, which is highly prevalent in the heart. A gamma camera that is capable of picking up radioactivity is placed over the heart where it produces an image on the monitor.

It is important that the thallium be injected at peak heart rate. The patient must exercise for 1 more minute after initial injection so the tracer can be picked up by the myocardium and maintained there. There is a time limit of 20 to 30 minutes in which imaging should be completed so a contrast between hot and cold areas can be made. A hot area would indicate good perfusion where a cold spot indicates a lack of perfusion.

Together with thallium-201 being considered as one of the most commonly used isotopes, there is technetium-99m. Technetium-99m is most often used for nuclear cardiology studies or for myocardial scanning. There are usually no reactions to these chemical tracers and they deliver very low radiation.

Myocardial Perfusion With Exercise

These studies are done mainly to demonstrate ischemia in patients who have known cardiac disease or those in whom such disease is being ruled out. In order to maintain a successful study, the patient should be pushed to his maximum and the thallium then injected. A false negative test can occur if thallium is injected too soon, regardless of what level is achieved. After exercise the patient is brought to the table where imaging is begun. No more than 5 to 10 minutes should elapse after the patient stops exercising and imaging is begun. Three or four images are obtained. An image with the patient in the LAO position is the first to be obtained. Four hours later the patient is usually brought back for redistribution studies that would show infarctions if present. The actual exercise test is done the same way as a regular stress test in that the ECGs and blood pressures are recorded throughout exercise. The only main difference is that fasting should be for 12 hours, rather than 4 hours.

Radionuclide Ventriculography

For stress ventriculography, technetium is injected to tag the red blood cells, preexercise. A rest study is performed, then the ptaient exercises in a supine position with a bicycle. During peak exercise, data acquisition begins and continues for approximately 2 to 4 minutes until an interpretable image with adequate counts appears. Ejection fraction is determined by this gated blood pool study, which must increase by 5% or more in order to be a normal response. An abnormal response would be failure of the ejection fraction to rise, or a "flat" response, or a fall in the ejection fraction.

Myocardial perfusion imaging as well as radionuclide ventriculography provide a variety of information depending on the degree of ischemia. Thallium studies of perfusion mainly show the degree of the coronary disease and are fairly reliable for location. Gated blood pool studies demonstrate ventricular function or dysfunction secondary to ischemia. The sensitivity of both these tests range from 85% to 90%, depending, of course, on the capabilities of the laboratory.

Bibliography

Ellestad HM: Stress Testing—Principles and Practice, 2nd ed. Philadelphia, FA Davis, 1980

Fox K, IIsley C: The Essentials of Exercise Electrocardiography. London, Current Medical Literature Ltd., 1984

Chapter 9

Basic Echocardiography

Linda Martin

Today, ultrasound is used for many diagnostic procedures. Ultrasound has been in use for many years, and only minor procedural changes have been made over the past 15 years. The echocardiogram is very useful in cardiac laboratories because it is easy to perform, painless for the patient, and completely noninvasive. The cardiac echo gives the physician useful information relating to chamber size, valvular functions, cardiac muscle functions, and general anatomical orientation. The principle of ultrasound will not be described in this chapter. Rather, our purpose is to acquire basic knowledge necessary for the performance of an echocardiogram, and understanding of normal echoes as well as disease states, and, finally, how to diagnose them.

Types of Echocardiography

There are several so-called "types" of echocardiography; the m-mode technique, two-dimensional echocardiography, and the Doppler principle of echocardiography.

The m-mode echocardiogram is a one-dimensional mode for viewing cardiac structures in one plane or with an "ice-pick" approach. Recordings are usually on a strip chart printout with the horizontal axis representing time and the vertical axis representing the distance to the structures from the transducer (Figure 9-1). The speed of the paper usually varies from 50 to 75 mm per second. The two-dimensional echo exam, also known as *real time echocardiography* or *cross sectional echocardiography*, uses two planes. A mechanical transducer or electronically phased array type gives an image of the cardiac structures on a viewing screen. Various views or images can be obtained by using the two-dimensional echocardiogram. Most two-

172 Basic Echocardiography

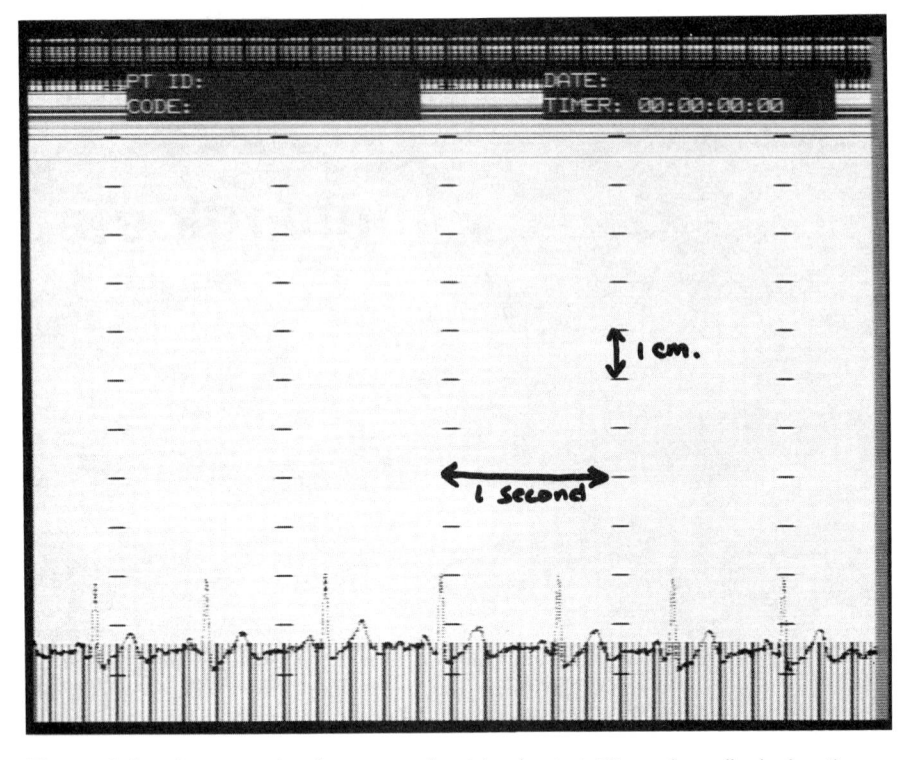

Figure 9-1 An example of an m-mode strip chart at 50 mm/sec displaying time versus depth.

dimensional echo machines can drive m-modes directly off the cardiac image on the viewing screen. Simultaneous recordings of both m-modes and 2-D's may also be obtained by some of the newer echo machines. The cardiac Doppler examines changes in the frequency of reflected sound from moving objects (usually red blood cells in motion). Audible analysis of these changes is also a helpful factor when using the Doppler for diagnostic purposes.

Machine and Instrument Control

Basically, echo machines are similar in their functions and operations, even though manufacturers may add little extras to make their products more appealing (Figure 9-2).

Ultrasound is emitted from a transducer that penetrates the patient's chest wall it reaches various cardiac structures. (A transducer is a device that converts energy from one form to another.) Once the ultrasound has reached its destination, it returns to the transducer and is converted into a recognizable image on the viewing screen. Various transducers are used, depending on the age of the patient and his body build. Megahertz is a term used to describe the frequency of the transducer. In adult echocardiography, generally, a 2.0, 2.25, or 2.5 megahertz (MHz) transducer is used, giving the

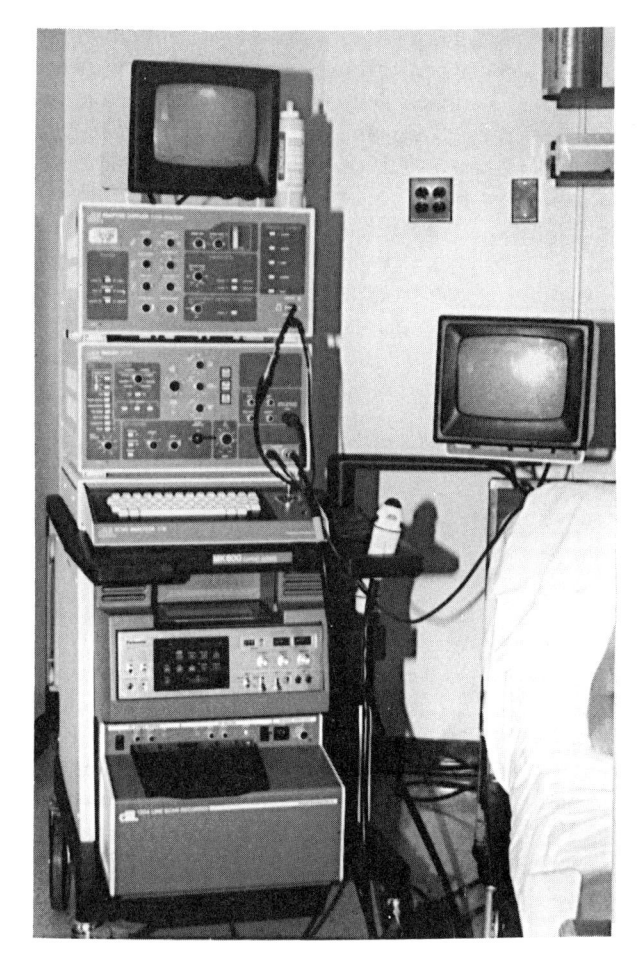

Figure 9-2 A two-dimensional/m-mode machine with the viewing screen, transducer, and added features that vary with each manufacturer.

appropriate penetration and resolution needed. Resolution is the ability to define or clarify structures clearly. Pediatric echocardiography requires a higher frequency transducer, usually a 3.5 or 5.0 MHz. A shorter penetration depth is needed in pediatric echocardiography because the heart is closer to the chest wall, whereas an adult's heart is set deeper in the chest cavity. The lower the frequency transducer, the greater penetration received; however, in such cases, there will be less resolution.

Echoscape Controls

A glossary of terms most frequently encountered in the echocardiography process will aid in understanding the technique.

1. *Coupling Gel*: A liquid that has been semisolidified into a gel, enabling an airtight seal between the transducer and the patient's chest.
2. *Transducer*: A device that converts energy into a recognizable image on a viewing screen. Transducers are of different frequencies, qualitated in megahertz (MHz). Adult transducers have a frequency of about 2.0 to 3.5 MHz, whereas pediatric transducers range from 3.5 to 7.5 MHz. The lower the frequency of the transducer, the deeper the penetration; however, less resolution results. Resolution means the ability to define certain structures one from another. A higher frequency transducer gives less penetration but greater resolution.
3. *Overall Gain*: Controls the number of overall echoes desired. This setting helps control far-field amplification. If this control is set too low, structures can be eliminated and poor definition may result. If its setting is too high, poor clarification and structure due to the excessive brightness will result.
4. *Neargain*: Controls the anterior echoes or the ultrasound waves close to the chest wall. If the neargain echoes are too strong, the right ventricle, for example, will not be clearly differentiated.
5. *Paper Speed*: Usually at 50 mm/sec. Paper speed may be adjusted for the appropriate need. Paper speed can range from 10 mm/sec to 100 mm/sec.
6. *ECG Amplitude and Position*: A simplified three lead ECG is routinely hooked up to the patient. (Usually a lead 11 is monitored.) Distinct visualization of the P wave, QRS, and T waves should be seen to help differentiate cardiac cycles for timing. This can be changed by adjusting the amplitude. Position of the ECG complex should also be adjusted to the top or bottom of the screen, clear of the cardiac image.
7. *Reject*: This control is used to eliminate low amplitude signals, such as weak echoes and artifact. Caution must be used, however, not to eliminate the *necessary* weak echoes or to lessen the intensity of fibrotic lesions by turning down the reject.
8. Time Gain-Compensation (TGC) or depth compensation: Anterior or proximal echoes appear much stronger than far-field echoes. This occurs because the ultrasound has to travel a greater distance to reach many posterior structures, losing many necessary echoes. Depth compensation is used to reserve this process, by minimizing the near-field echoes and enhancing the far-field structures. TGC controls vary with different brands of equipment. A "ramp" is one type of control that can be adjusted by changing the slope of the ramp to alter the echoes. A second type is a panel of "slide" controls that also can be adjusted to suppress or enhance echoes.

Types of Real-Time Echocardiography

There are two basic types of real-time echocardiography—mechanical and electronic. A mechanical system uses a probe with either an oscillating head or a rotating head. An oscillating transducer generally has one element and the rotary type generally has three or four elements, all encased in a liquid medium. The oscillating mechanical transducer produces a vibration that patients often feel when the transducer is placed on their chests. The mechanical rotating transducer does not produce this vibration, because the elements are mounted in a wheel, causing a smooth, rotating action.

Phased array is the most popular electronic real-time scanner. This unit uses a multielement transducer, creating a single ultrasound beam. Electronic real-time scanners are composed of computer components. As a result, this type of scanner can cover a wider angle than other types of scanners. Defining and clarifying fine details is not as precise with this unit as with the mechanical type, but there is less distortion of the image being viewed. These electronic systems are oftem more expensive.

Linear array is another type of electronic system containing a multielement transducer that is fired repetitively. The scanner in which these elements is fired causes the ultrasound beam to move linearly. Various types of transducers are illustrated in Figure 9-3.

The Examination

When performing the echocardiogram, the patient, as well as the technician, should be comfortable. If the environment is not ideal, an inadequate study will by obtained, making correct interpretation impossible. The cardiac laboratory must by large enough for either a bed or an examining table for the patient, the machine itself, and space for the physician and technician. Patients often are nonambulatory and must come to the laboratory on a stretcher; consequently, adequate space must be considered for such contingencies. A simplified three lead ECG should be hooked up to the patient so that the cardiac cycles can be differentiated. The ideal position would find the patient resting on his left side, enabling his heart to drop out of the lung field. If possible, the patient should raise his left arm up and under his head, thus helping spread the rib somewhat for a clearer image (Figure 9-4). Patients unable to turn on their left sides should remain in the supine position. Elevation of the head of the bed may also help clear up the cardiac image. A routine echo exam takes approximately 20 to 45 minutes. Every hospital has its own interpretation form that the attending physician must complete (Figure 9-5). M-mode measurements, as well as an overall interpretation, are made.

M-Mode Examination

M-mode examination used to be the only technique employed to visualize heart structures. Today, the two-dimensional examination has the capability of obtaining m-modes directly from the 2-D image, making sole m-mode exams obsolete. However, the m-mode exam should be described, to provide an understanding of the structural orientation and manipulation of the trans-

176 Basic Echocardiography

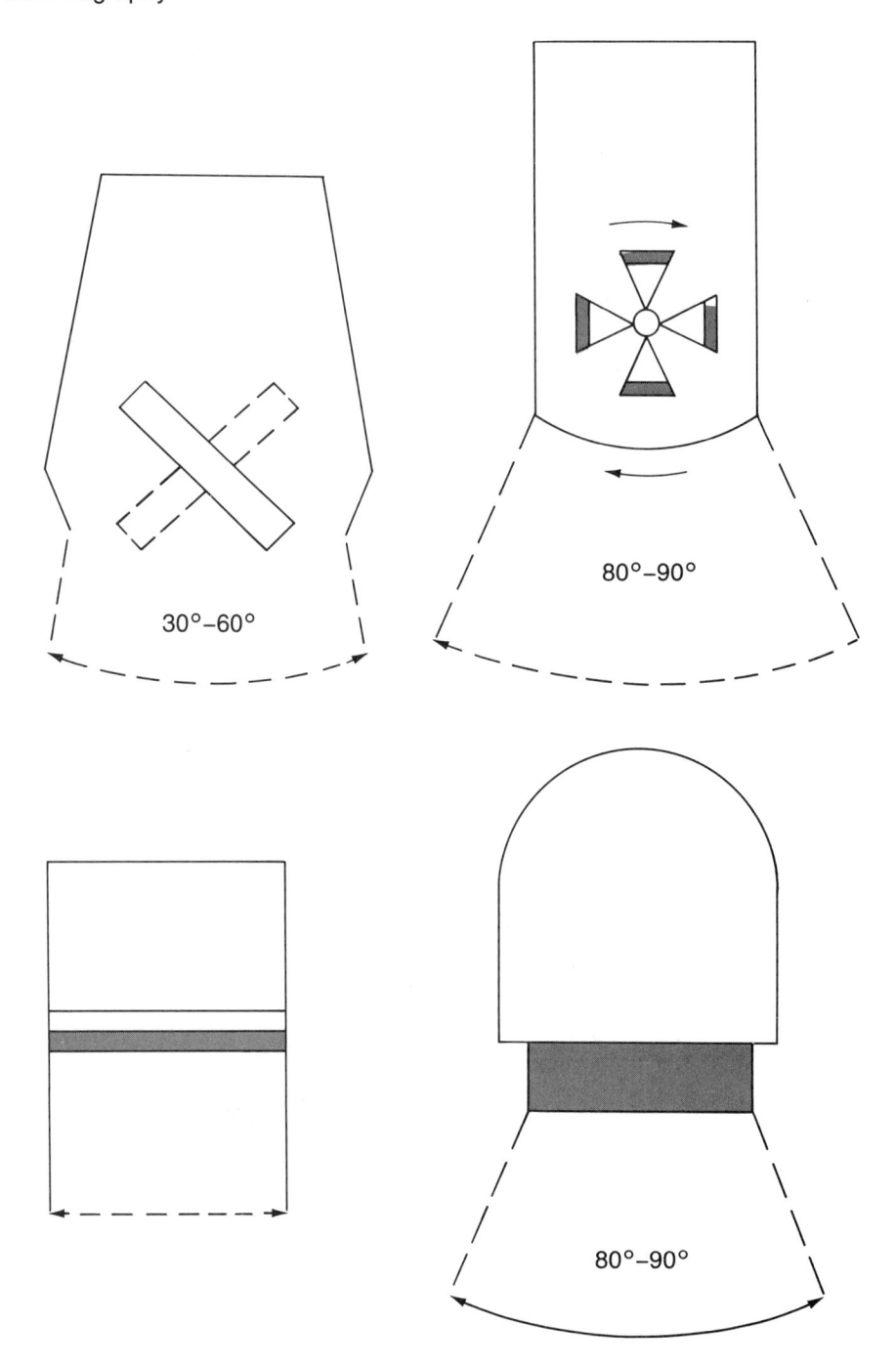

Figure 9-3 Diagram demonstrating the various types of transducers.

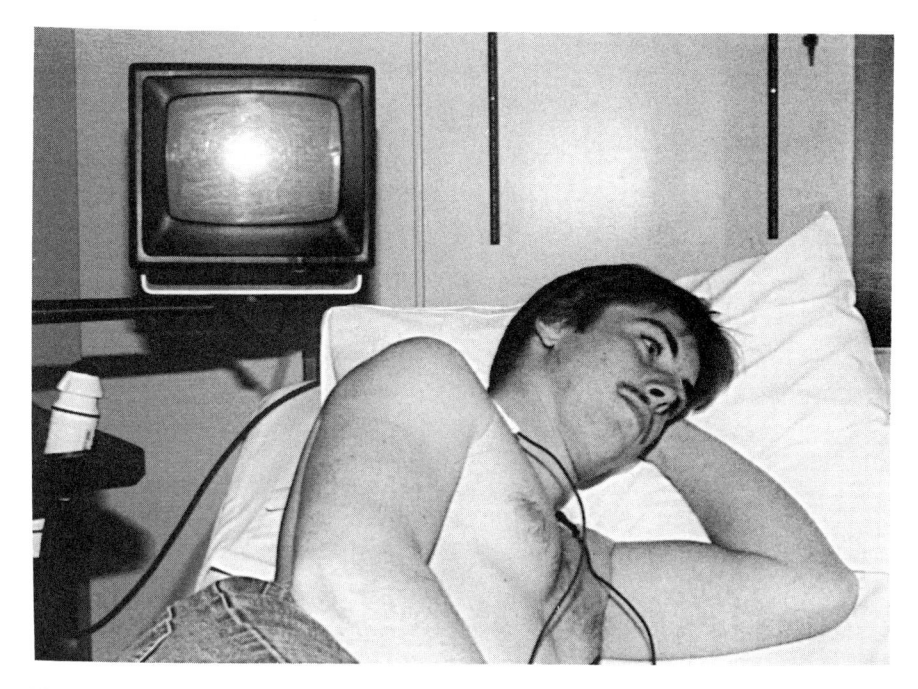

Figure 9-4 Positioning the patient on his left side may help the heart drop away from the lung field, providing a clearer cardiac image.

ducer (Figures 9-6 and 9-7). The two-dimensional and m-mode exams are quite similar. The transducer is placed between the third and fourth intercostal spaces, two to three centimeters from the left sternal border on the chest. To help the ultrasound penetrate, an aqueous gel or coupling gel is placed on the transducer. Depending on the patient's anatomy, the transducer may have to be moved up or down one or two intercostal spaces. Once a relatively clear image is obtained, the so called "cardiac window" has been found, meaning that there is no lung or rib interference. With the transducer directed posteriorly, an image of the mitral valve should be visualized. The anterior mitral valve leaflet resembles an "M" in shape and the posterior mitral valve leaflet resembles a "W" in shape (Figure 9-8). Certain "points" are designated on the mitral valve (A, C, D, E, and F), representing various motions (Figure 9-9). The A point coincides with the P wave on the electrocardiogram, indicating atrial contraction. The C point represents mitral valve closure (the end of diastole or beginning of systole) and occurs at the end of the QRS complex on the ECG. The D point is the end of systole or the beginning of diastole, and occurs directly following the T wave. The E point is the most anterior portion of the mitral valve complex and represents maximum leaflet separation. The F point follows the E wave, coinciding with a semiclosure of the valve leaflets.

A patient's heart rate and rhythm can affect the appearance of the m-mode. The mitral valve, in particular, can change in configuration. Sinus

178 Basic Echocardiography

MORRISTOWN MEMORIAL HOSPITAL
Morristown, New Jersey
<u>DIVISION OF CARDIOLOGY ECHOCARDIOGRAM REPORT</u>

NAME: _____ AGE: _____ DOB: _____ DATE: _____

LOG #: _____ U#: _____ TAPE #: _____ LOCATION: _____

MEDICATIONS: _____ REFERRING PHYSICIAN: _____

CLINICAL DIAGNOSIS: _____

<u>PERICARDIAL EFFUSION:</u>	ANTERIOR	POSTERIOR	
Estimated Amount	_____	_____	

<u>MITRAL AND TRICUSPID VALVES</u>	MITRAL	TRICUSPID	NORMAL
E-F Slope	_____	_____	80–120 mm/sec
Total Excursion	_____	_____	20–30 mm/sec
Abnormal Movement	_____	_____	
Thickness	_____	_____	
Prosthetic Opening Vel.	_____	_____	
Prosthetic Closing Vel.	_____	_____	

<u>AORTIC VALVE AND ROOT</u>		MEASUREMENT	NORMAL
Aortic Root Diameter		_____	2.0–3.7 cm
Aortic Leaflet		_____	1.5–2.6 cm
Excursion		_____	
Thickness		_____	

<u>DIMENSIONS</u>	MEASUREMENT	NORMAL
Right Ventricular Diameter (diastole)	_____	.7–2.3 cm
Left Ventricular Diameter (diastole) m^2	_____	2.1–3.2
Left Ventricular Diameter (diastole)	_____	3.7–5.4 cm
Left Ventricular Diameter (systole)	_____	————
Left Ventricular Diastolic Volume (d^3)	_____	Less than 160 cc
Ejection Fraction	_____	.67 or greater
Left Ventricular Posterior Wall Thickness	_____	.7–1.1 cm
Septal Thickness	_____	.7–1.1 cm
Left Ventricular Outflow Tract	_____	2.0–3.5 cm
Left Atrial Diameter (systole)	_____	1.9–4.0 cm
Left Atrial Diameter /m^2	_____	1.2–2.2 cm

<u>INTERPRETATION</u>

_____ M.D.

Figure 9-5 An example of an interpretation form used in an echo laboratory for measurements and an overall interpretation. Note the normal ranges for chamber sizes and valvular excursions. (Figures may vary slightly in different institutions.)

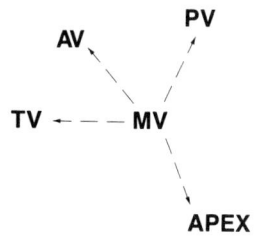

Figure 9-6 The transducer is angled inferiorly, superiorly, laterally, and medially to image various cardiac structures and valves. Using the mitral valve as a central landmark, the diagram at left helps show the orientation to nearby structures.

bradycardia will spread out the D, E, F, A, and C points of the mitral valve (Figure 9-10). A patient in sinus tachycardia would exhibit a single opening excursion. The E and A points merge, due to the rapid heart rate (Figure 9-11). Since atrial fibrillation causes a varied ventricular response, the m-mode depicts varied irregular cardiac cycles. In diastole the mitral valve may show "course fluttering" in long diastolic intervals, representing short opening motions. The A wave is usually absent in the presence of atrial fibrillation (Figure 9-12). VPC's and APC's would cause an early contraction, disturbing the normal distance between each normal ventricular contraction (Figure 9-13 and 9-14). The transducer must then be directed laterally, medially, or inferiorly to visualize other cardiac structures. An image of the aortic valve can be obtained by directing the transducer superiorly from the position of the mitral valve to the patient's right shoulder. The aortic root is characterized by two parallel lines moving together and arising anteriorly in ventricular systole. The aortic valve is within the root and excursion of the valve visualized. The left atrium is directly beneath the root (Figure 9-15). The left ventricle can be imaged by directing the transducer inferiorly, then laterally towards the patient's left hip. The intraventricular septum (IVS) and left

(Text continues on page 185)

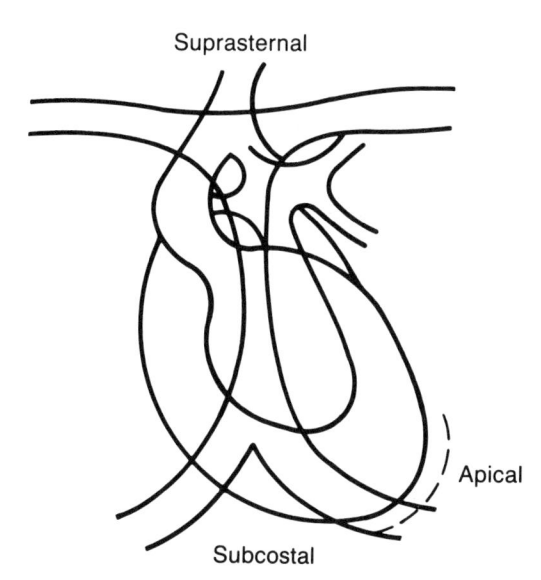

Figure 9-7 A diagram exhibiting the heart positioned in the chest cavity, behind the sternum.

180 Basic Echocardiography

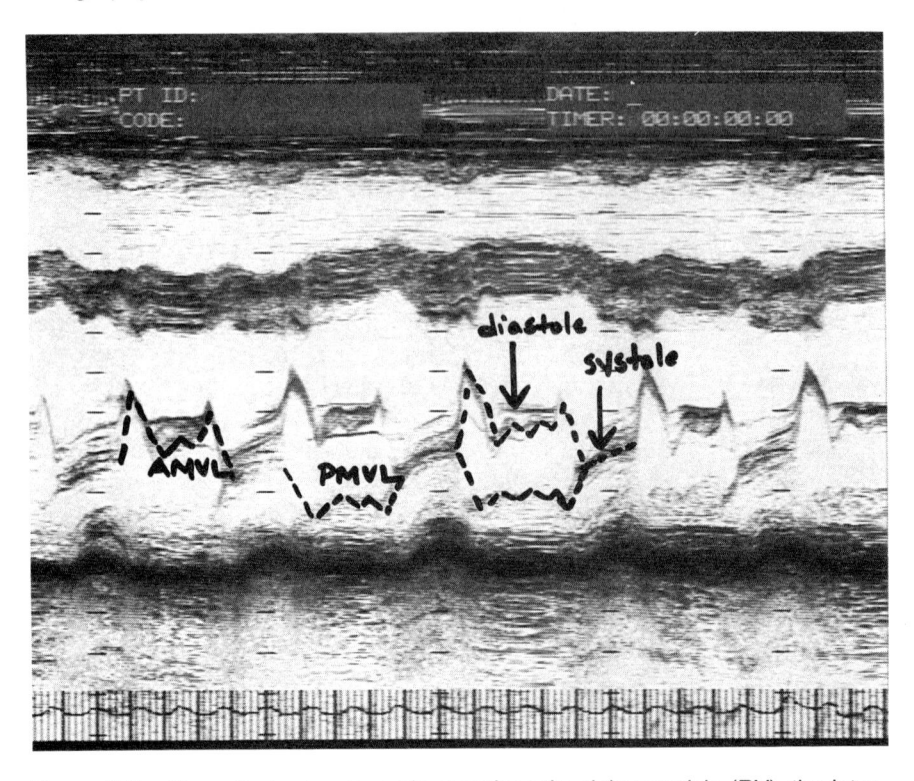

Figure 9-8 The mitral valve m-mode examines the right ventricle (RV), the intraventricular septum (IVS), the mitral valve (MV), and the left ventricular posterior wall (LVPW). Both the anterior and posterior mitral valve leaflets are seen (AMVL-PMVL). Ventricular diastole occurs when the MV leaflets are separate, and systole occurs when they join together, forming a closure line.

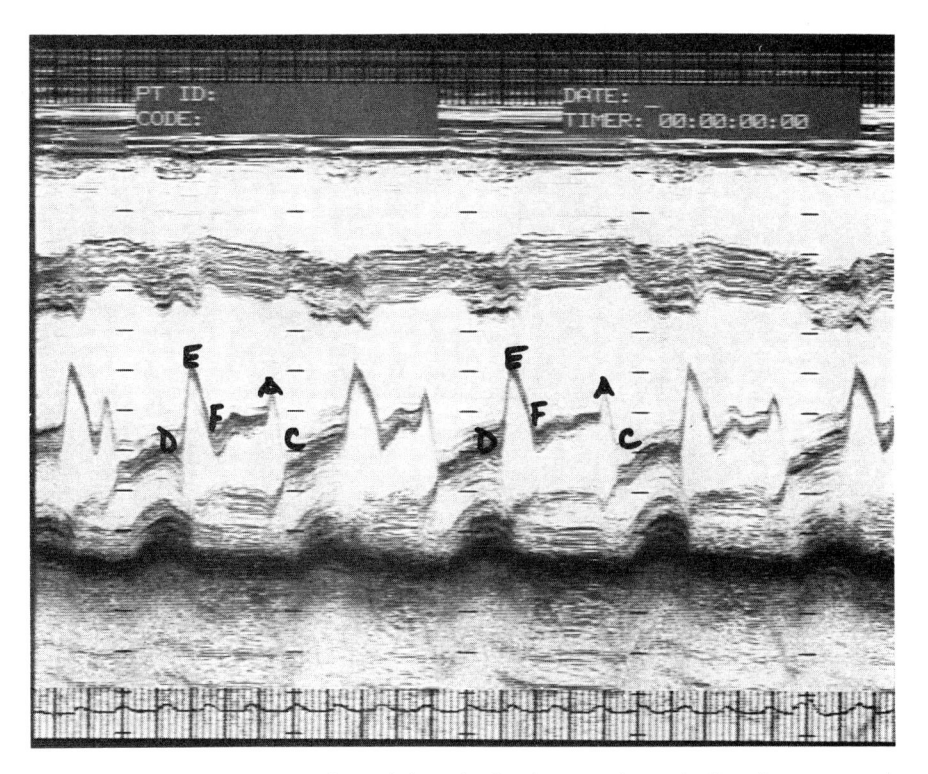

Figure 9-9 The various points of the mitral valve are shown in the above m-mode.

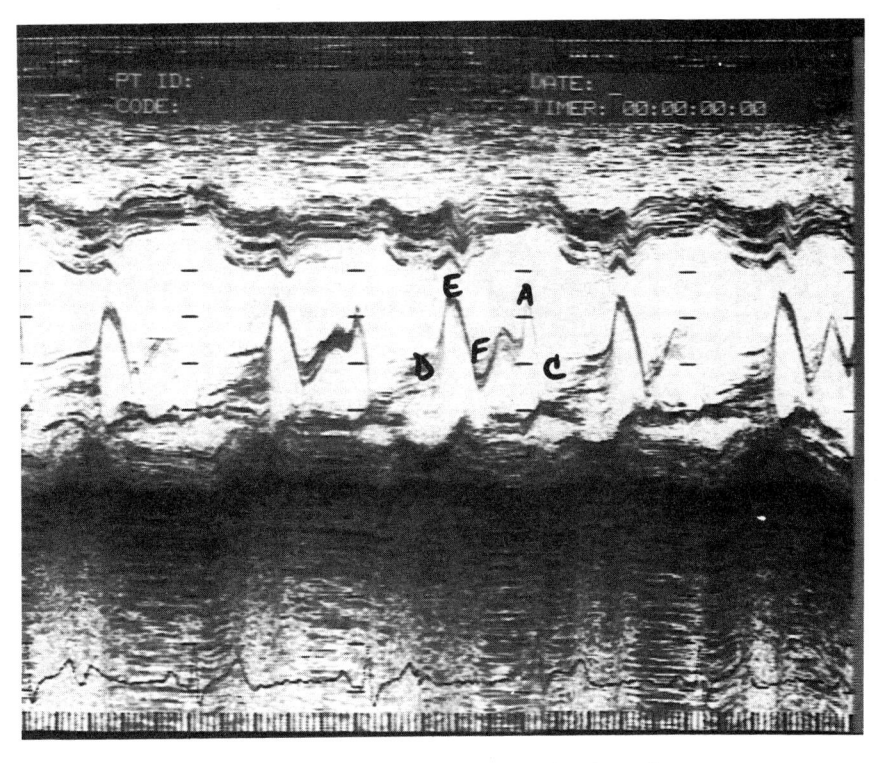

Figure 9-10 Mitral m-mode of a patient in sinus bradycardia.

181

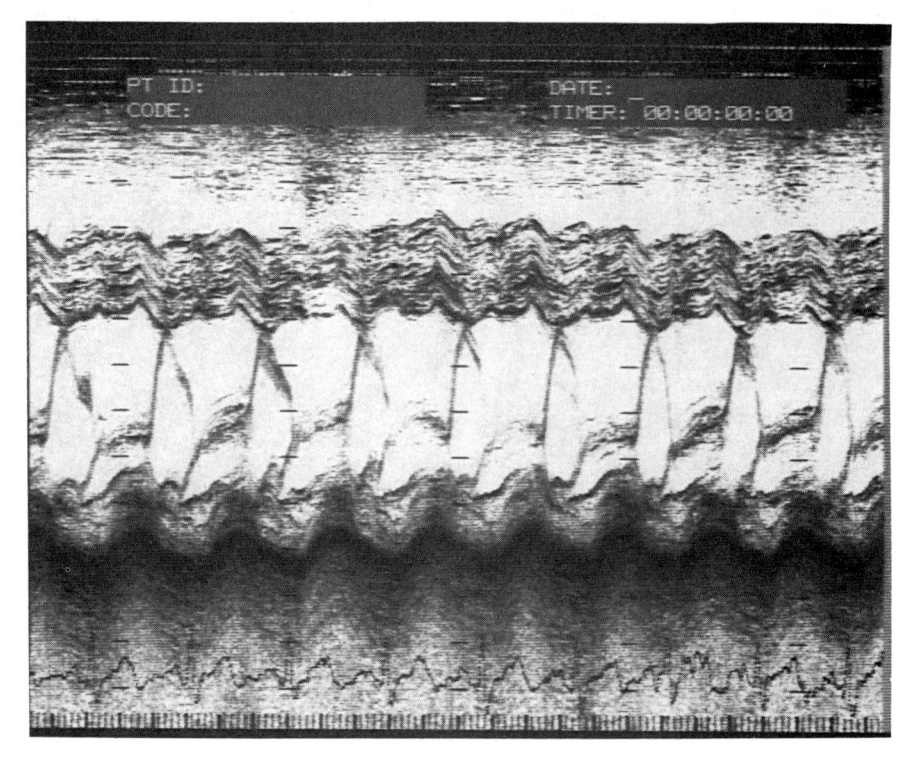

Figure 9-11 M-mode of the mitral valve, demonstrating a patient in sinus tachycardia. Notice the single opening in diastole.

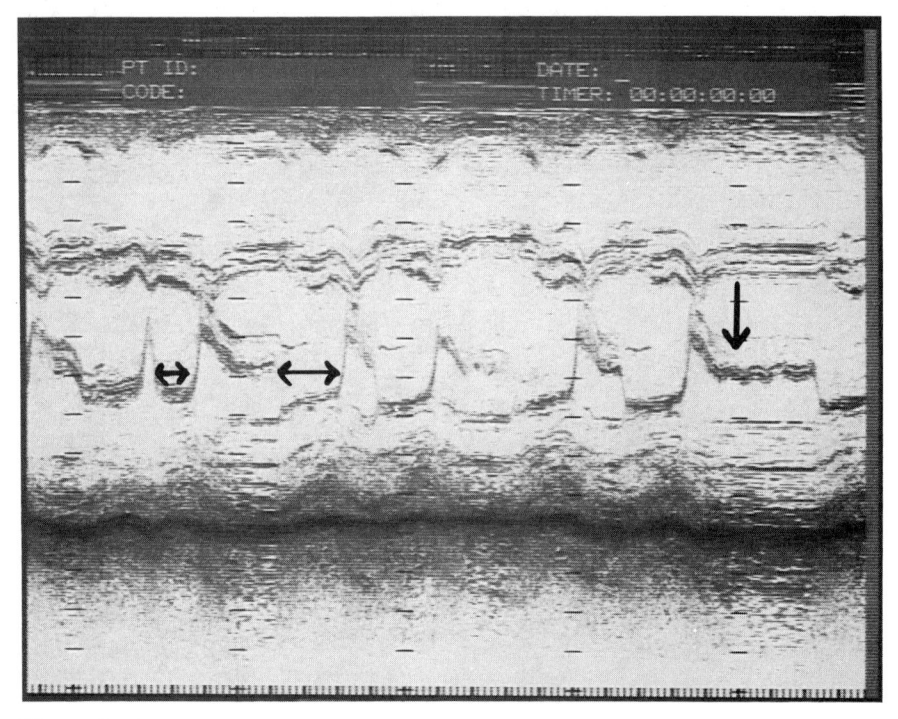

Figure 9-12 A patient in atrial fibrillation would register the above mitral appearance.

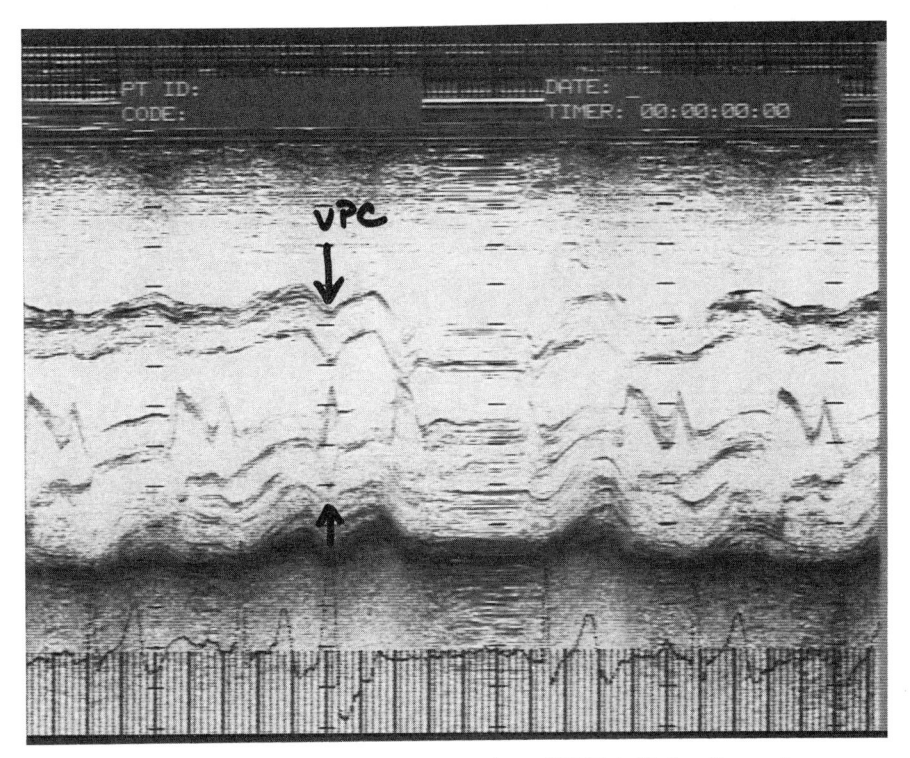

Figure 9-13 Ventricular premature contractions (VPC's). Notice the early complex followed by a pause.

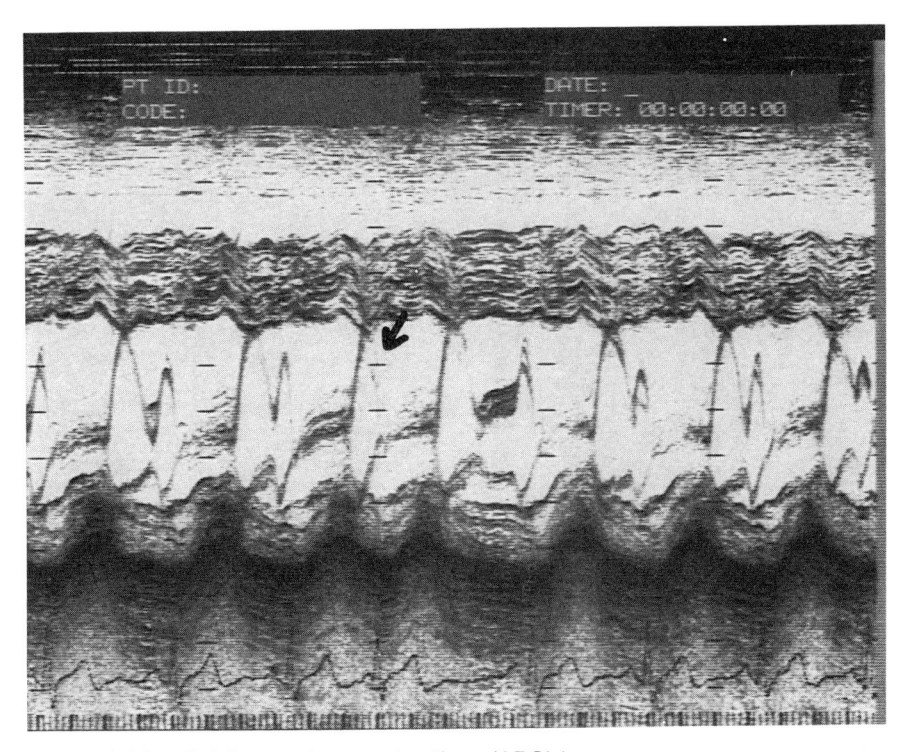

Figure 9-14 Atrial premature contractions (APC's).

183

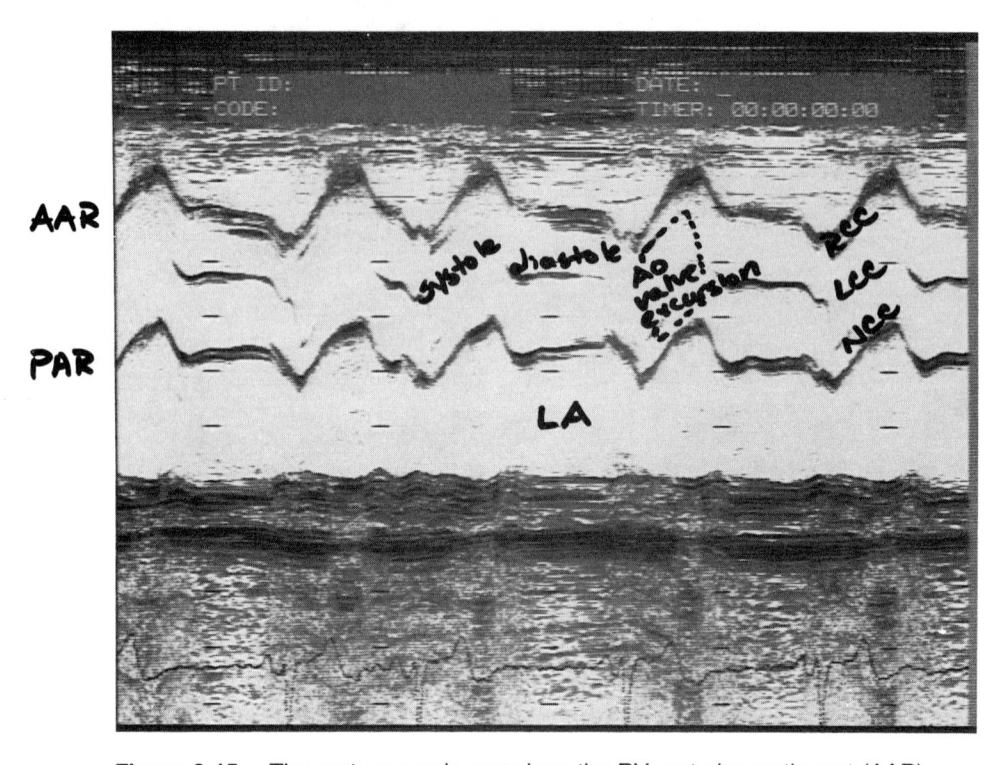

Figure 9-15 The aorta m-mode examines the RV, anterior aortic root (AAR), posterior aortic root (PAR), the valve leaflets, and the left atrium (LA). There are three aortic valve leaflets: the right coronary cusp (RCC), the left coronary cusp (LCC) and the non-coronary cusp (NCC). The RCC and NCC are visualized in systole; however, the LCC is parallel with the ultrasound beams so it cannot be seen. Diastole is the closure of all valvular leaflets.

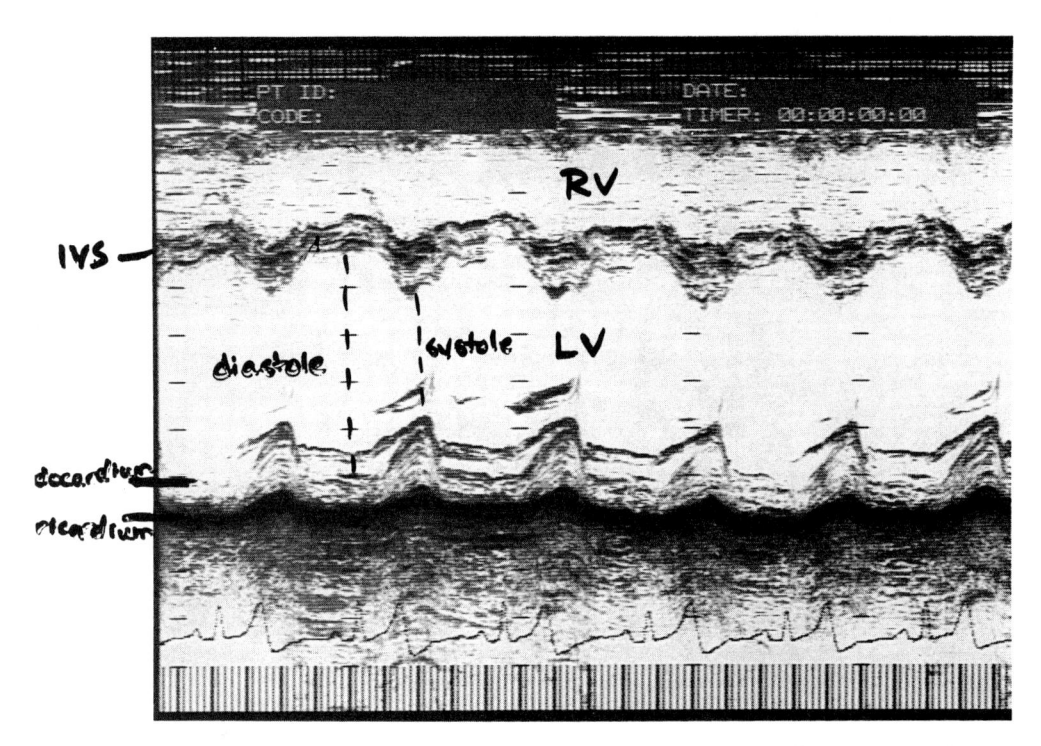

Figure 9-16 The left ventricular m-mode images the RV, IVS, the left ventricular cavity, and the LVPW.

ventricular posterior wall (LVPW) move together in ventricular systole and move apart in diastole. The LVPW is composed of three distinct layers: the pericardium (represented as the darkest band of echoes within the LVPW), the epicardium (moving with the LVPW), and the endocardium (moving with the LVPW but rising more rapidly in ventricular systole than does the epicardium—Figure 9-16). An example of an m-mode scan obtained from this technique shows the aortic position turning into the mitral, and then into the left ventricular position (Figure 9-17). The pulmonic and tricuspid valves are usually difficult to visualize. From the mitral valve, the tricuspid valve can be recorded by directing the transducer medially and the pulmonic valve by directing the transducer superiorly. The tricuspid valve m-mode also resembles an "M" shape, and is set high on the strip chart (Figure 9-18). The pulmonic valve resembles somewhat the aortic valve. Usually only the closure line of the valve is seen and the A wave is visualized (Figure 9-19).

The disadvantage of using the m-mode exam alone, without the two-dimensional exam, lies in its "ice-pick" or one-dimensional effect. The single plane visualization is not fully accurate because the echocardiographer has no way of knowing the location of the ultrasound beam.

(Text continues on page 188)

186 Basic Echocardiography

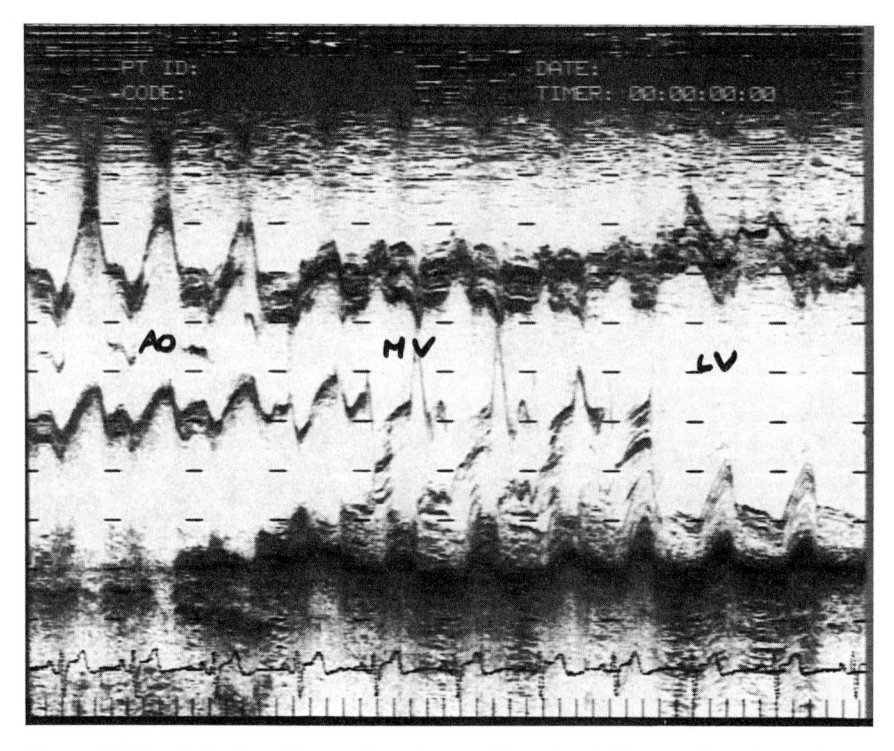

Figure 9-17 Note from the aortic valve position, the AAR turns into the IVS and the PAR turns into the AMVL. Scanning further into the left ventricle, the mitral valve disappears. (Paper speed at 25 mm/sec)

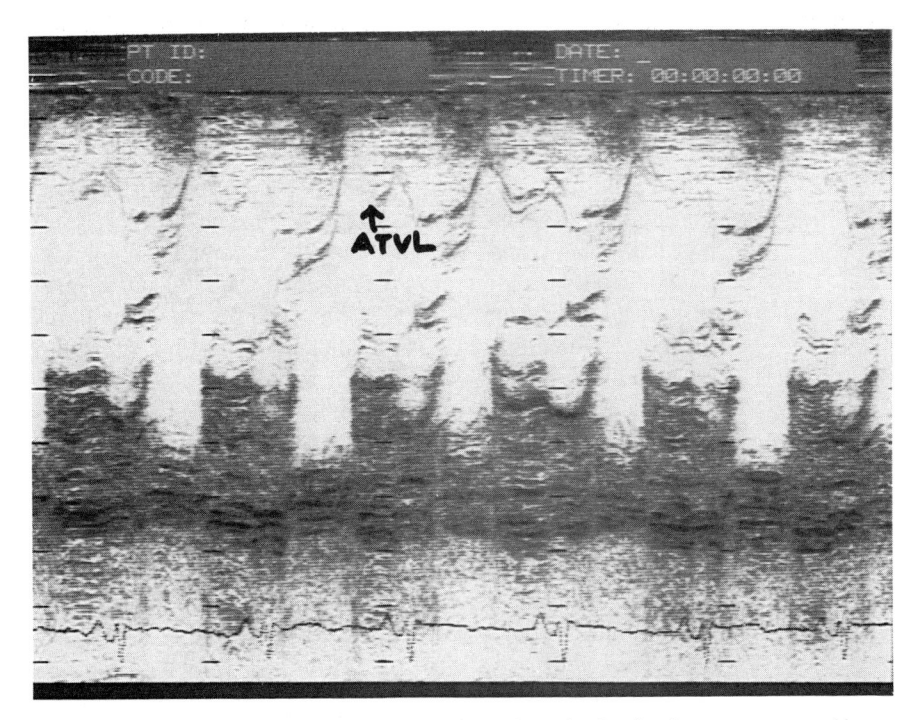

Figure 9-18 The tricuspid valve resembles the mitral valve in appearance. Usually only the anterior tricuspid valve leaflet is recorded.

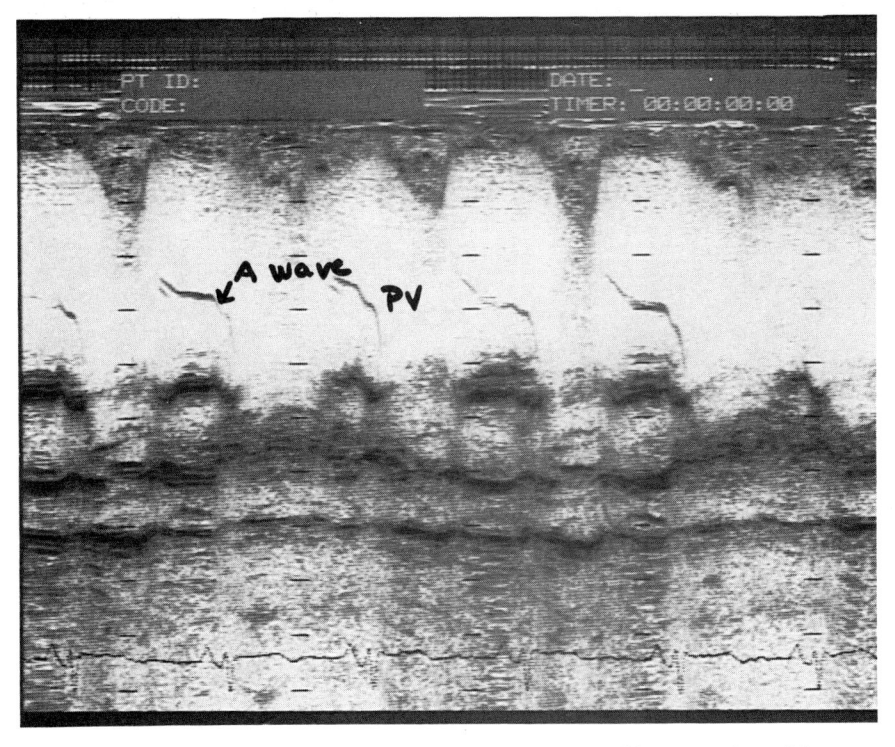

Figure 9-19 Notice the pulmonic A wave and the resemblance to that of the aortic valve m-mode.

Two-Dimensional Examination

Because the two-dimensional echo records a tomogram, there are several areas on the chest used for each specific image (Figures 9-20 through 9-23). The first is termed the *parasternal long-axis view*, and is obtained by positioning the transducer in the same manner as when performing an m-mode exam. The transducer is placed in a parallel position on the chest, on the left sternal border between the third and fourth intercostal spaces. A so-called "notch" (common to all transducers) has to be rotated to obtain the various two-dimensional views. Each brand of machinery has a different location for this notch, which transects the heart into its various planes. An image of the heart from the base to the apex is visualized in the parasternal long-axis view (Figure 9-24). The parasternal long-axis view visualizes the following structures: the left atrium (LA), the mitral valve (MV), the left ventricle (LV), the intraventricular septum (IVS), the right ventricle (RV), the aortic root, and the aortic valve (Figures 9-25 and 9-26). This view is used in many disease states as well as when imaging left ventricular function. It is ideal for obtaining m-modes, which will be discussed later. Another view is the *parasternal short-axis view*. Rotation of the transducer 90° from the long-axis position gives the short-axis view. (The following short-axis views are cross-

(Text continues on page 192)

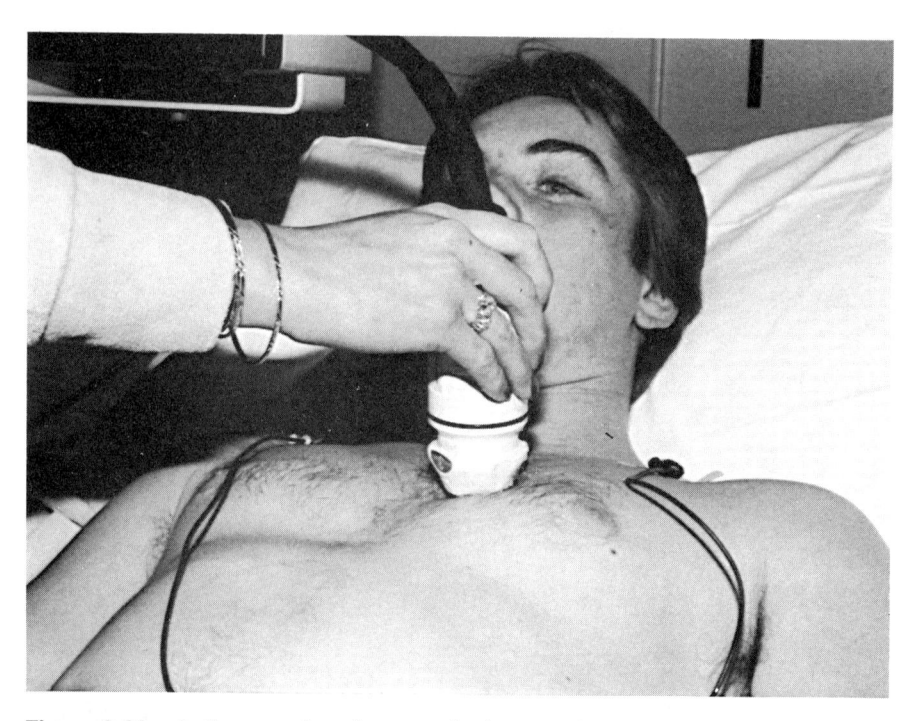

Figure 9-20 In the parasternal approach, the transducer is placed on the left sternal border.

The Examination 189

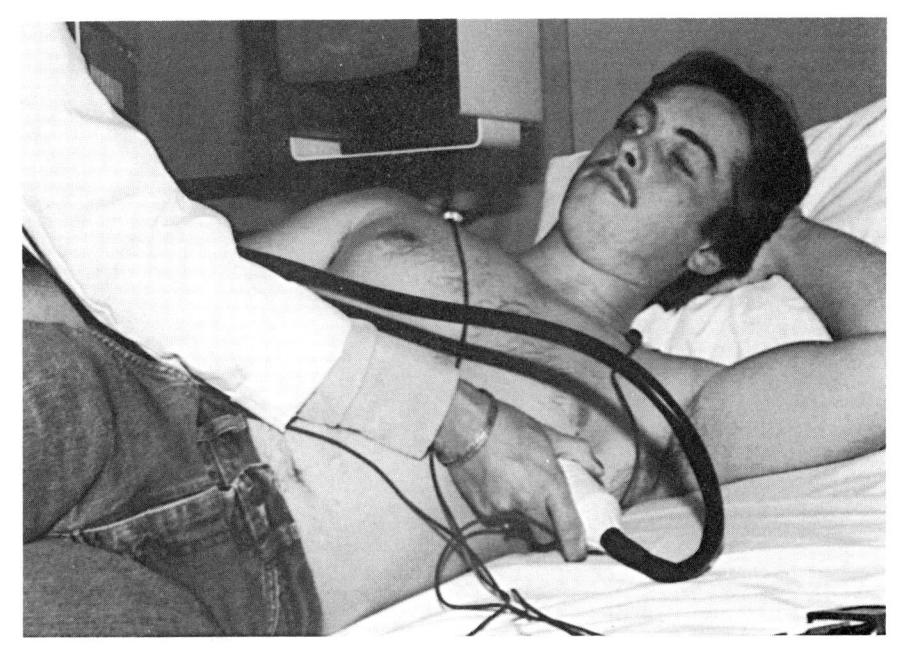

Figure 9-21 In apical approaches, the transducer in repositioned at the apex, where the palpable pulse is felt.

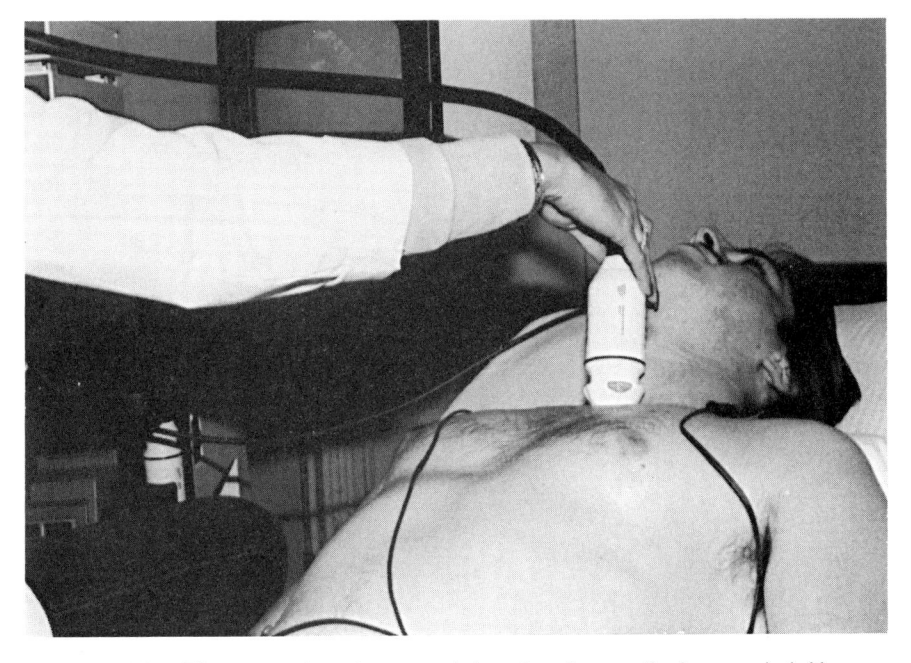

Figure 9-22 The suprasternal approach is not a view routinely recorded. However, at times it is necessary. The transducer is placed in the suprasternal notch.

190 Basic Echocardiography

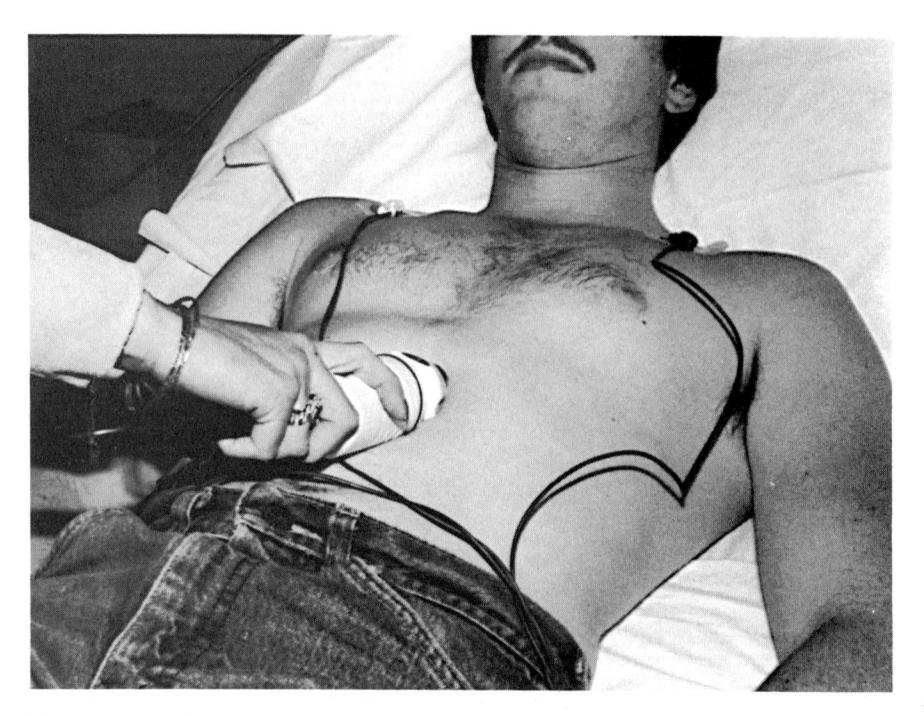

Figure 9-23 The subcostal view is an excellent technique when parasternal and apical views are unobtainable. The transducer is placed beneath the zyphoid process, aiming the transducer toward the heart.

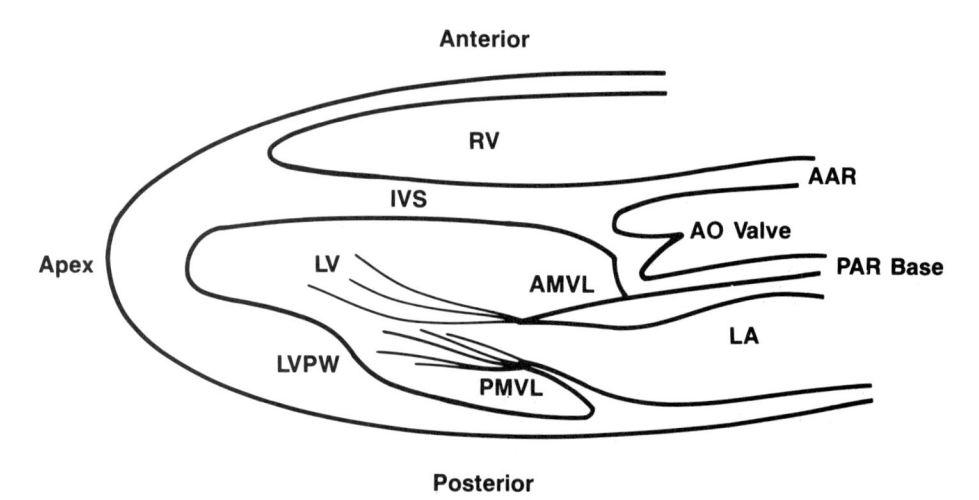

Figure 9-24 A schematic representation of a parasternal long-axis view (right ventricle = RV; left ventricle = LV; mitral valve = MV; aortic valve = AO; left atrium = LA; intraventricular septum = IVS; left ventricular posterior wall = LVPW).

The Examination 191

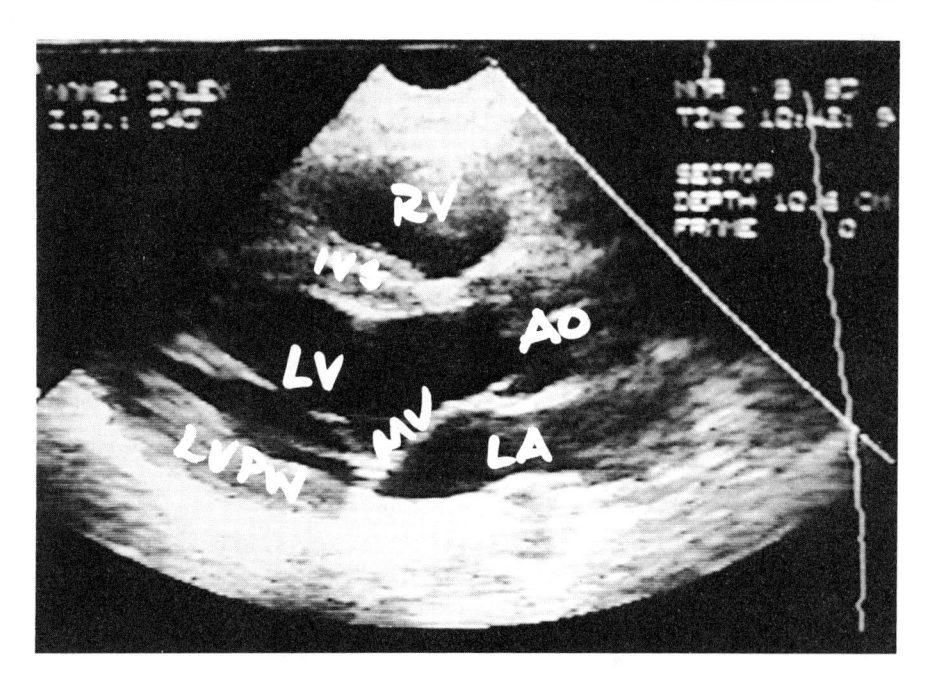

Figure 9-25 The two-dimensional parasternal long-axis view in systole shows that the MV is closed as the AO valve is open.

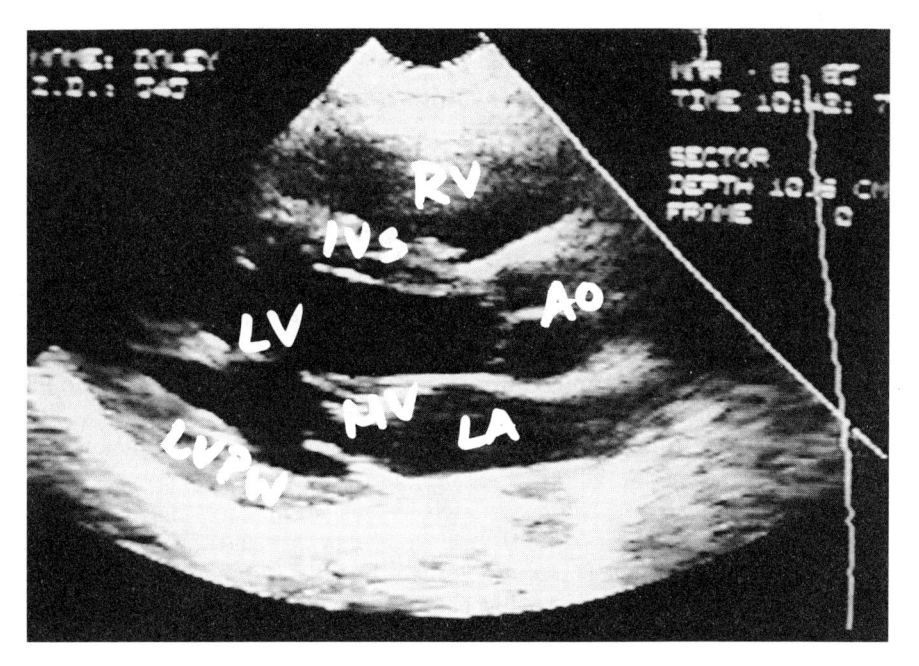

Figure 9-26 In ventricular diastole, note that the MV is open, whereas the AO valve is closed.

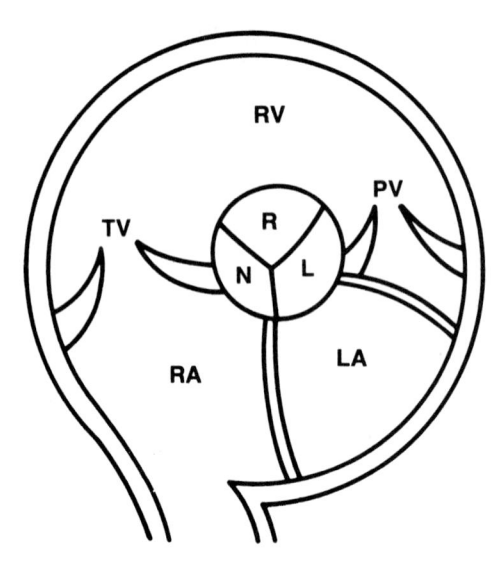

Figure 9-27 A schematic representation of a parasternal short-axis view at the level of the aortic valve. (Tricuspid valve = TV; pulmonic valve = PV; pulmonary artery = PA; right atrium = RA; Aortic valve = AO.)

sectional cuts of the heart.) Three images are demonstrated from this position by a slight movement of the transducer. Angling the transducer superiorly towards the right shoulder gives the short-axis view at the level of the aortic valve (Figure 9-27). In this view, a cross-sectional cut of the aortic valve with all three leaflets (right, left, and noncoronary cusp) is imaged as well as the LA, the intra-atrial septum (IAS), the right atrium (RA), the RV, the tricuspid valve, and the pulmonic valve (Figure 9-28). This view is particularly useful in assessing aortic valve disease and visualizing the right-sided valves. Positioning the transducer more medially and directing the ultrasound beam posteriorly gives the short-axis view of the mitral valve level (Figure 9-29). The mitral valve, which resembles a "fish-mouth" configuration, is surrounded by the doughnutlike appearance of the left ventricle. The mitral valve orifice can be seen clearly, and evidence of any leaflet restriction is easily recognized (Figure 9-30). Angling the transducer inferiorly and toward the left hip gives the image of the left ventricle and the short-axis plane. As mentioned above, the left ventricle appears as a doughnut (Figure 9-31). At the base of the LV, both papillary muscles can be imaged (Figure 9-32). This cross-sectional view is one of the best views used to evaluate left ventricular function as well as thickness of the ventricle. The IVS, true anterior wall, lateral wall, and LVPW are all seen. A small portion of the right ventricle is also seen bordering the IVS (Figure 9-33). By repositioning the transducer toward the apex of the ventricle and parallel to the chest, a view termed the *apical four-chamber view* is seen. Visualization of all four cardiac chambers, as well as the atrioventricular valves is imaged (Figure 9-34). Left ventricular function can be evaluated in the apical four-chamber view, as can estimated chamber size, mitral and tricuspid valve

(Text continues on page 197)

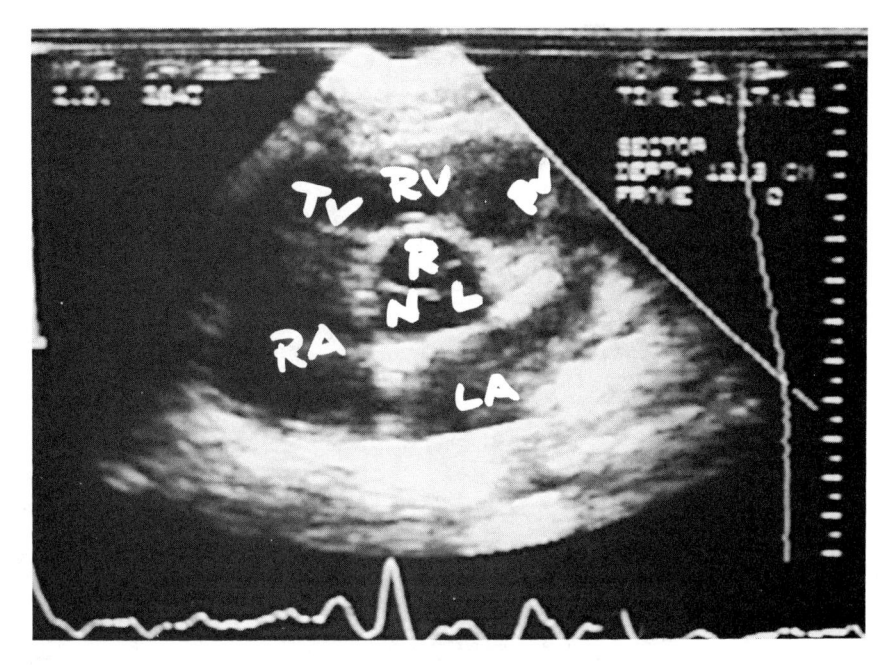

Figure 9-28 A two-dimensional parasternal short-axis view at the AO level in diastole exhibits both the aortic and pulmonic valves closed. Note the aortic valve forms a "peace sign" or a "Y." In ventricular systole, the semilunar valves open and the atrioventricular valves close.

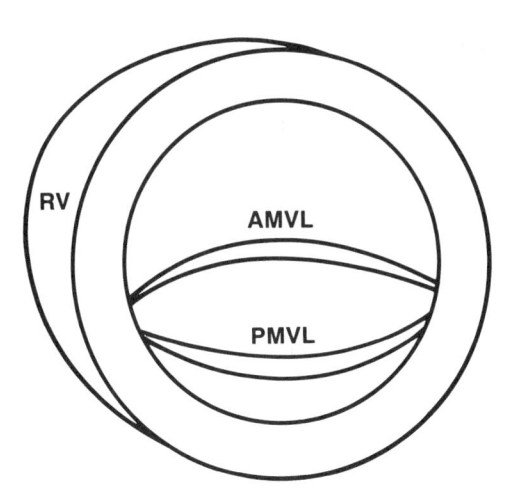

Figure 9-29 A schematic figure of the MV at the parasternal short-axis level. The AMVL/PMVL are set within the left ventricular cavity.

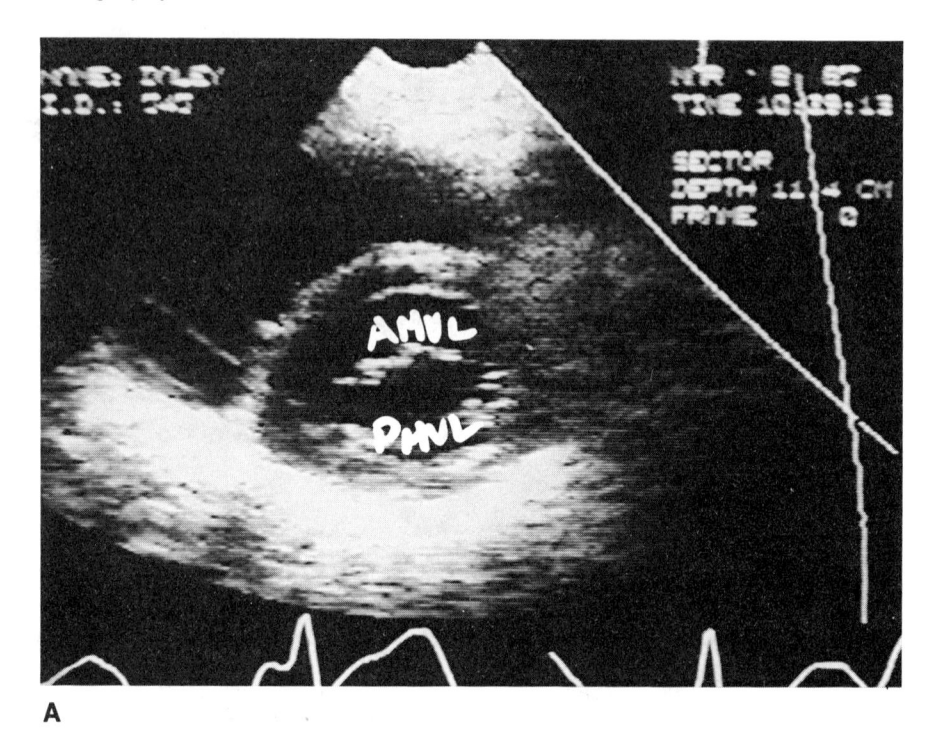

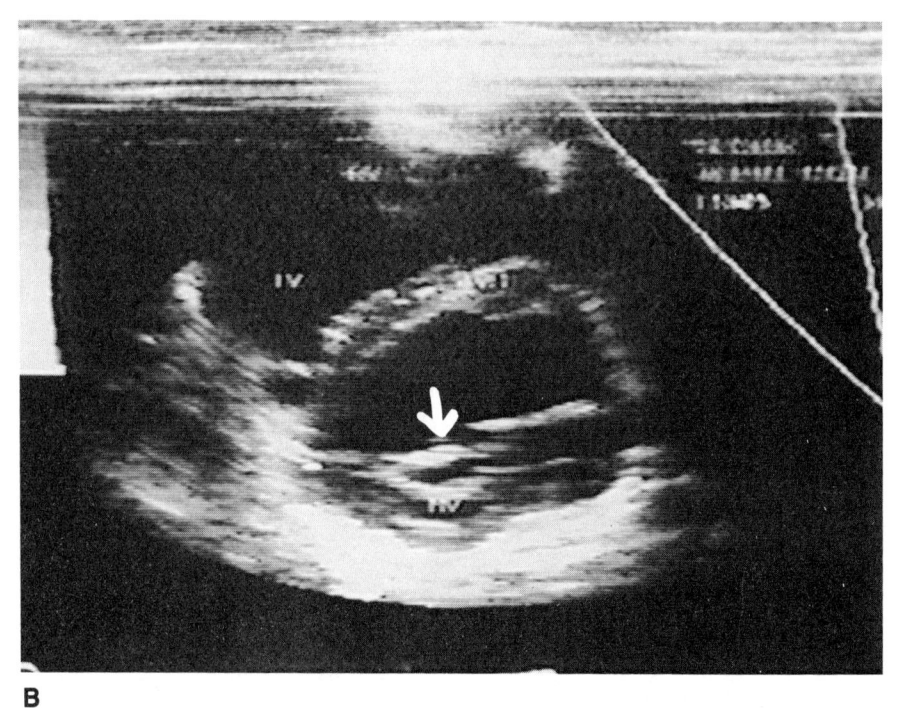

Figure 9-30 *(A)* A two-dimensional parasternal short-axis view at the MV level exhibits a "fish-mouth" configuration in diastole when the valve is fully open. *(B)* In systole, the valve leaflets close, creating a single closure line.

The Examination   195

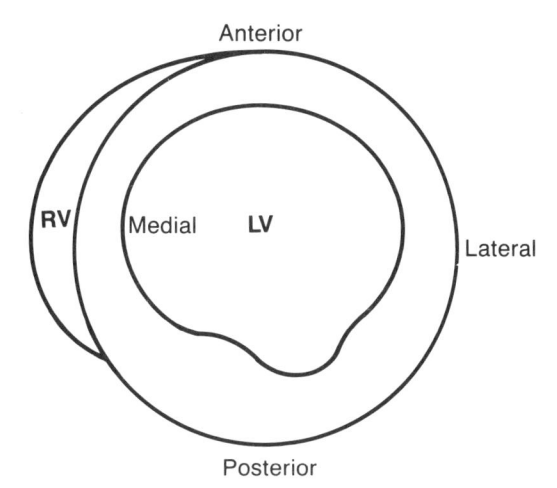

Figure 9-31 A schematic image of the left ventricle at the papillary muscle level. Left ventricular walls are labeled.

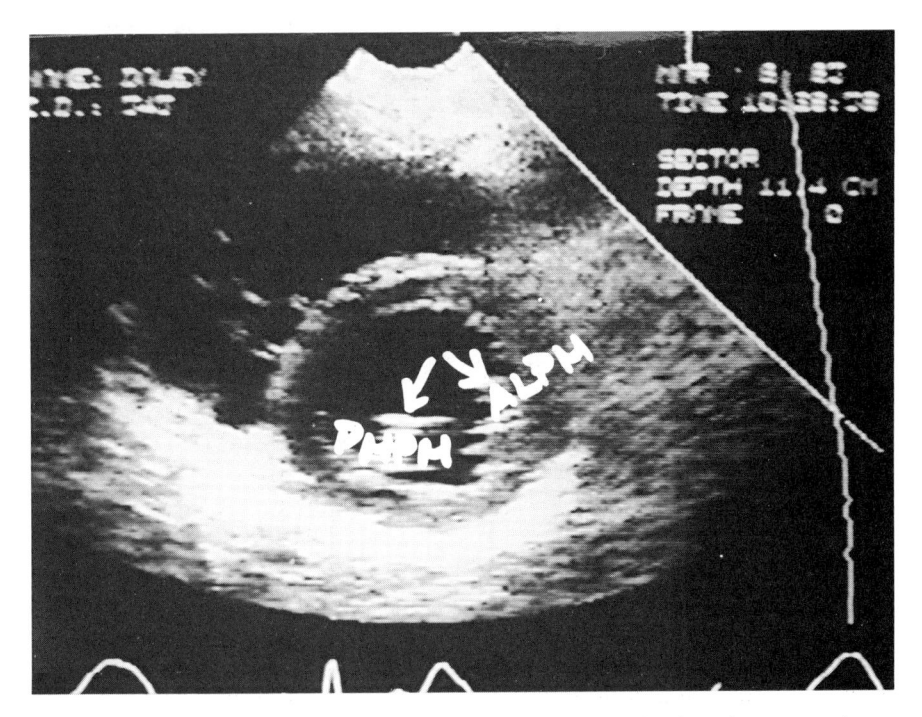

Figure 9-32 A two-dimensional LV image in the short-axis plane is seen at the papillary muscle level. Both the anterior lateral papillary muscle (ALPM) and the posterior medial papillary muscles (PMPM) are seen.

196 Basic Echocardiography

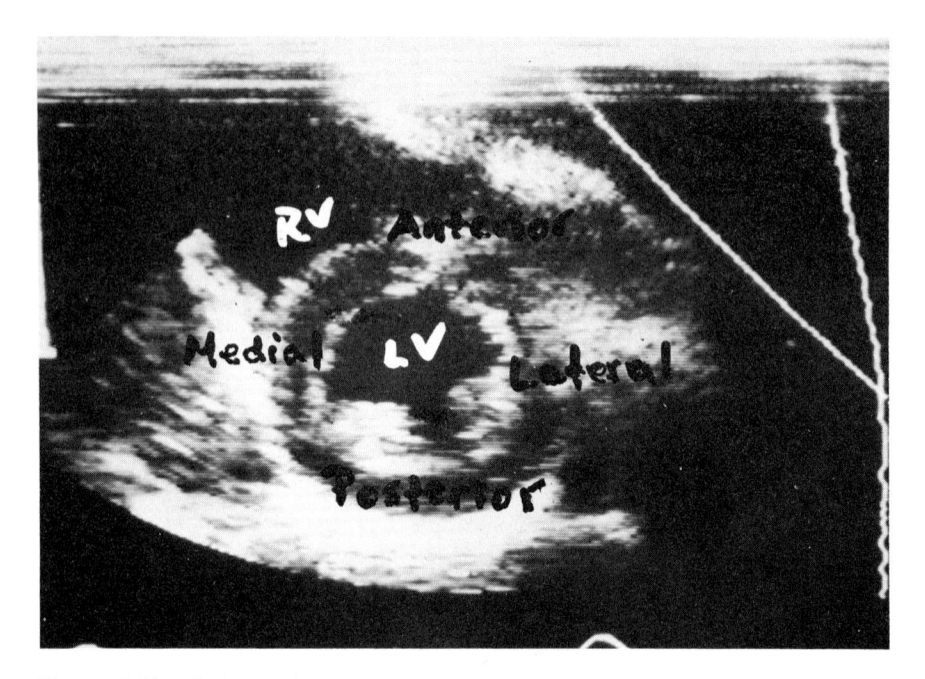

Figure 9-33 Left ventricular walls are shown in this two-dimensional LV image. This view is useful in evaluating left ventricular function.

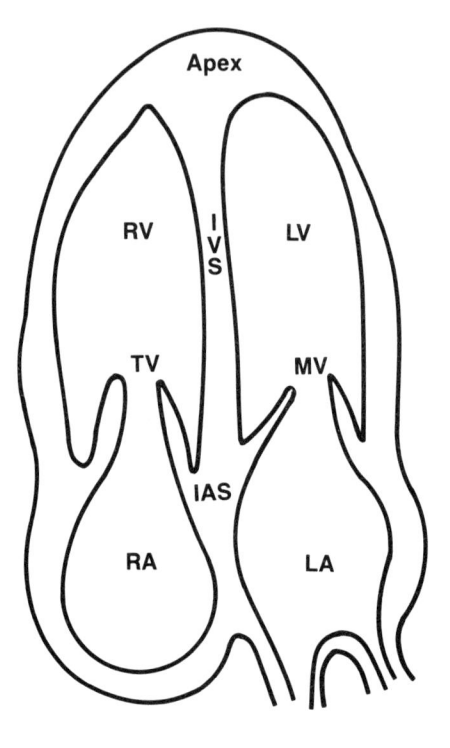

Figure 9-34 A schematic diagram showing the apical four chamber view, visualizing all four cardiac chambers as well as both atrioventricular valves.

diseases; it can also be used for the detection of left ventricular clots (Figures 9-35 and 9-36). Another view termed the *apical five-chamber view* is obtained by angling the front portion of the transducer superiorly from the apical four-chamber position. The aortic valve is visualized in the middle of the four cardiac chambers. This view is used when visualization of the aortic valve from the parasternal views is unobtainable (Figure 9-37). Keeping the transducer at the apex and rotating it in the same direction as the parasternal long-axis view gives a view termed the *apical two-chamber view* or the *apical long axis view* (Figure 9-38). This view shows the same structures as the parasternal long-axis view, except that the left ventricle is tipped up vertically. The "true inferior" wall is visualized and this view is similar to the right anterior oblique (RAO) view used in the catheterization laboratory (Figure 9-39). The *subcostal four-chamber* or subxiphoid view is obtained by once again repositioning the transducer under the xiphoid process, and angling it toward the heart. This image is similar to the apical four-chamber view (Figure 9-40). This view is often used for a patient with a barrel-chested configuration or with any lung disorder such as emphysema, because these patients usually do not have parasternal windows. M-modes can be derived from this view for approximate measurements. The *suprasternal approach* is one that is not often used but sometimes necessary for a specific diagnosis.

(*Text continues on page 201*)

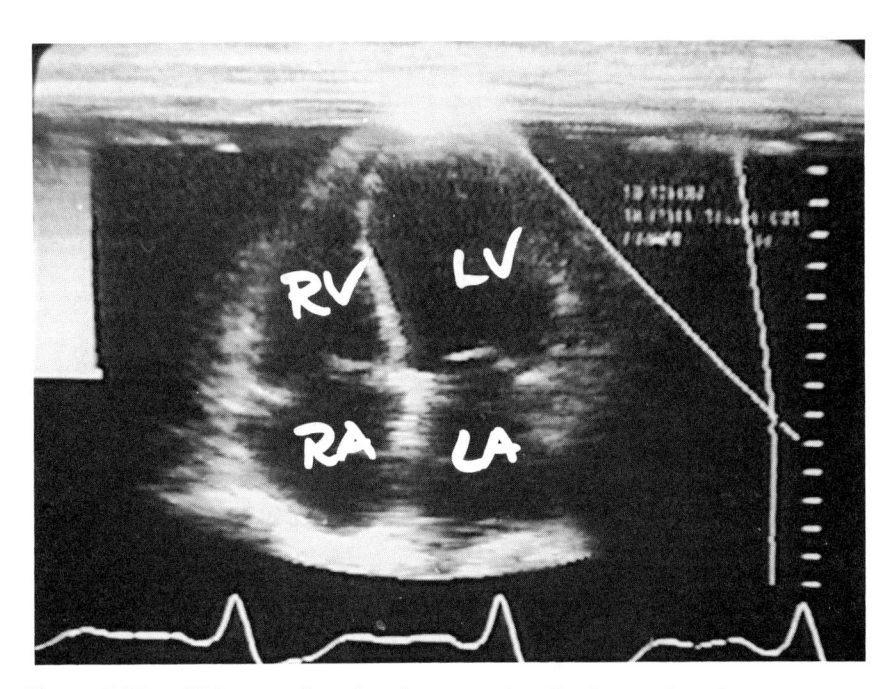

Figure 9-35 All four cardiac chambers are visualized as well as the atrioventricular valves (AV). In ventricular systole, the AV valves are closed.

198 Basic Echocardiography

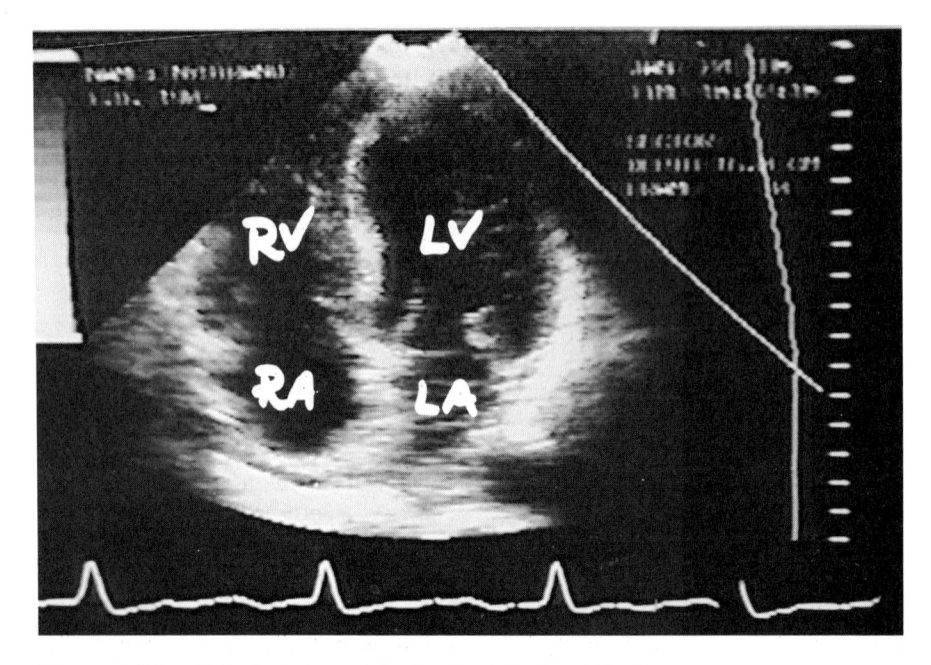

Figure 9-36 Note that, in ventricular diastole, the AV valves are open.

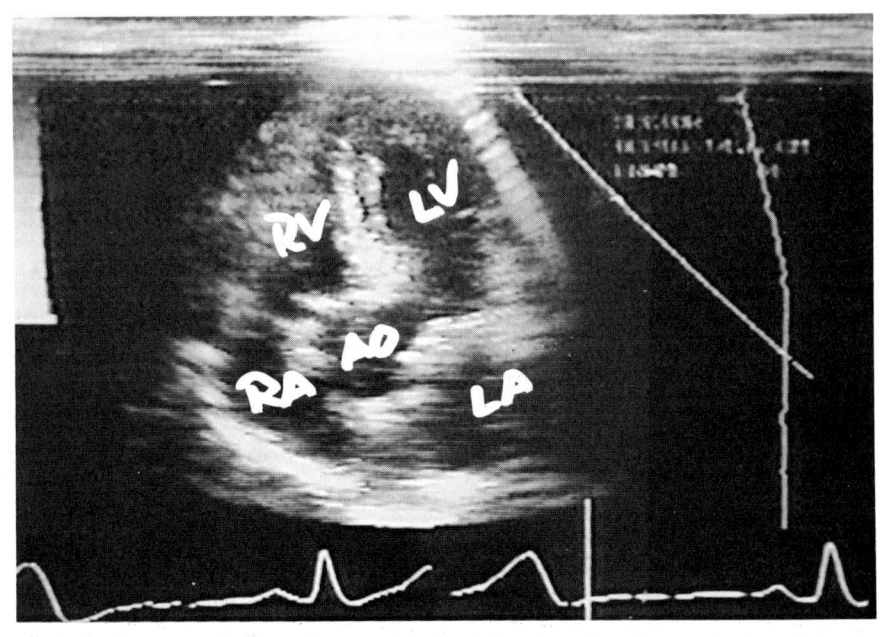

Figure 9-37 A two-dimensional apical five-chamber view demonstrating all four chambers with the aortic valve in the center, leaving the left ventricular outflow tract.

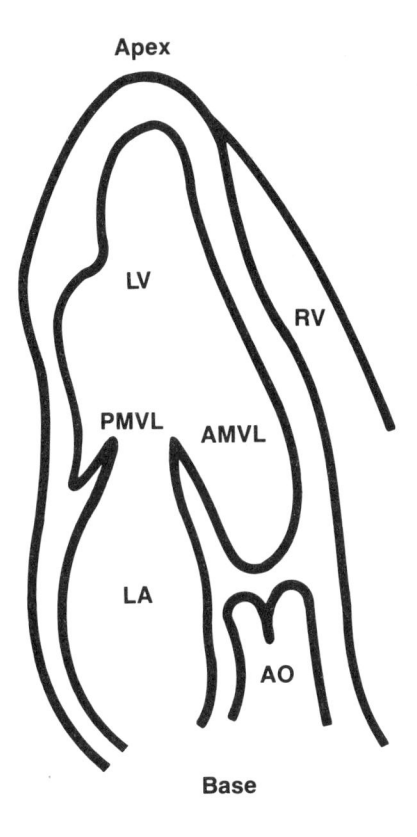

Figure 9-38 A schematic diagram of an apical two-chamber view. Notice the similarity to the parasternal long axis view.

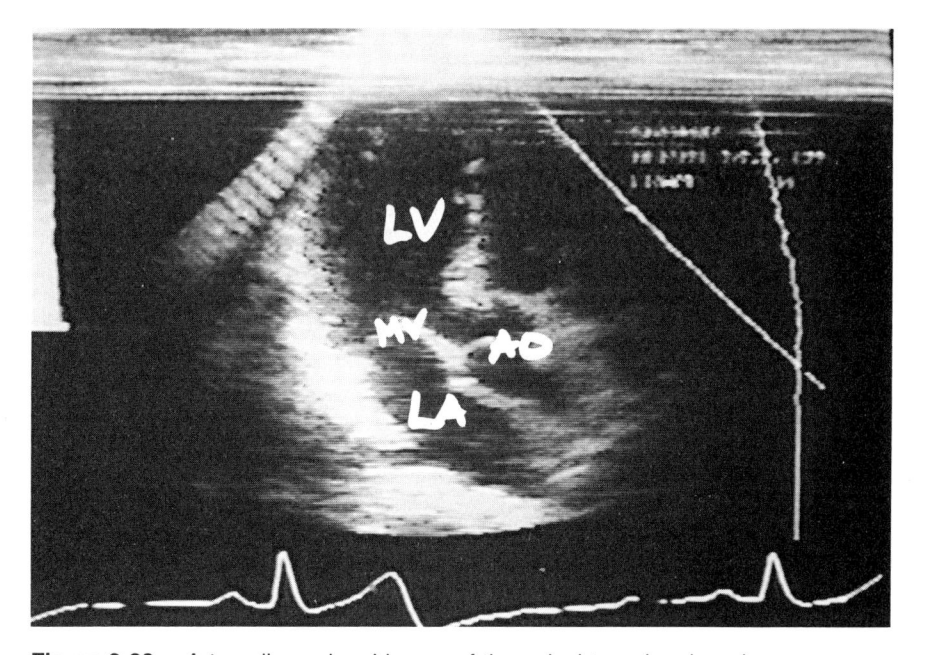

Figure 9-39 A two-dimensional image of the apical two-chamber view.

200 Basic Echocardiography

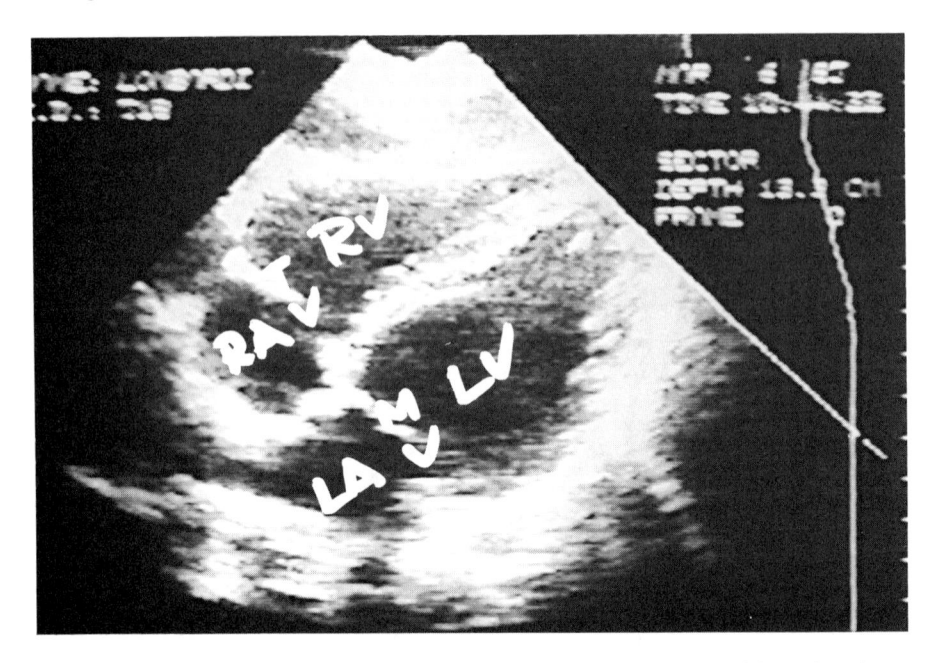

Figure 9-40 Similar to the apical four-chamber view, the subcostal four-chamber view examines all cardiac chambers and both atrioventricular valves.

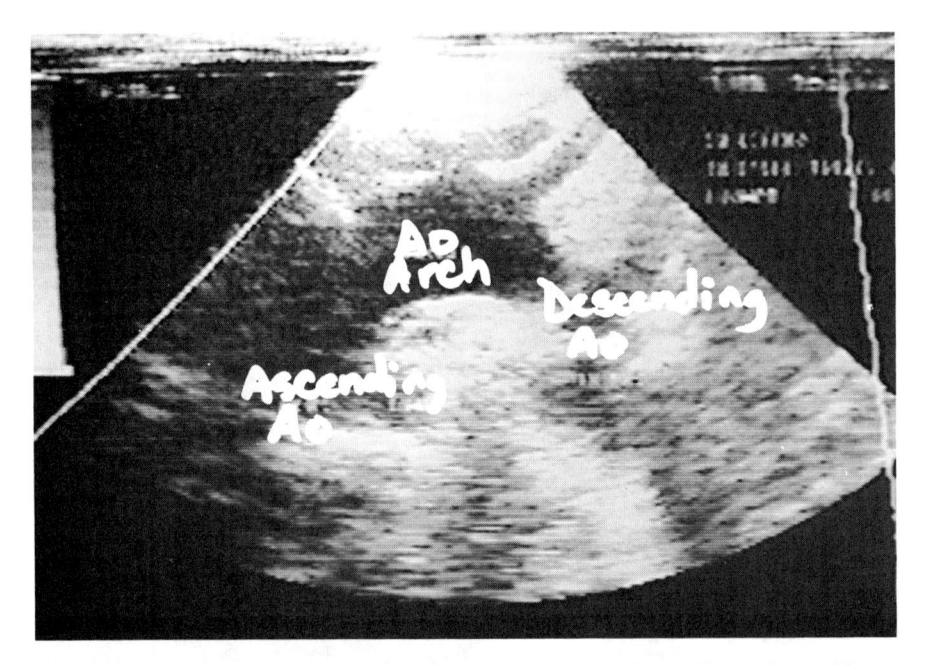

Figure 9-41 This view is commonly used in pediatric echocardiography and is especially useful in conjunction with the cardiac Doppler.

The transducer is placed in the "notch" of the neck, above the sternum level. This view is sometimes uncomfortable for the patient and not routinely recorded. It is mainly used in pediatric echocardiography for visualization of the ascending aortic, the arch itself, the descending aorta, as well as the vessels arising from the arch (Figure 9-41). In order to achieve an adequate two-dimensional examination, the patient has to be somewhat "echogenic," meaning that an adequate cardiac window must be found. The patient's anatomy and chest configuration are also important factors when performing an echo exam. Again, proper instrument control can also affect the quality of the image.

Deriving M-Modes From Two-Dimensional Examinations

Most two-dimensional echo machines have the capability of obtaining m-modes by means of the two-dimensional exam. By visualizing the actual image in two dimensions, the m-mode is more precise for interpretation as well as for measuring. By moving a "cursor" or "ice pick" to a designated area on the two-dimensional image, an m-mode is obtained. An aortic valve m-mode echo can be derived from either the parasternal long-axis view or the parasternal short-axis view at the aortic valve level. The m-mode can be achieved by directing the cursor through the aortic root, including the aortic valve leaflet, and the left atrium (Figure 9-42). Aortic valve/left atrium m-modes are important because they reflect many disease states. Direct assessment of the aortic root is important for determining the size as well as the motion of the root. Dilatation of the root may represent a disease state such as aortic insufficiency or Marfan's Syndrome. Aortic root motion is important for assessing left ventricular function. The actual aortic valve recording is important for pliability of the valve leaflets, presence of calcification, or possibly left ventricular dysfunction. The right and noncoronary cusp is recorded; however, the left coronary cusp is not seen (Figure 9-43). The left atrium, and particularly its size, is important because it may reflect a mitral valve disease.

A mitral valve m-mode can be derived in the same manner as the aortic/left atrium m-mode; however, the parasternal short-axis view at the mitral valve level is used rather than at the aortic valve level (Figure 9-44). By moving the cursor to the designated area on the two-dimensional image, a mitral valve m-mode can be obtained. The cursor is placed through the anterior and the posterior mitral valve leaflets. As a result, an m-mode including the RV, IVS, MV, and LVPW is obtained (Figure 9-45). Recording of the posterior mitral valve leaflet is important and is easily accessible with the actual visualization of the two-dimensional image. Mitral valve m-modes can visualize valve abnormalities such as mitral stenosis, mitral valve prolapse, and aortic insufficiency, and can indicate left ventricular dysfunction. The mitral valve is also useful in a finding for idiopathic hypertrophic subaortic stenosis. These disease states will be discussed later in this chapter.

(Text continues on page 205)

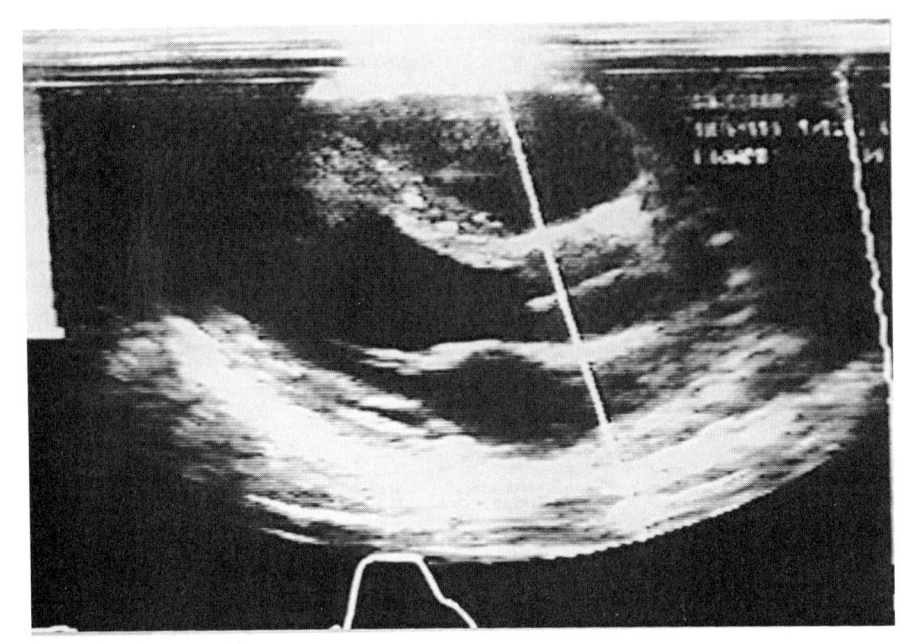

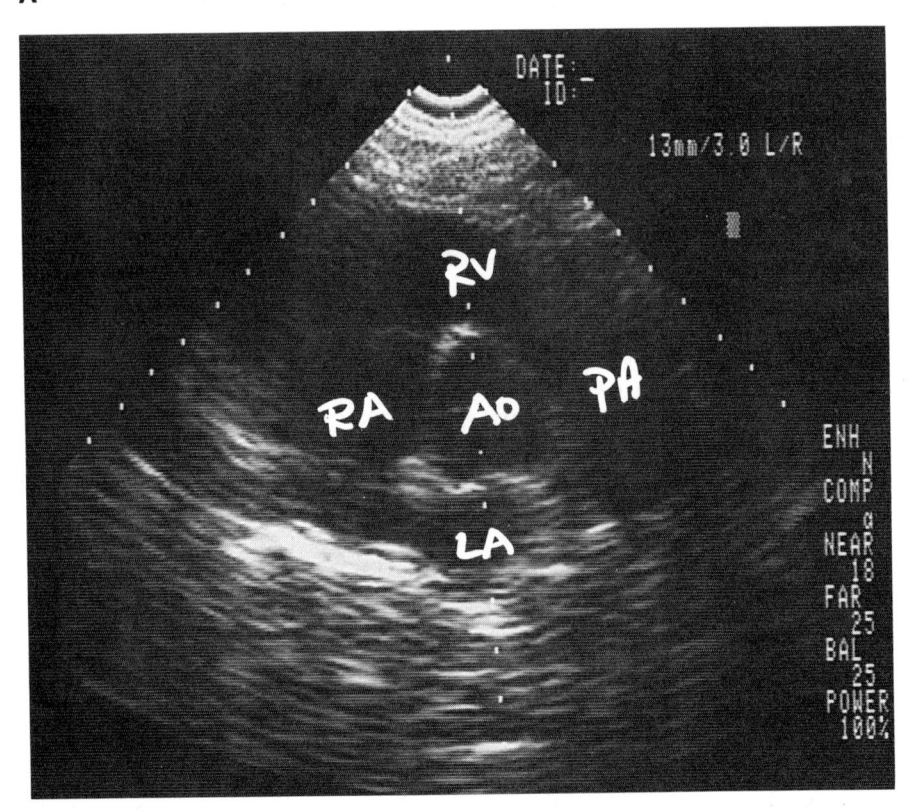

Figure 9-42 (A) Directing the cursor through the aortic valve in the parasternal long-axis view gives an aortic m-mode. (B) The cursor can also be placed through the aortic valve in the parasternal short-axis view.

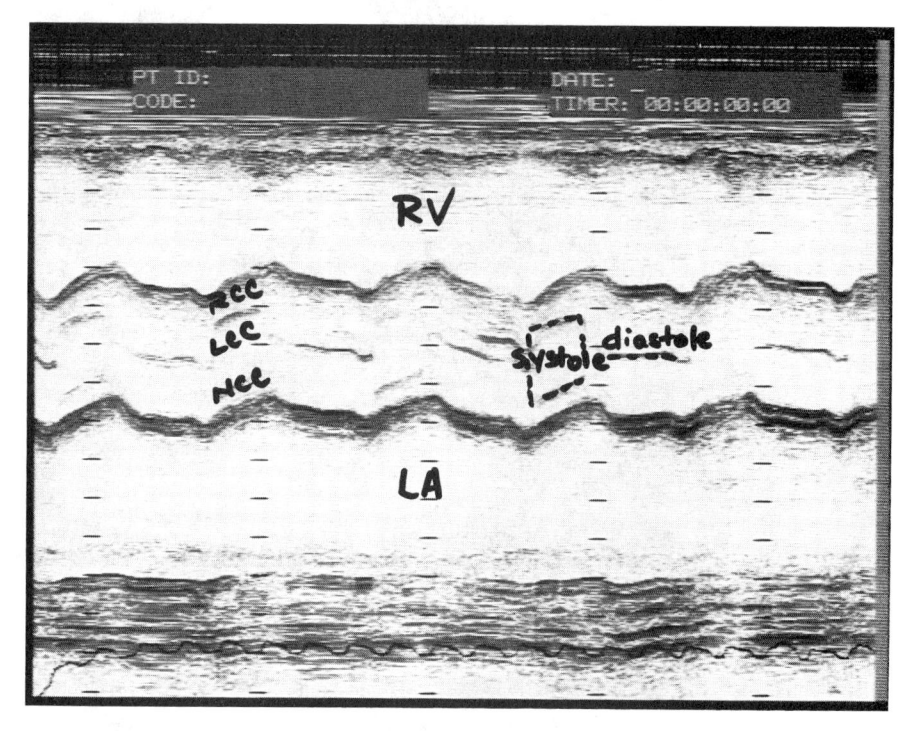

Figure 9-43 Notice that the right and non-coronary cusps are visualized but the left coronary cusp is not.

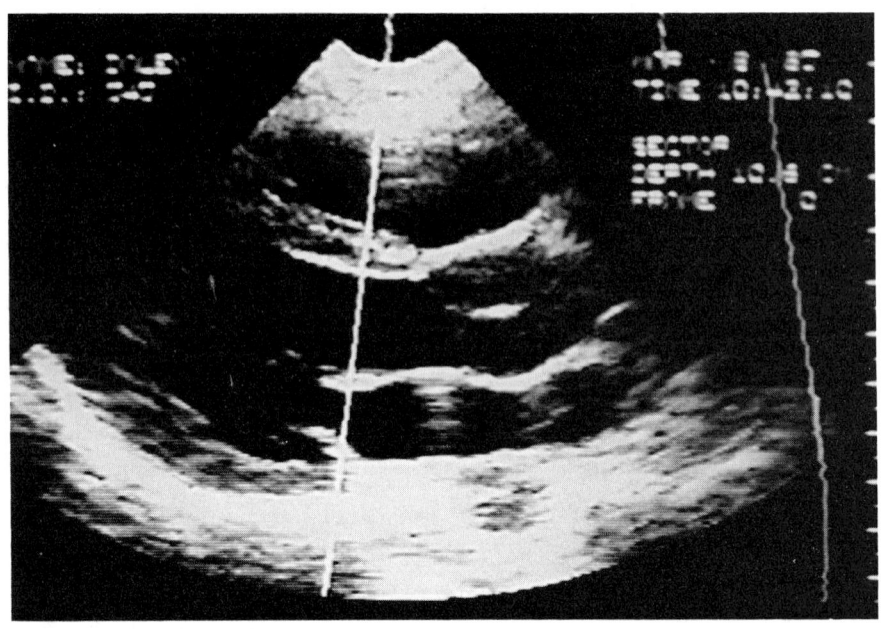

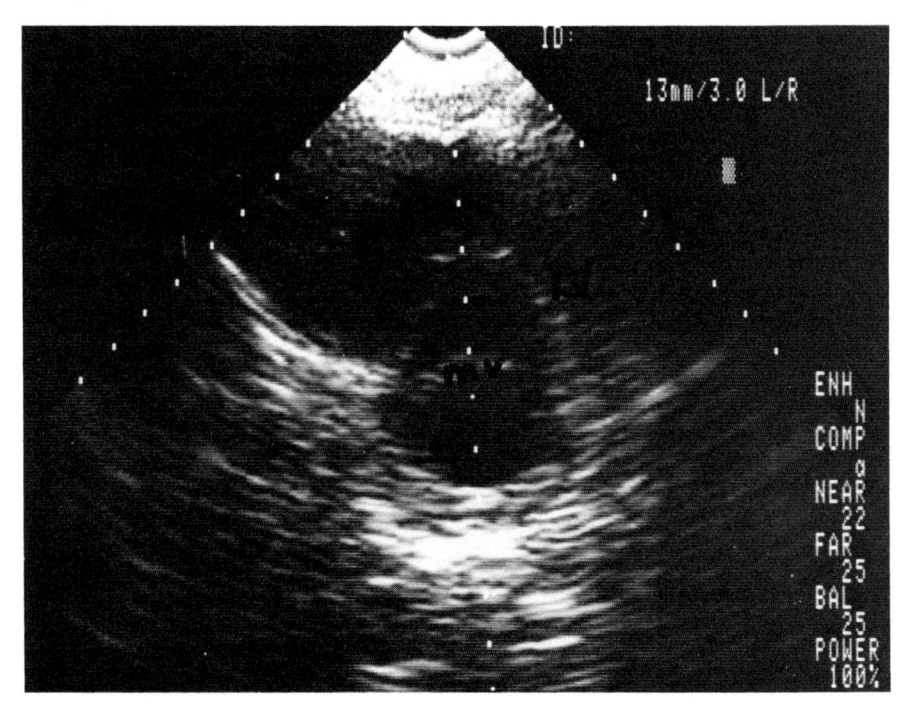

Figure 9-44 *(A)* A mitral valve m-mode can be obtained by directing the cursor through the MV leaflet in a parasternal long-axis view. *(B)* In a parasternal short-axis view at the MV level, a mitral valve m-mode can be obtained.

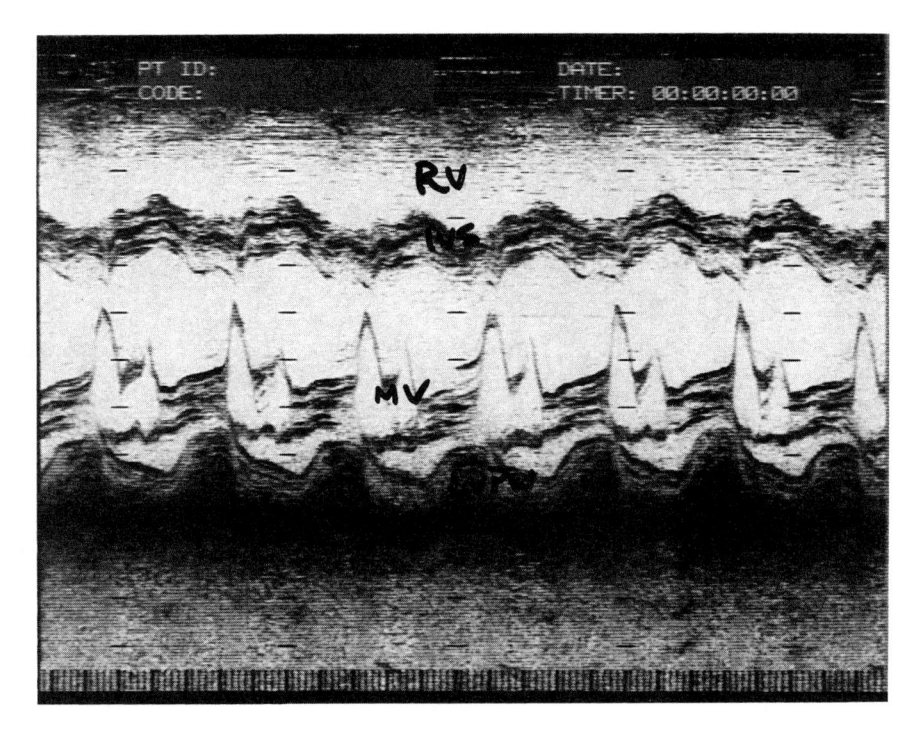

Figure 9-45 The above mitral valve m-mode resembles an "m" in shape, making it easy to recognize.

The left ventricle (LV) m-mode is obtained by moving the cursor to the left ventricle chamber in either the parasternal long-axis view or the parasternal short-axis view at the level of the LV, at the papillary muscle level (Figure 9-46). A left ventricular m-mode is extremely important for measuring left ventricle internal dimensions in both systole and diastole. In this m-mode, the RV, IVS, LV chamber, and LVPW are all visualized (Figure 9-47). Left ventricular functions can be assessed, as can wall thickness, chamber dilatation, left ventricular dysfunction, and many more abnormalities.

Both the tricuspid valves and pulmonic valves can be derived from the parasternal short-axis view at the level of the aortic valve.

An m-mode recording of the tricuspid valve is important if an abnormality is detected by the two-dimensional image. Routinely, this m-mode is not taken because it is often difficult to obtain. Disease states such as tricuspid valve prolapse and tricuspid stenosis can be detected by m-mode.

The pulmonic valve is also difficult to visualize by m-mode and is not routinely recorded. The pulmonic A wave is a key factor when imaging this m-mode. The absence of the A-wave may indicate pulmonary hypertension. On the other hand, an exaggerated A wave may indicate pulmonic stenosis.

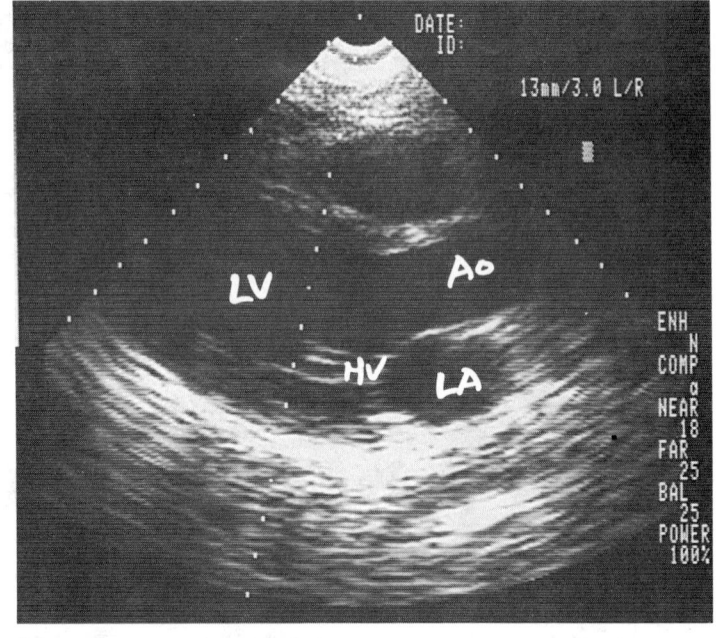

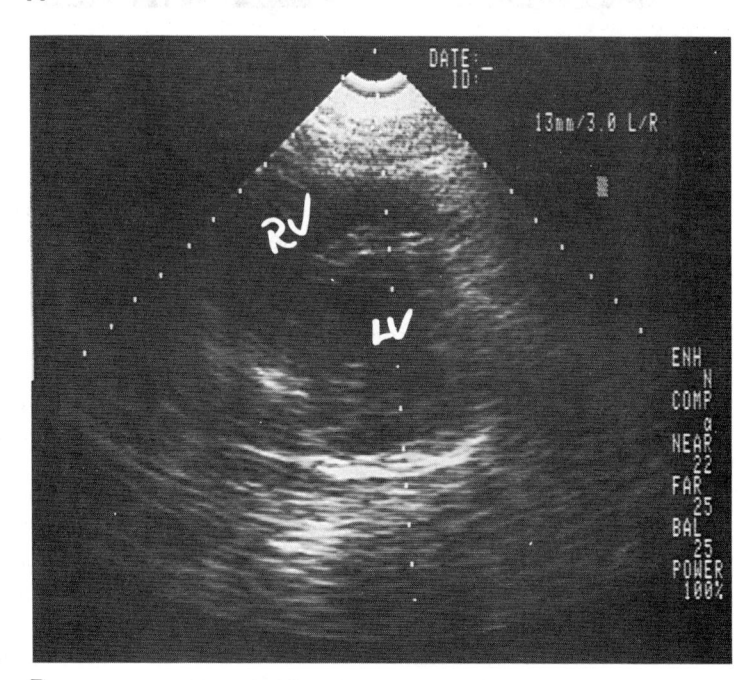

Figure 9-46 (A) An LV m-mode can be obtained in the parasternal long-axis view. (B) A parasternal short-axis view at the LV level can also be used for deriving LV m-modes.

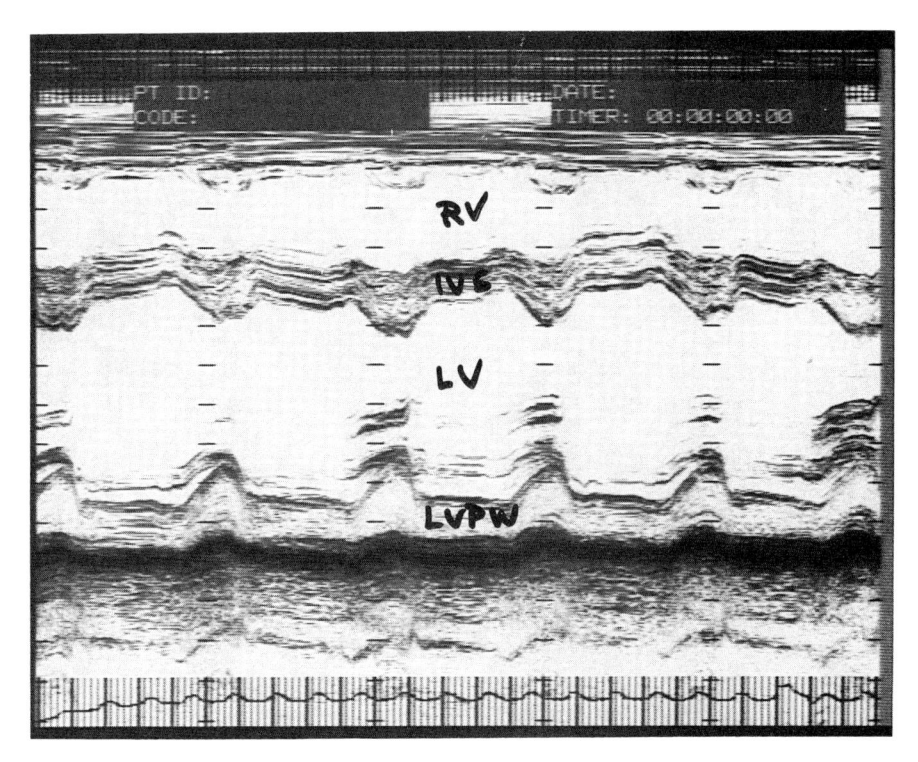

Figure 9-47 The left ventricular m-mode is comprised of the following structures: RV, IVS, LV, and LVPW.

Measuring M-Mode Echocardiograms

Once m-mode echoes have been derived, measurements must be taken to evaluate chamber sizes as well as valvular functions. It is important to obtain legible and accurate m-modes for proper measurements. When examining the aorta/left atrium m-mode, the following measurements are made: the aortic root, aortic valve excursion, and the left atrial size. All of the above components must be seen for an adequate aortic m-mode. The following measurements are obtained in centimeters, by using the centimeter markings on the m-mode.

The aortic root is measured when it is most anterior in systole. Measuring from the top of the anterior aortic root to the top of the posterior aortic root provides an accurate aortic root size. Measuring from bottom to bottom of the root is also adequate. The aortic valve excursion is measured in systole, representing the valve opening at its fullest. Measuring from the right coronary cusp to the noncoronary cusp gives this dimension. Left atrial size can be obtained by measuring in systole from the inner surface of the posterior aortic wall to the innermost portion of the left atrial wall (Figure 9-48).

208 Basic Echocardiography

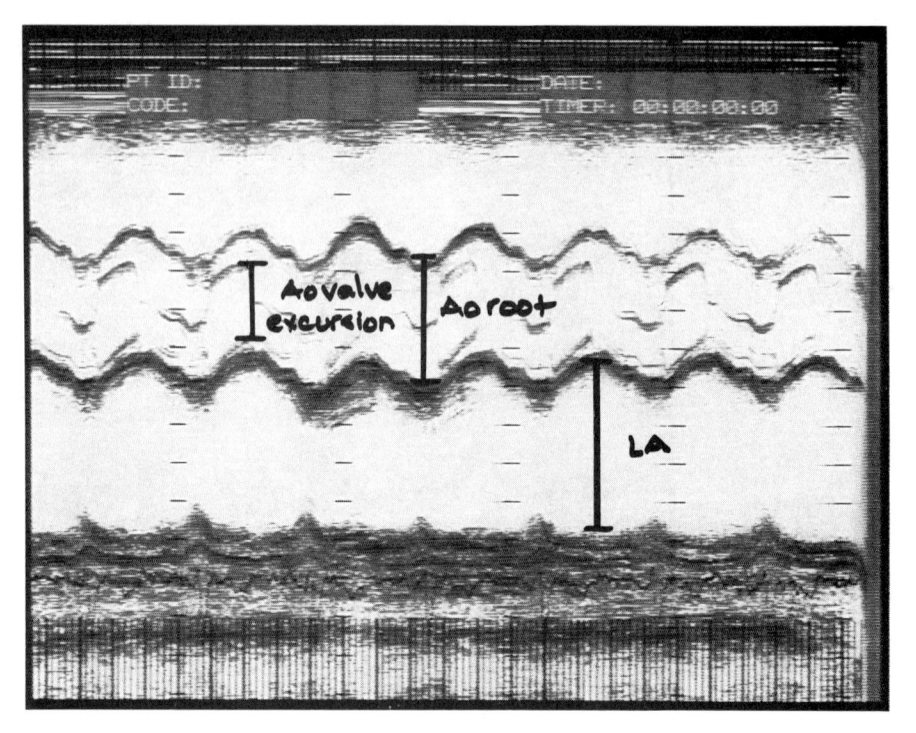

Figure 9-48 From the above AO/LA m-mode, the following measurements can be obtained: LA size = 4.5 cm; aortic root = 3.3 cm, and the aortic valve excursion = 2.0 cm.

The mitral m-mode has two measurements that must be made. One is called the *D-to-E slope*, representing the diastolic descent rate or the rate at which the atrium enters the ventricles. Mitral measurements are measured in millimeters. (Multiply centimeters by 10.) The D-to-E slope is measured at the end of systole or the beginning of diastole and is derived by measuring the D-to-E excursion and multiplying by 10, deriving a number in millimeters. The E-to-F slope is a bit more complicated and the following procedure should be helpful (Figure 9-49).

The LV m-mode has five measurements that are made: LV systole, LV diastole, RV, IVS, and the LVPW thickness. Good clarification of the IVS and the LVPW are essential when measuring this m-mode.

A vertical line is drawn in ventricular diastole. Four out of the five measurements can be obtained from here. RV size is measured from the inner portion of the anterior RV wall to the RV side of the IVS. The IVS is measured from the RV side of the IVS to the left ventricle side of the IVS. The LV diastolic dimension is measured from the LV side of the IVS to the endocardium of the LVPW. The LVPW is measured from the anterior portion of the LVPW to the pericardium. If another vertical line is drawn in

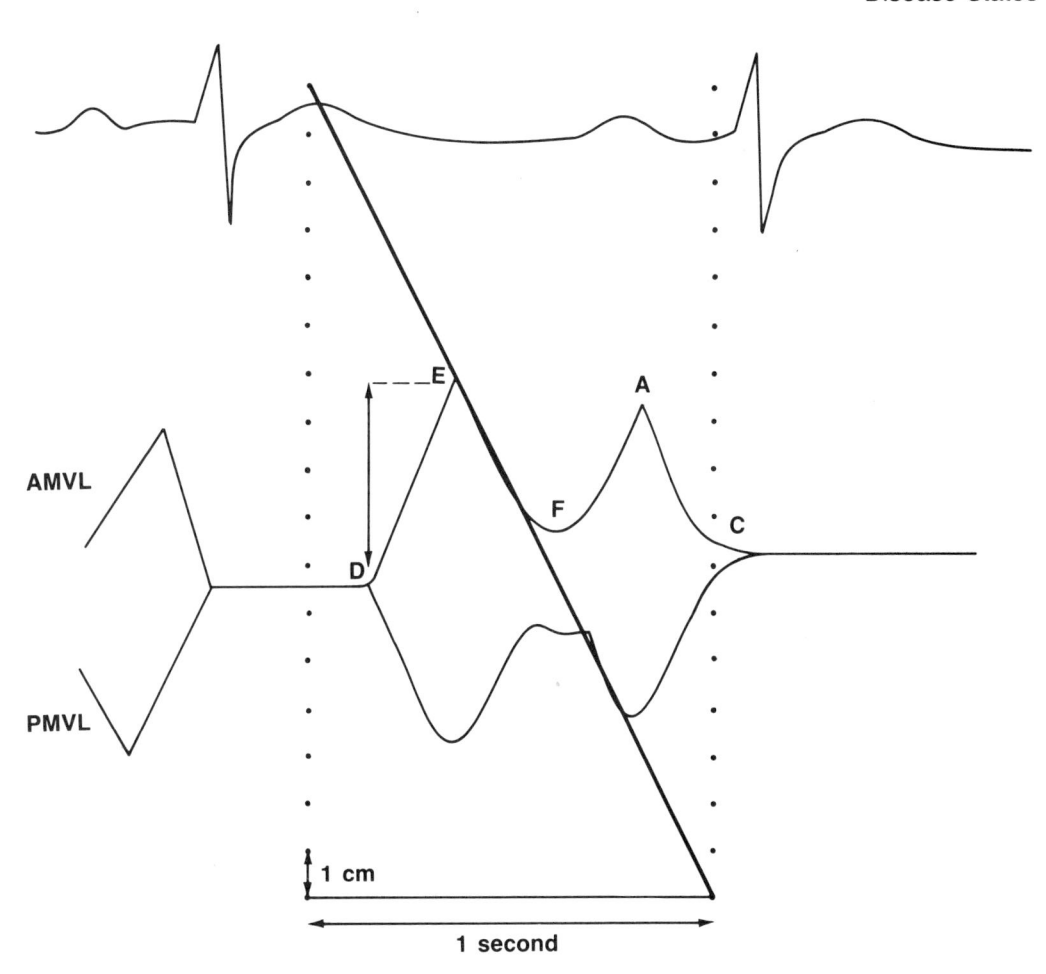

Figure 9-49 DE slope represents the maximum mitral valve leaflet excursion. This is obtained by measuring the D to E distance in mm. The EF slope represents the diastolic descent rate of the MV leaflets. An extended EF slope is drawn. A horizontal line is drawn (representing 1 second) to meet the extended slope. A vertical line is now drawn to meet the initial slope drawn. This measurement is in mm.

ventricular systole, this measurement can be obtained. The LV in systole is measured from the LV side of the IVS to the endocardium in systole in its most anterior position (Figure 9-50).

Disease States

The main purpose of this portion of Chapter 9 is to provide a brief description of the following disease states that actually focus on the m-mode and two-dimensional findings.

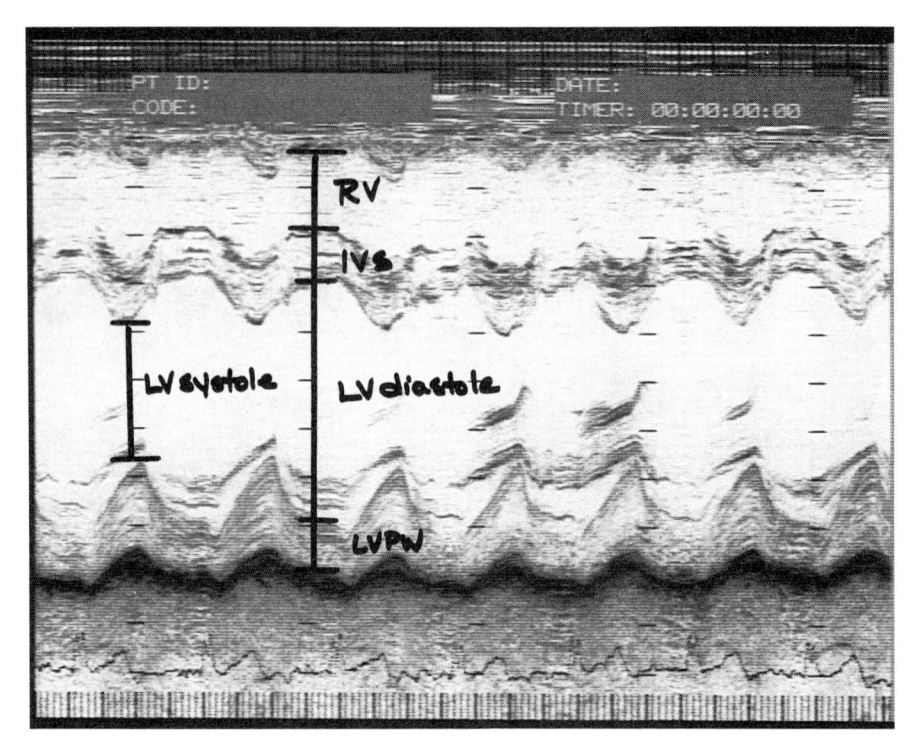

Figure 9-50 From a left ventricular m-mode, the following measurements are made: LV (systole) = 2.8 cm; LV (diastole) = 4.8 cm; RV = 1.6 cm; IVS = 1.0 cm, and the LVPW = 1.0 cm.

Aortic Sclerosis

Aortic sclerosis is a process that produces a buildup of calcium on the valve leaflets. The aortic valve leaflets remain pliable and there is an adequate excursion. Any or all of the leaflets can be affected and this disease state is usually considered a disease of the elderly. Although it is seen with the natural aging process, persons of any age can develop this calcium buildup. On the two-dimensional image, there are bright white spots (representing calcium) that adhere to the leaflets and move with the opening and closing of the valve (Figures 9-51 and 9-52). The m-mode echo shows some extra echoes around the valve excursion or within the aortic root itself. The valve excursion is somewhat reduced, but sufficiently adequate to allow blood flow to move freely through the orifice with no restriction (Figure 9-53).

Mitral Valve Prolapse

Mitral valve prolapse, also termed *Barlow's syndrome*, is a common disorder of the mitral valve. It tends to be more common in females and, in particular, in tall, thin females. It causes a number of symptoms such as chest pains and

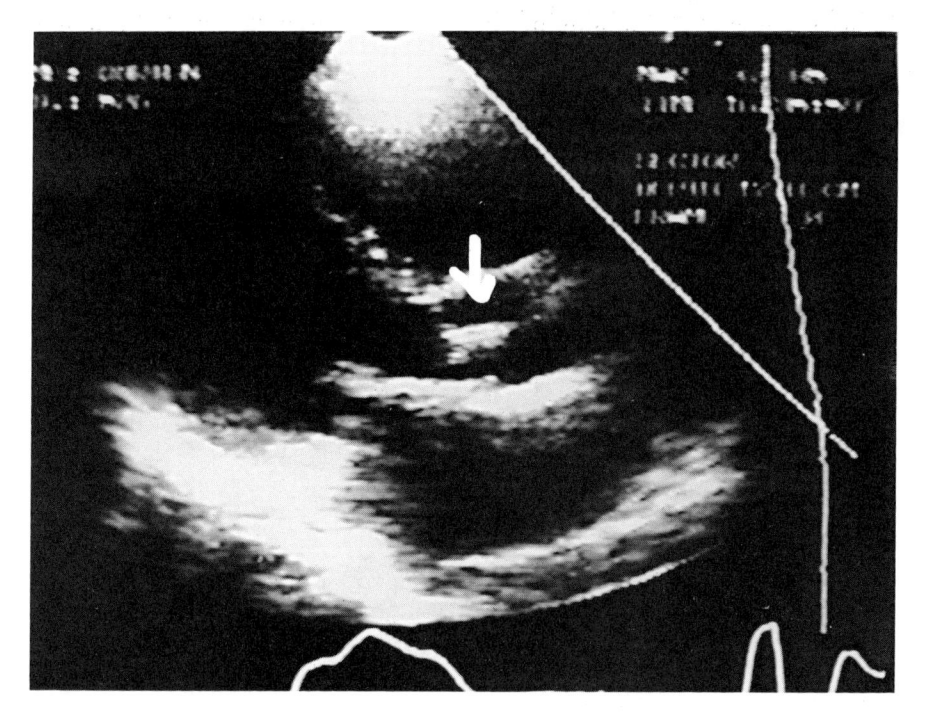

Figure 9-51 Parasternal long-axis view showing the calcium buildup in the aortic valve region. The valve leaflets remain pliable.

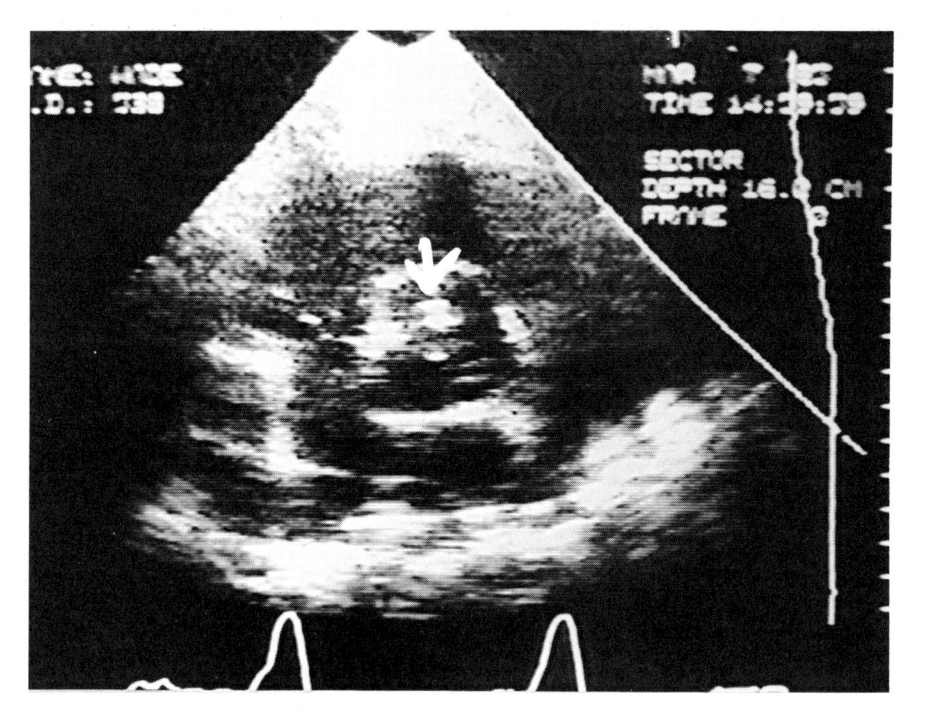

Figure 9-52 Parasternal short-axis view depicting calcium on the valvular regions.

212 Basic Echocardiography

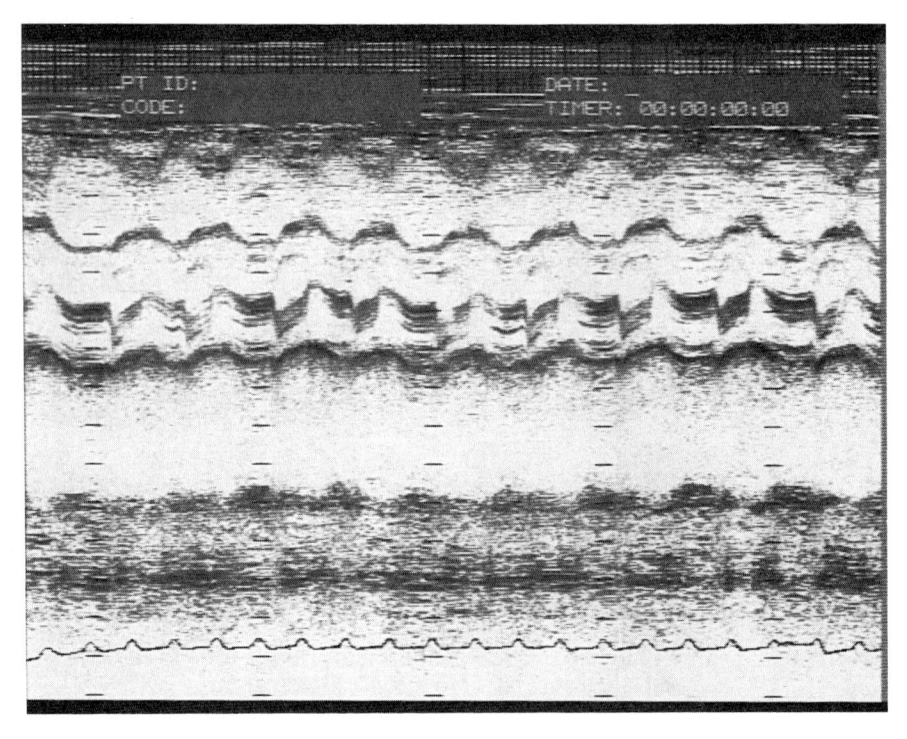

Figure 9-53 The above m-mode displays "extra echoes" within the aortic root and valve, somewhat reducing the valve excursion.

palpitations. Mitral valve prolapse occurs when the valve does not close properly, causing a "bowing back" of the mitral valve in systole into the left atrium. There are different degrees of mitral valve prolapse, from mild to moderate to severe, depending on how displaced the leaflets are from the coapt point into the left atrium. Mitral valve prolapse can affect the anterior leaflet only, the posterior mitral valve leaflet only, or both mitral valve leaflets.

On two-dimensional echo, mitral valve prolapse can be detected in all views. The parasternal short-axis view at the level of the mitral valve is not an accurate means of evaluating mitral valve prolapse. In this view, the ultrasound beam is parallel with the valve, making it difficult to detect. In all other views, mitral valve prolapse is noted when the mitral valve leaflets prolapse into the atrium beyond the natural coapt point (Figures 9-54 and 9-55).

The m-mode would demonstrate a sagging or posterior displacement of the mitral valve in systole. Angulation can produce mitral valve prolapse on m-mode echo. The valve must be scanned carefully; this sagging should be seen on the majority of the beats (Figure 9-56).

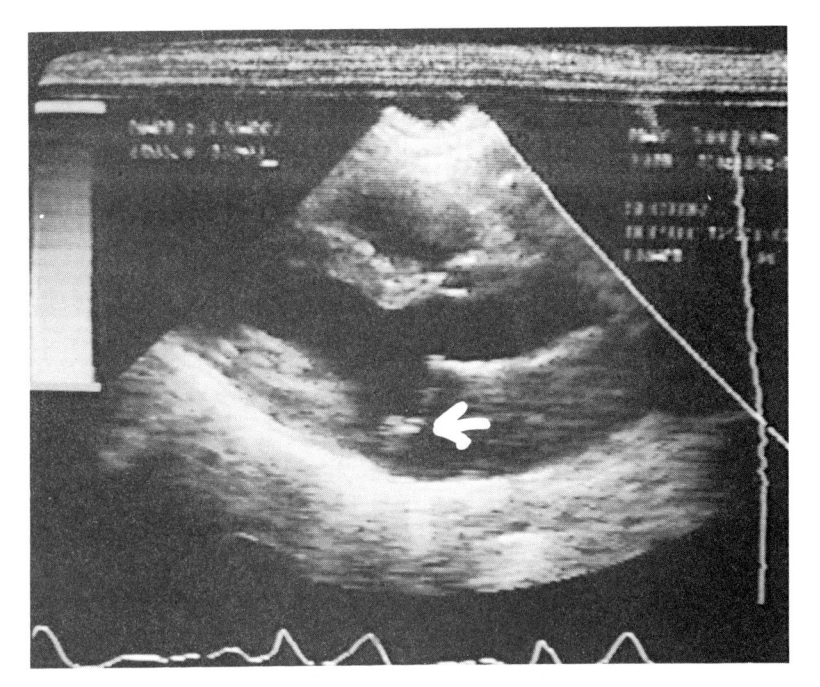

Figure 9-54 The posterior displacement of the MV leaflet (anterior, posterior, or both) into the left atrium is consistent with MVP in this parasternal long-axis view (PLAV).

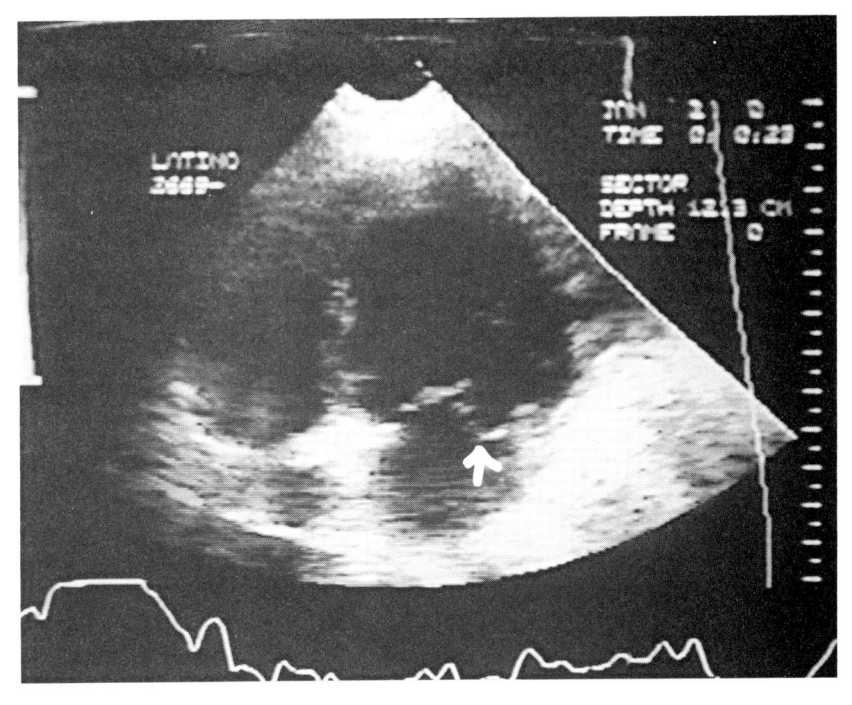

Figure 9-55 The apical four-chamber view is useful when evaluating MVP; notice the posterior MV leaflet "bowing" into the left atrium.

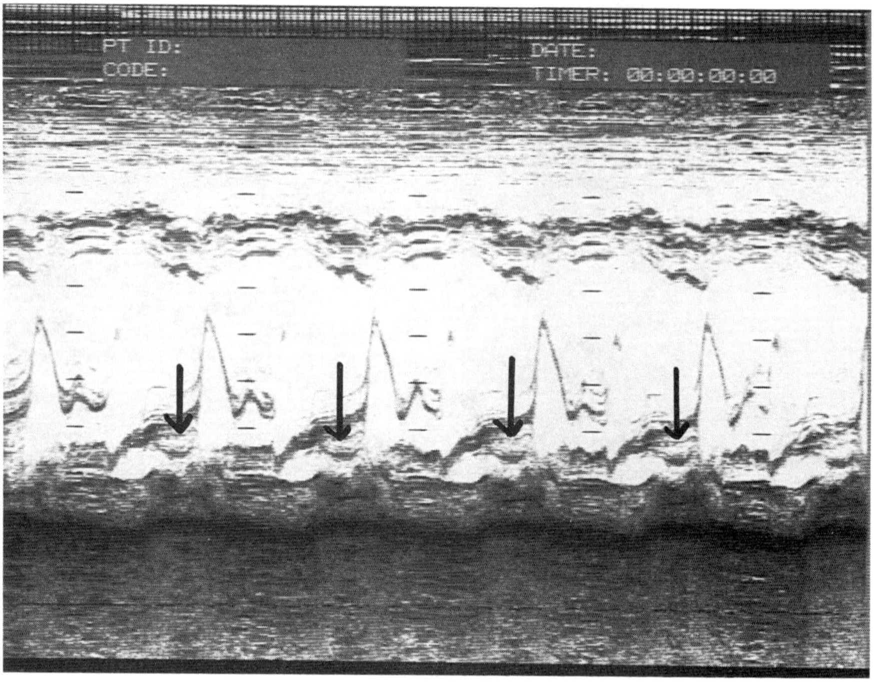

Figure 9-56 The arrows point to the posterior sagging of the MV leaflets in ventricular systole.

Mitral valve prolapse is considered an innocent finding; however, in some cases, it may cause mitral regurgitation, a flail mitral valve leaflet from ruptured chordae tendineae or, in rare instances, sudden death.

In many cardiac laboratories, amyl nitrate may be used to detect MVP or simply to exaggerate the findings. Amyl nitrate is a drug that is inhaled by the patient, causing a rapid increase in the heart rate and thus allowing this abnormality to be detected.

Bicuspid Aortic Valve

A bicuspid aortic valve is probably the most common congenital anomaly. As the term indicates a valve has only two leaflets, rather than the normal three. This may be seen on the two-dimensional echo with an echogenic patient in the parasternal short-axis view, at the level of the aortic valve (Figure 9-57). On m-mode, the eccentric closure of the aortic valve in diastole may be seen. Eccentric closure occurs when the diastolic closure line within the aortic root is displaced, either too high or too low. Normally, the diastolic closure line cuts the root into equal sizes. Eccentric closure causes a dis-

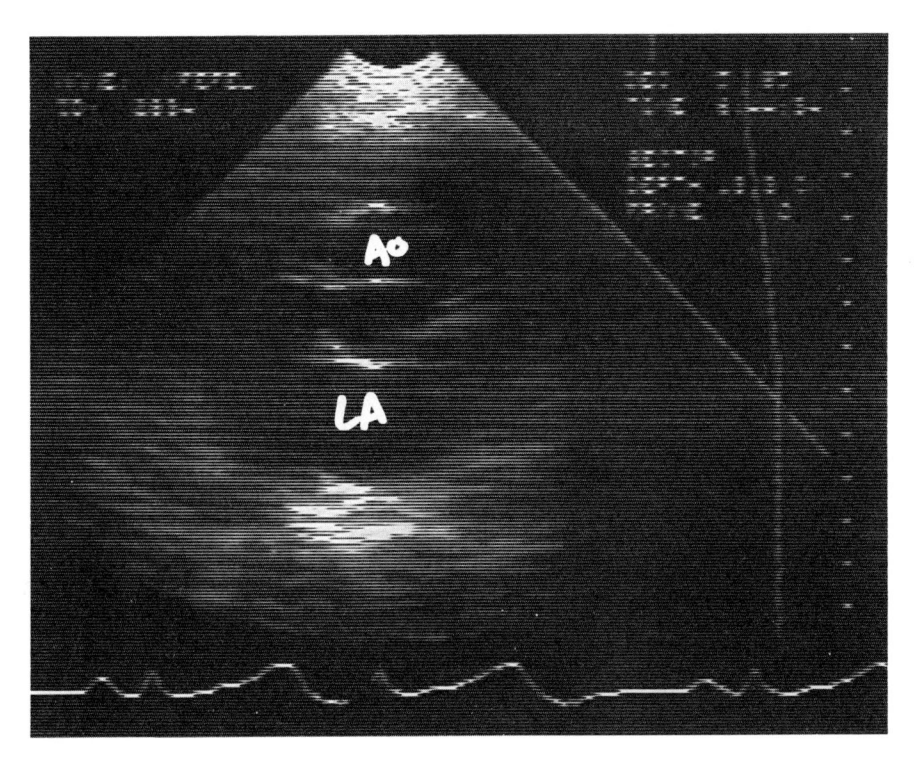

Figure 9-57 In the parasternal short-axis view notice only two aortic valve leaflets cutting the root in half, instead of three equal sections.

proportionate ratio between both sides (Figure 9-58). A bicuspid aortic valve should not be diagnosed by this criteria alone; there tends to be a high incidence of false positives. Because of angulation, this eccentricity can be created. As a patient ages, calcium, may build up on the bicuspid valve more readily than on a normal valve. The valve may also become incompetent, resulting in aortic insufficiency. On the other hand, the valve function may be normal and never acquire these secondary problems.

Calcified Mitral Valve Annulus

Calcified mitral valve annulus is usually a finding in older patients and is considered a disease of the elderly, as is aortic sclerosis. The annulus supporting the mitral valve calcifies with age, particularly near the posterior mitral valve leaflet. Depending on the severity of the calcium buildup, mitral regurgitation may develop and actual restriction of the valve excursion may result.

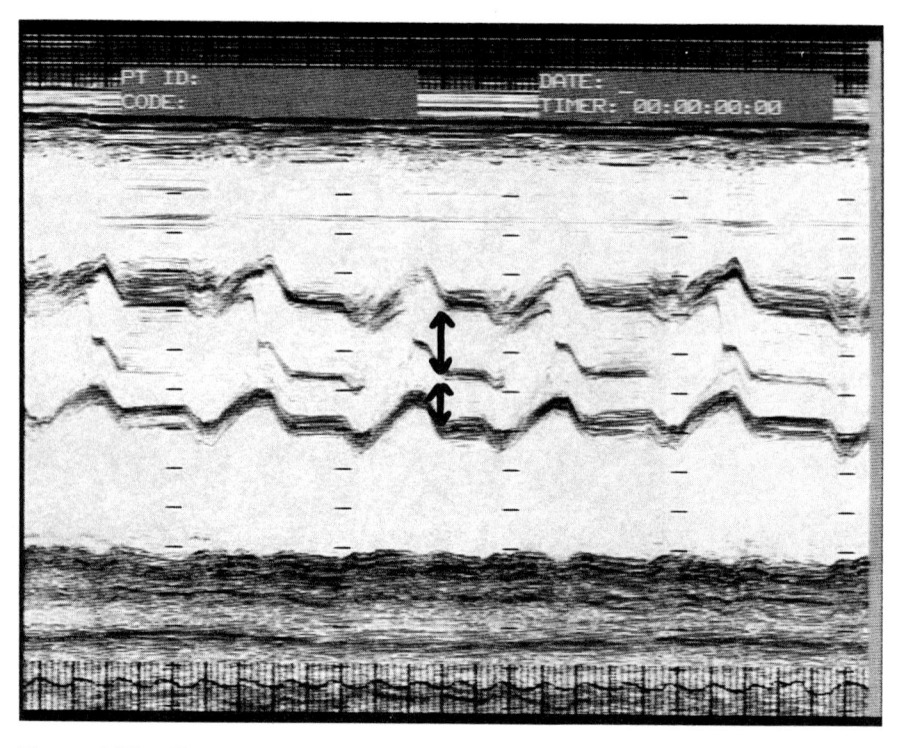

Figure 9-58 Eccentric closure of the aortic valve could indicate a bicuspid aortic valve. Notice the unequal diastolic closure line.

On two-dimensional echo, a bright area of calcium would be noted near the posterior mitral valve leaflet at the annular region (Figures 9-59 and 9-60).

On m-mode echo, a dark, rigid band of echoes would run parallel with the posterior left ventricle wall. The annular band located directly under the mitral valve is separated from the left ventricular wall (Figure 9-61).

Aortic Stenosis

Aortic stenosis can be a congenital defect or it can be acquired. Aortic stenosis can also result from rheumatic fever. (Rheumatic fever may lead to a scarring of the heart valves, causing actual restriction in the pliability of the valve.) With congenital aortic stenosis (meaning that an individual is born with the defect), the aortic valve excursion may be reduced. The valve leaflets may be thickened or they may be fused, enabling the valve to open fully. A distinct doming of the aortic valve in the parasternal long-axis can be noticed. An m-mode echo may reveal a relatively normal-looking aortic valve.

Acquired aortic stenosis occurs when there is a gradual accumulation

Disease States 217

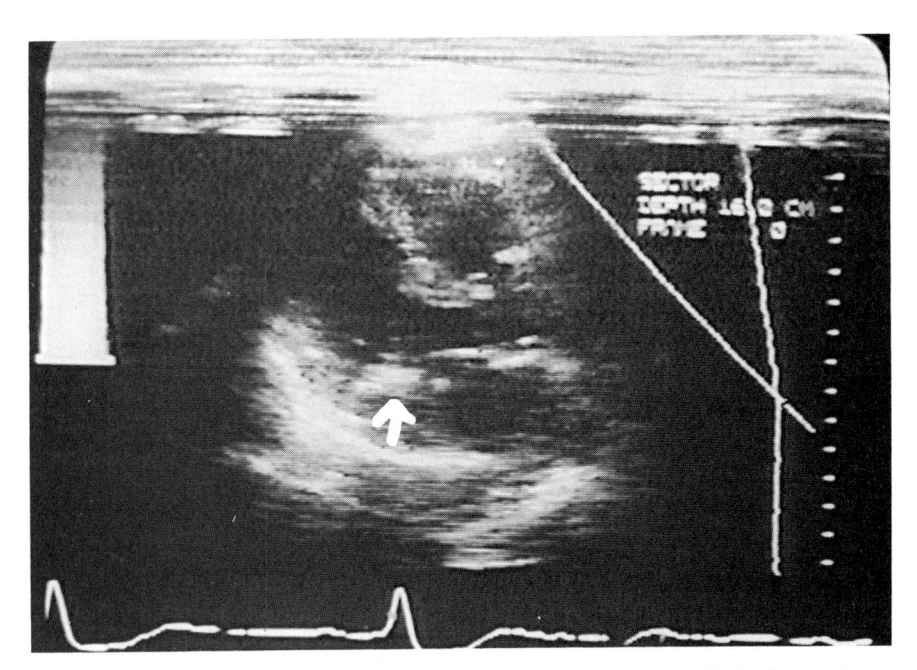

Figure 9-59 A parasternal long-axis view demonstrating a calcified mitral valve annulus (arrow).

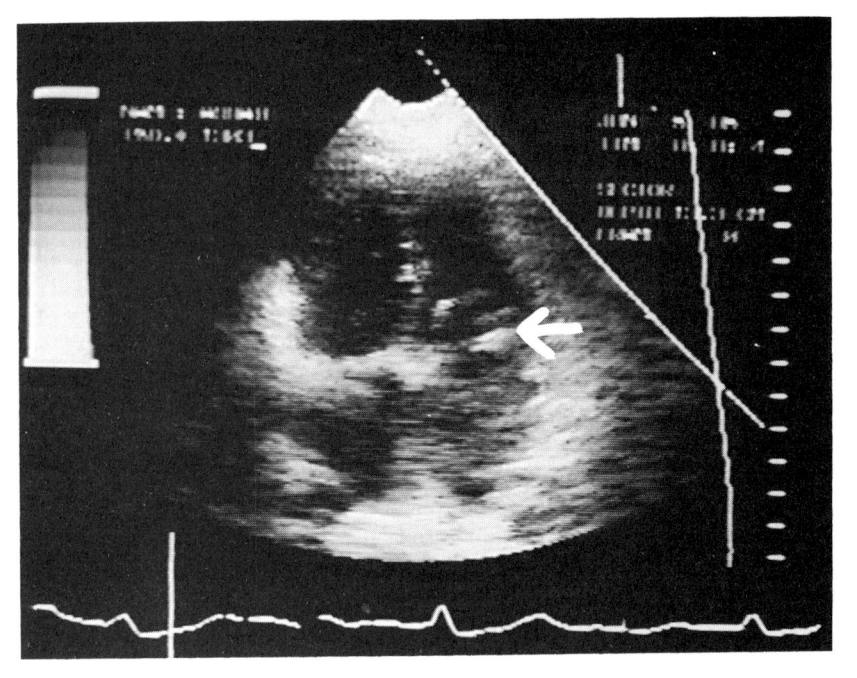

Figure 9-60 An apical four-chamber view exhibiting annular calcification (arrow).

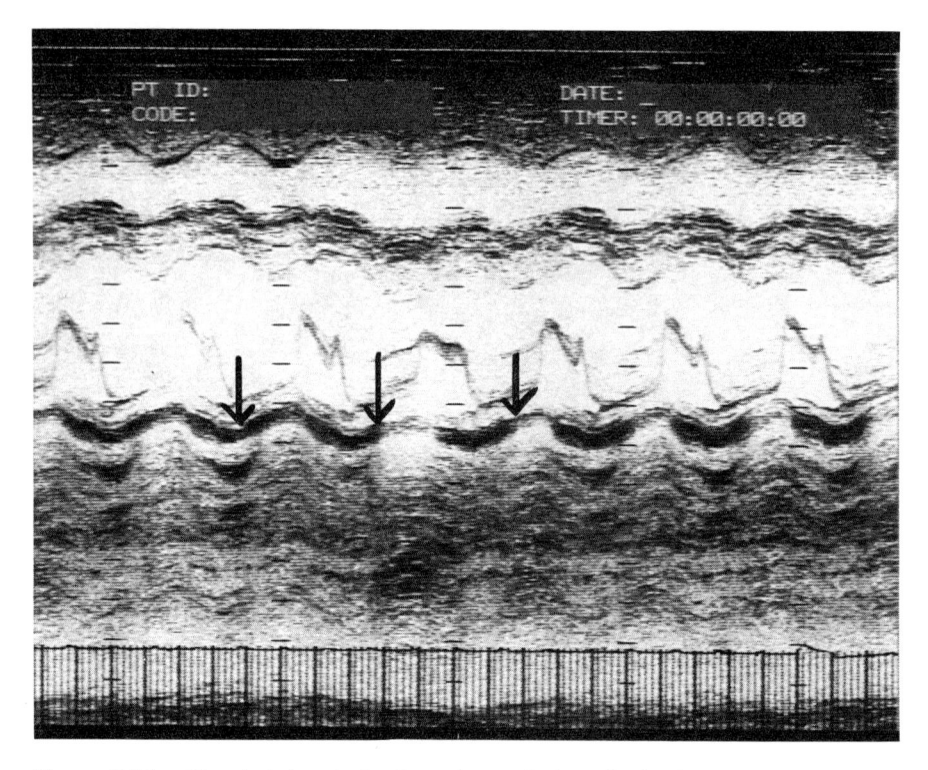

Figure 9-61 The dark band of echoes beneath the mitral valve coincides with a calcified mitral valve annulus.

of calcium on the valve leaflets, as well as on the aortic root. The valve pliability is reduced and becomes very rigid, giving a "rocklike" appearance on two-dimensional echo. Echocardiography is not an accurate means of diagnosing aortic stenosis. There are usually degrees of severity: mild, moderate, and severe, depending on the valvular excursion. The ultrasound beam can exaggerate or underestimate the severity of aortic stenosis. The cardiac Doppler, and in particular, continuous wave Doppler, has been more accurate in quantitating the gradient across the valvular lesion. As mentioned previously, on two-dimensional echo, there will be white clumps of calcium on the aortic valve leaflets and within the root, giving it a rocklike appearance (Figures 9-62 and 9-63). In severe aortic stenosis, the left ventricle may become concentrically hypertrophied, due to the excess force that must be maintained to try and empty the left ventricle through this stenotic lesion. The aortic m-mode appearance would show a heavily calcified valve with a reduced excursion (if one can even be seen), as well as heavy bands of echoes within the aortic root (Figure 9-64). The LV m-mode may show concentric left ventricular hypertrophy (LVH) in moderate to severe cases of aortic stenosis.

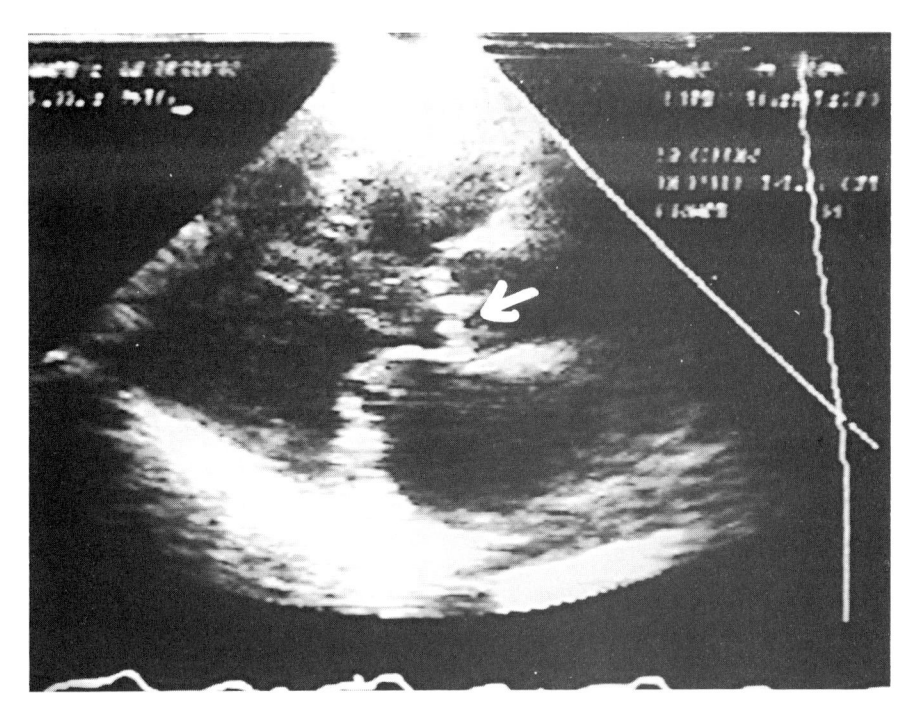

Figure 9-62 A heavily calcified aortic valve in the above parasternal long-axis view is consistent with aortic stenosis.

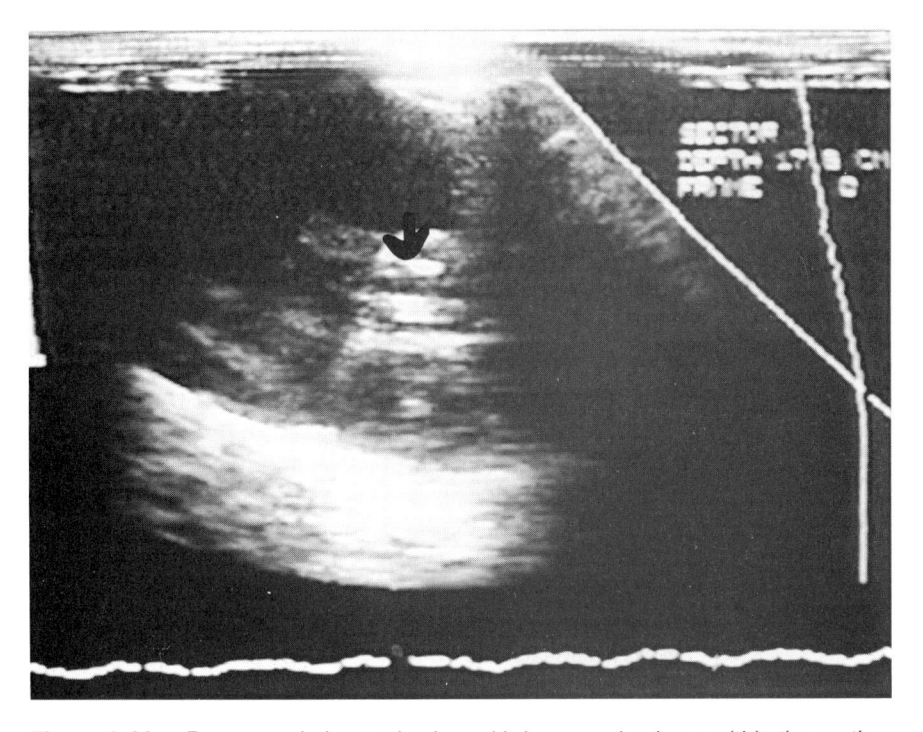

Figure 9-63 Parasternal short-axis view with increased echoes within the aortic valve region, which actually restricts valvular mobility.

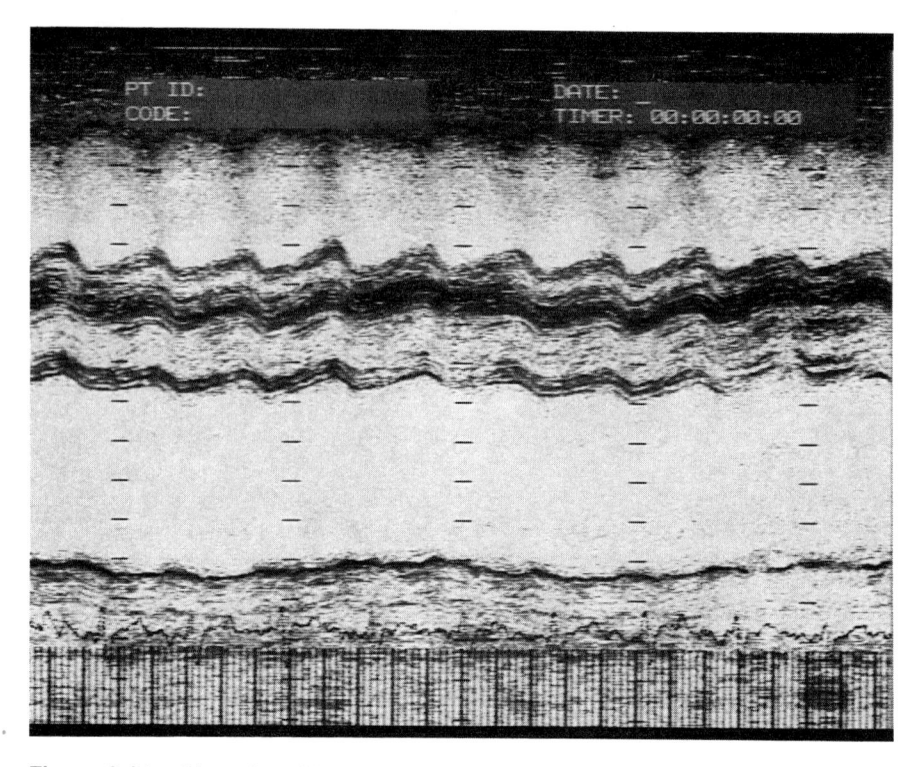

Figure 9-64 M-mode exhibiting a heavily calcified aortic root and valve, where the valvular excursion is barely visible.

Aortic Insufficiency

Aortic insufficiency (AI) occurs when the aortic valve does not close properly and allows blood to flow back into the left ventricle in diastole. (Note that the aortic valve may appear normal, even in the presence of aortic insufficiency). The main way in which to diagnose aortic insufficiency is by m-mode echo. Fine fluttering of the anterior mitral valve leaflet can be seen. This fluttering may also occur on the intraventricular septum on the left ventricular side. The fluttering occurs because a surge of blood returns to the left ventricle during diastole; incidentally, the left atrium empties into the left ventricle in the normal cardiac cycle. The mitral valve opens in diastole and is affected by the regurgitation flow (Figure 9-65).

In addition to the mitral valve fluttering that can be seen on the m-mode, a dilated, hypercontractile left ventricle can be noticed. The mor severe the aortic insufficiency, the more dilated and the more hypercontractile the left ventricle becomes. This occurs because of the excessive back flow of blood and because of the force needed to eject the extra blood volume out of the left ventricle.

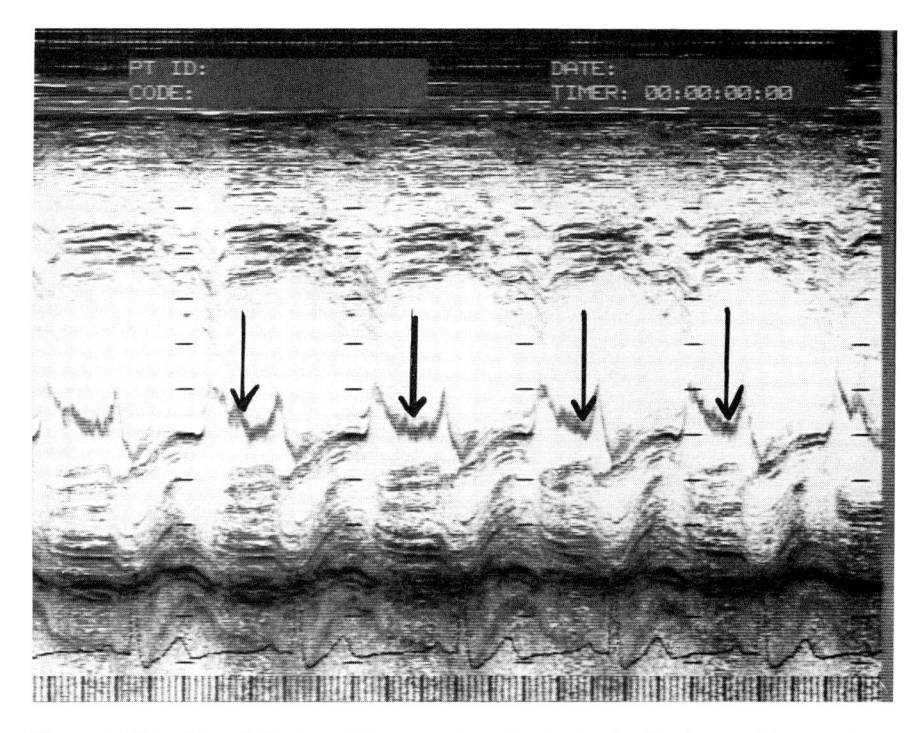

Figure 9-65 Fine fluttering of the anterior mitral valve leaflet (arrows) is consistent with aortic insufficiency.

Diagnosing aortic insuffiency by two-dimensional echo is extremely difficult. With a trained eye, one may see the fine fluttering of the anterior mitral valve leaflet, or notice a dilated left ventricle. The most accurate technique that can be used to confirm the diagnosis of aortic insufficiency is the cardiac Doppler.

Idiopathic Hypertrophic Subaortic Stenosis—IHSS

This disease state can be inherited, and children may want to be studied to rule out any abnormalities associated with this disease. Once the left ventricular outflow tract becomes obstructed, the term *hypertrophic obstructive cardiomyopathy*, or *IHSS*, can be used. Nonobstructive cardiomyopathy occurs when the left ventricular outflow tract is not interrupted. Echocardiography is quite sensitive in confirming the diagnosis of this disease and, in particular, m-mode echocardiography is effective. In order that this diagnosis may be made by echo, all of the following criteria should be present:

222 Basic Echocardiography

1. Systolic Anterior Motion—SAM—of the mitral valve (Figure 9-66)
2. Asymmetric Septal Hypertrophy—ASH—, in which the IVS/LVPW ratio is in excess of at least 1.3 : 1 (Figure 9-67)
3. Preclosure of the aortic valve (Figure 9-68)
4. Normal left ventricular contraction
5. A narrowed or obliterated left ventricular cavity

The only criterion that may not be seen is the preclosure of the aortic valve, which at times is hard to visualize. A patient having IHHS is often not echogenic, which makes the diagnosis even harder. Clear and measurable m-modes are essential.

SAM motion occurs when the mitral valve leaflets in ventricular systole move toward the IVS causing an obstruction in the left ventricular outflow tract. SAM motion can be seen more prominently on the m-mode echo than on the two-dimensional echo.

Two-dimensional echocardiography is not as accurate in finding the abnormalities associated with IHSS. One may notice ASH simply by viewing the IVS and the LVPW (Figure 9-69). As mentioned earlier, SAM is harder to detect by two-dimensional echo but, at times, it may be seen in the apical four-chamber view.

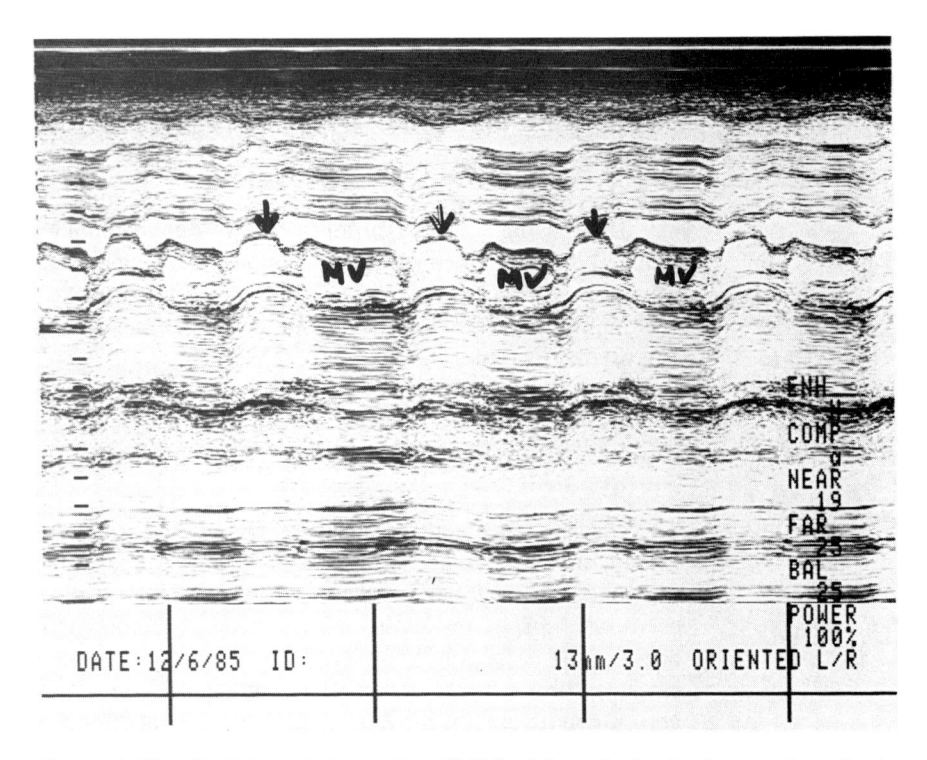

Figure 9-66 Systolic anterior motion (SAM) of the mitral valve is seen in patients with IHSS. Note the anterior movement towards the IVS (arrows) in systole.

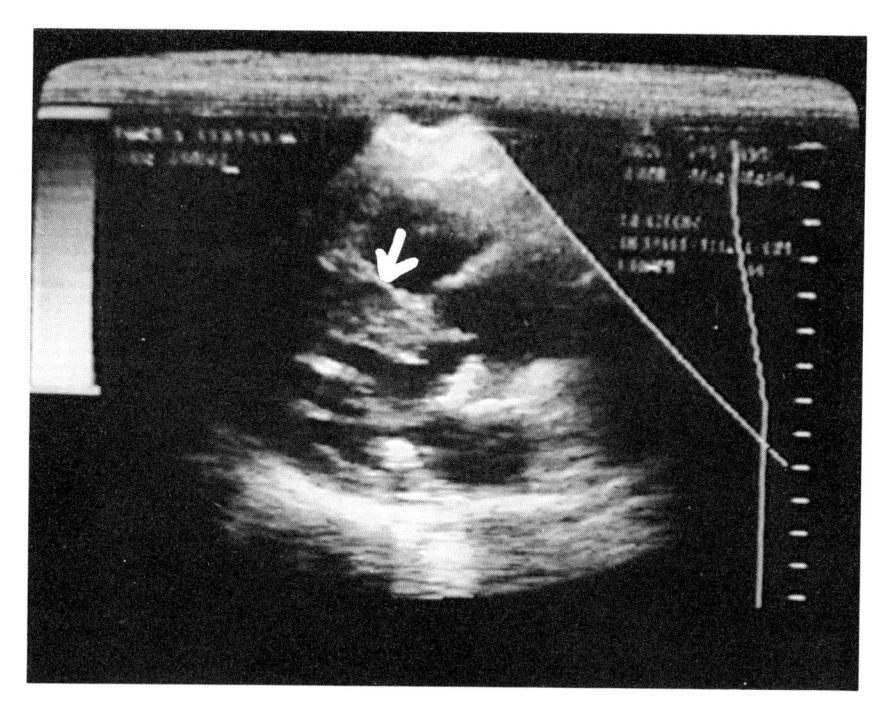

Figure 9-67 Asymmetric septal hypertrophy (ASH) occurs when the IVS is hypertrophied disproportionately compared to the LVPW.

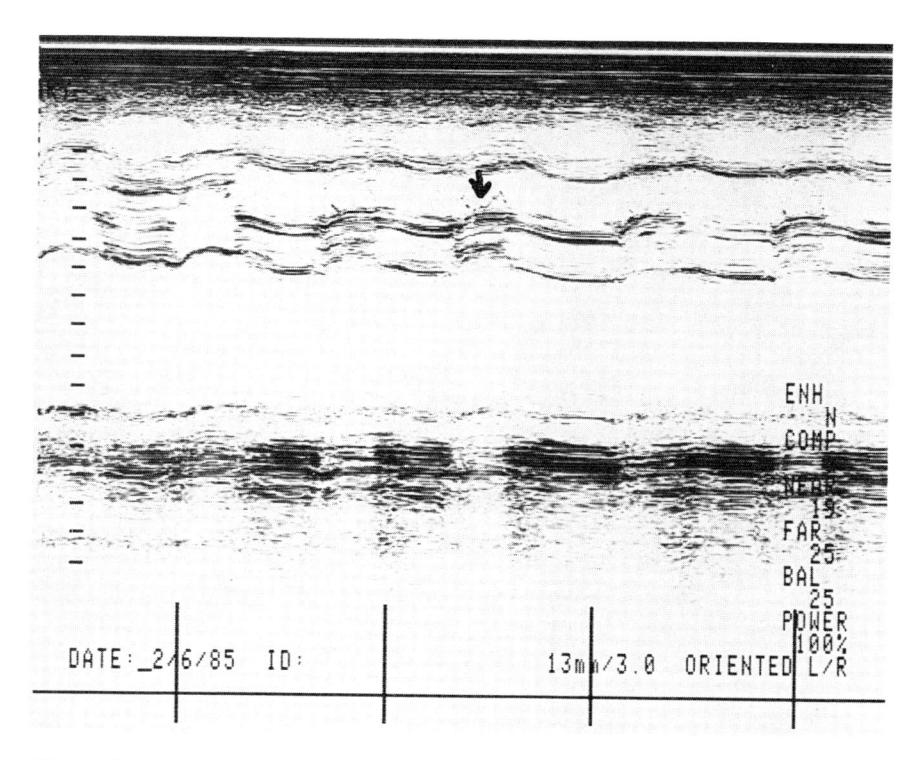

Figure 9-68 Preclosure of the aortic valve is sometimes seen in patients with IHSS (arrow).

223

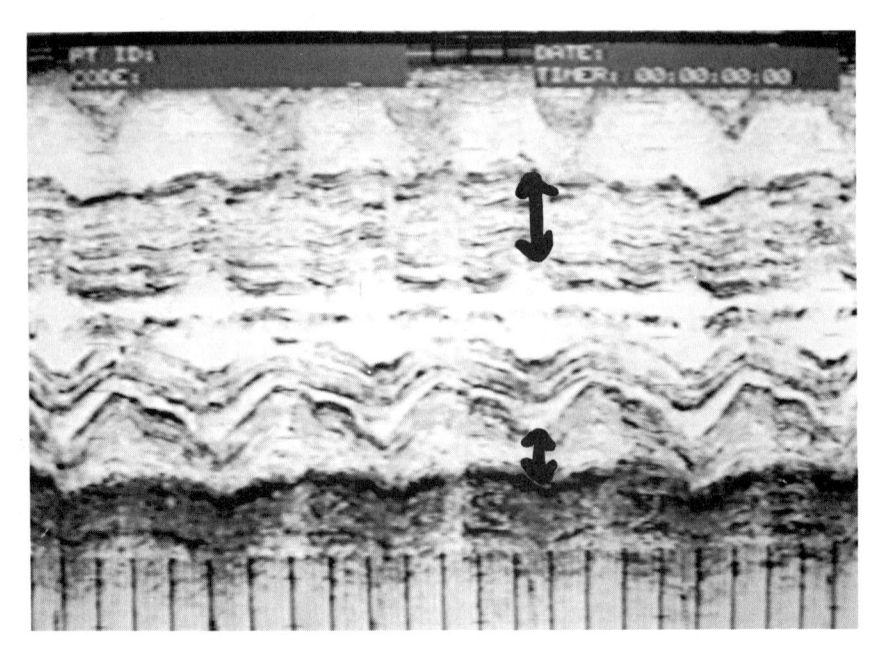

Figure 9-69 A parasternal long-axis view demonstrating ASH (arrow).

Amyl nitrate may be used to enhance SAM motion, as the heart rate increases.

M-mode echocardiography is more sensitive in diagnosing this disease. SAM motion should be seen clearly on m-mode echo, as should ASH. Preclosure of the aortic valve can also be seen on m-mode echo. Once all of these factors have been confirmed, the diagnosis of IHSS or obstructive hypertrophic cardiomyopathy may be made.

Bacterial Endocarditis (BE)

An infection in the body that may affect the heart is known as *bacterial endocarditis*, *infective endocarditis*, or *bacterial vegetations*. This disease may be acquired innocently or IV drug users may be suseptible. Ultrasound does not pick up vegetations until they reach a size of at least 2 to 3 millimeters. If a diagnosis of BE has been proven by blood cultures and possible vegetations have been noted by echo, the course of the valvular vegetations can be followed for further changes. A diagnosis should never be made by echo alone. Vegetations can imitate calcific or fibrotic lesions, which may make accurate diagnosis impossible. Evaluating for BE on prosthetic valves, once again, is not a sensitive method, because of excessive echoes within the prosthetic structure.

On two dimensional echo, vegetations would appear as dense "clumplike" growths on the valve itself, or on the valvular apparatus surrounding the valve. The vegetations move with the heart valve (not like a stenotic valve, which is rigid). Caution must be taken when making the diagnosis of BE by two-dimensional echo.

M-mode echocardiography is even less sensitive when evaluating BE. One may observe "shaggy," "thickened" valves. Remember: valvular mobility will remain pliable, in most cases, unlike that of a stenotic valve. The downfall in using this criteria is that BE can mimic many other abnormalties, such as left atrial myxoma, mitral stenosis, a left atrial clot, and many others.

Left Ventricular Dysfunction

Echocardiography, especially two-dimensional echo, is an excellent means of detecting left ventricular wall abnormalities. The exact area of the infarct and the actual amount of damage can be seen. However, if an infarct is small and not much damage has occurred, the echo may appear normal. Like brain cells, once the heart muscle has been damaged, it rarely repairs itself. Therefore, old myocardial infarctions as well as new ones can be detected. All two-dimensional views are used when evaluating left ventricular functions. This is generally done by comparing opposite walls for motion. (Example: If, in the parasternal short-axis view the lateral wall is thickening nicely in systole but the septal area does not thicken, the wall motion abnormality would be in the septal region.) Remember, all views should be used when evaluating left ventricular function.

There are several terms used to describe left ventricular function.

1. Dyskinetic: This term describes an area that moves in a direction that is opposite from normal. Instead of the normal thickening in systole, the area moves outward.
2. Akinetic: An akinetic area describes a wall motion abnormality that does not move at all.
3. Hypokinetic: A term describing an area that does not move as well as other walls. The area usually has little motion left as a result of a myocardial infarction or a muscle damaged area.
4. Hyperkinetic: A wall that is extra vigorous, usually compensating for a wall that is not moving as it should.

The m-mode is not as accurate for left ventricular function. Due to the "ice-pick" effect, the ultrasound beam has to be in the exact spot of the damaged area in order to be seen. (For instance, a patient may have a septal infarct involving the distal septum, but the m-mode may be taken higher up from the infarcted area, resulting in a normal left ventricular m-mode). The m-mode does not image all areas of the LV, such as the inferior wall, the lateral wall, and the apex. If a septal or posterior infarct is detected on m-mode, one would notice an area would be noticed that does not move when compared to the opposite wall (Figures 9-70 and 9-71).

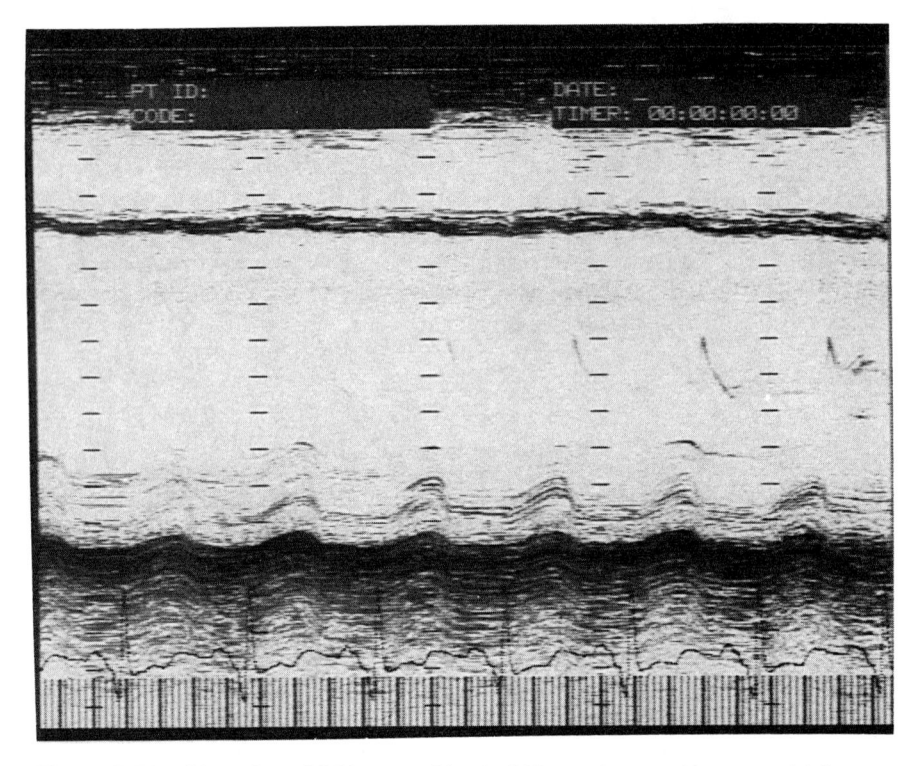

Figure 9-70 M-mode exhibiting an akinetic IVS consistent with a septal infarct.

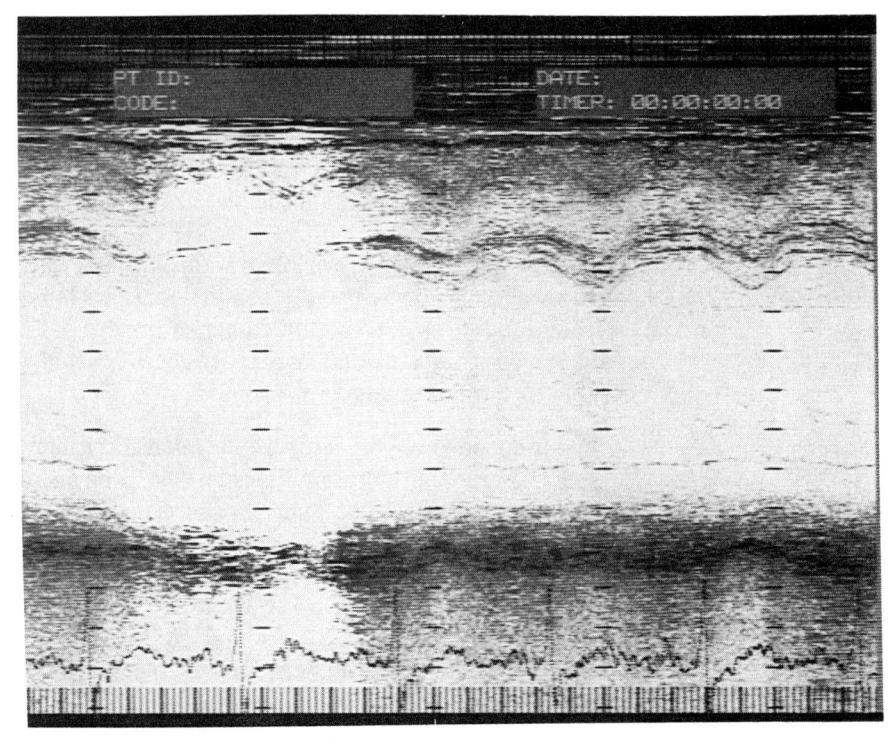

Figure 9-71 This left ventricular m-mode depicts an akinetic LVPW representing a true posterior infarct.

Pericardial Effusions

Echocardiography is one of the best methods of diagnosing pericardial effusions. A pericardial effusion is an excessive accumulation of fluid around the sac of the heart. This accumulation of fluid can occur because of pericarditis, trauma, injury to the heart, a tumor, renal disorders, or a number of other reasons. An echo-free space is seen between the pericardium and the posterior left ventricular wall when viewing either an m-mode or two-dimensional echo (Figures 9-72 through 9-75). Both methods are accurate in detecting this abnormality. The sizes of the pericardial effusions are judged simply by classifications: trivial, small, moderate, and large. Effusions can occur either anteriorly or posteriorly. An anterior effusion is an effusion that borders the right ventricle and chest wall. Usually an anterior effusion is seen only in the presence of a posterior effusion (which exists behind the left ventricle). An echo interpreter must be careful when noting an isolated anterior clear space. This may not be an anterior pericardial effusion but a pericardial fat pad.

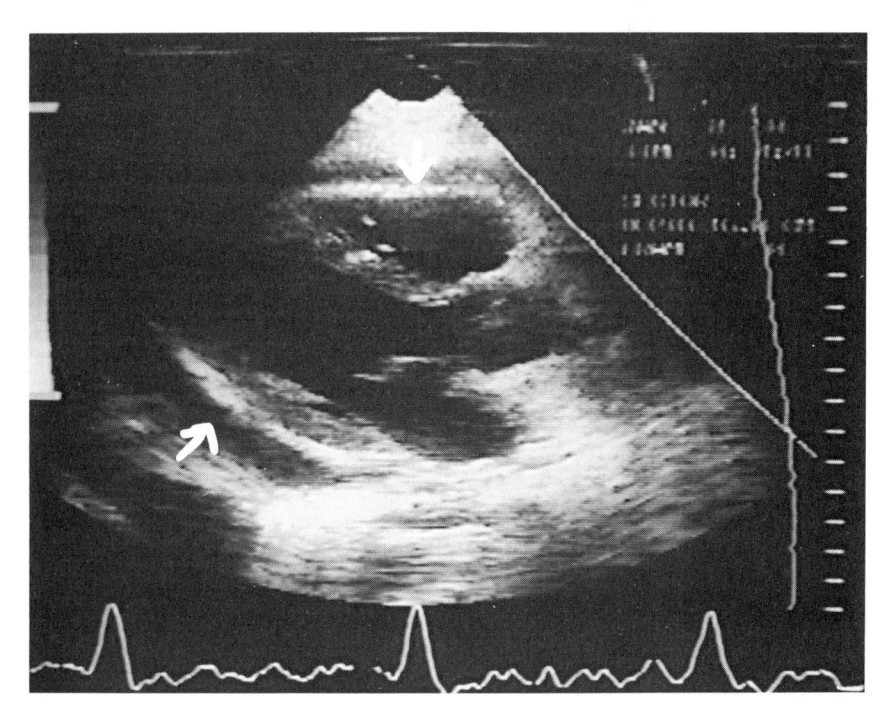

Figure 9-72 Parasternal long-axis view consistent with a posterior and anterior pericardial effusion. Note the posterior space just above the pericardium, as well as the anterior space above the right ventricular free wall.

228 Basic Echocardiography

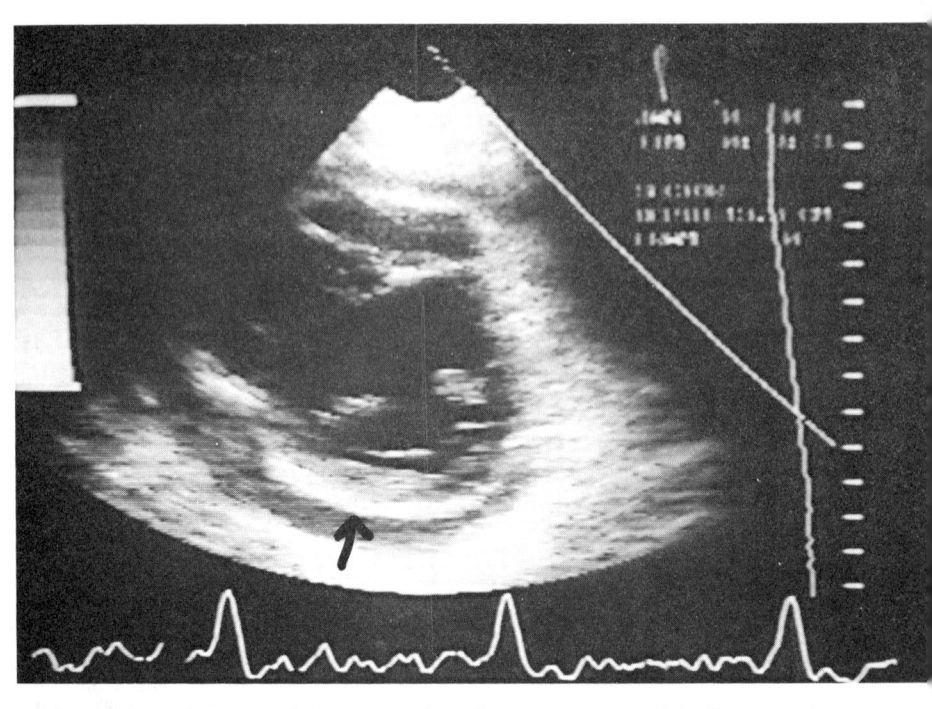

Figure 9-73 Parasternal short-axis view showing a pericardial effusion both anteriorly and posteriorly.

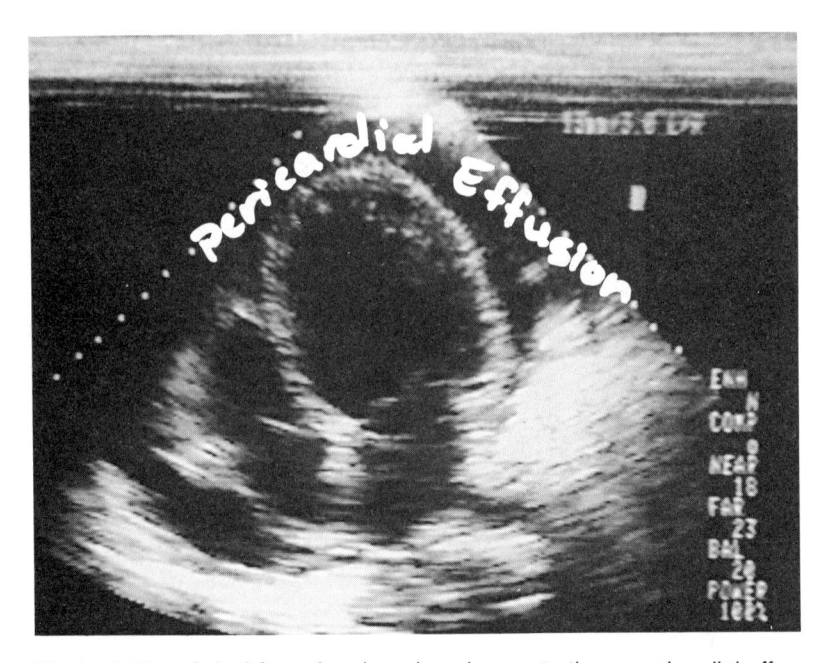

Figure 9-74 Apical four-chamber view demonstrating a pericardial effusion anteriorly and posteriorly surrounding the apex.

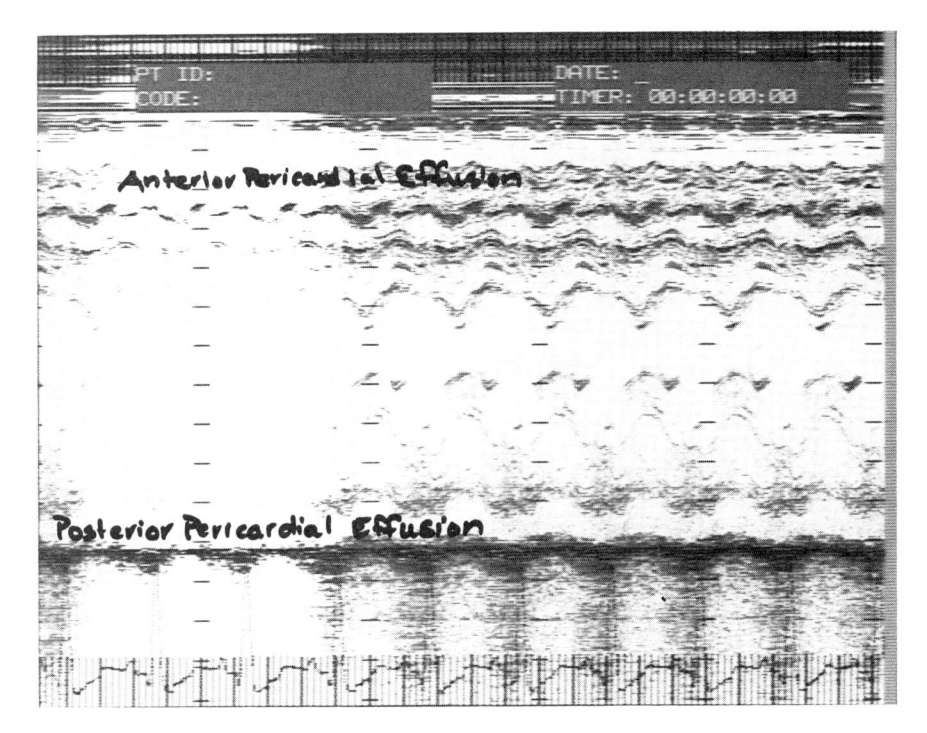

Figure 9-75 An anterior and posterior "clear space" indicates a pericardial effusion. By damping down the overall gain, the pericardium is clearly defined, clarifying the effusion.

Paradoxical Septal Motion

Parodoxical septal motion is an abnormal finding effecting the intraventricular septum. Normally, the IVS moves inward, toward the left ventricular wall in ventricular systole. When paradoxical septal motion is present, the IVS moves in the same direction as the LVPW. There are several reasons why this may occur

1. A right ventricular volume overload (RVVO). As a result, a dilatation and enlargement of the ventricle occurs, exceeding that of the left side. This increase in volume causes the IVS to move in the opposite direction. This volume overload may include tricuspid insufficiency, pulmonic insufficiency or an atrial septal defect.
2. Left bundle branch block (LBBB). A LBBB may cause paradoxical septal motion due to interference in the normal conduction pathway.
3. Valvular surgery. Valvular replacements may cause paradoxical septal motion due to a disturbance in the surrounding tissue.

When viewing the two-dimensional echo, one will actually notice the IVS can be noticed moving in the direction opposite to that normally expected in ventricular systole. LV views can be used to detect this abnormal-

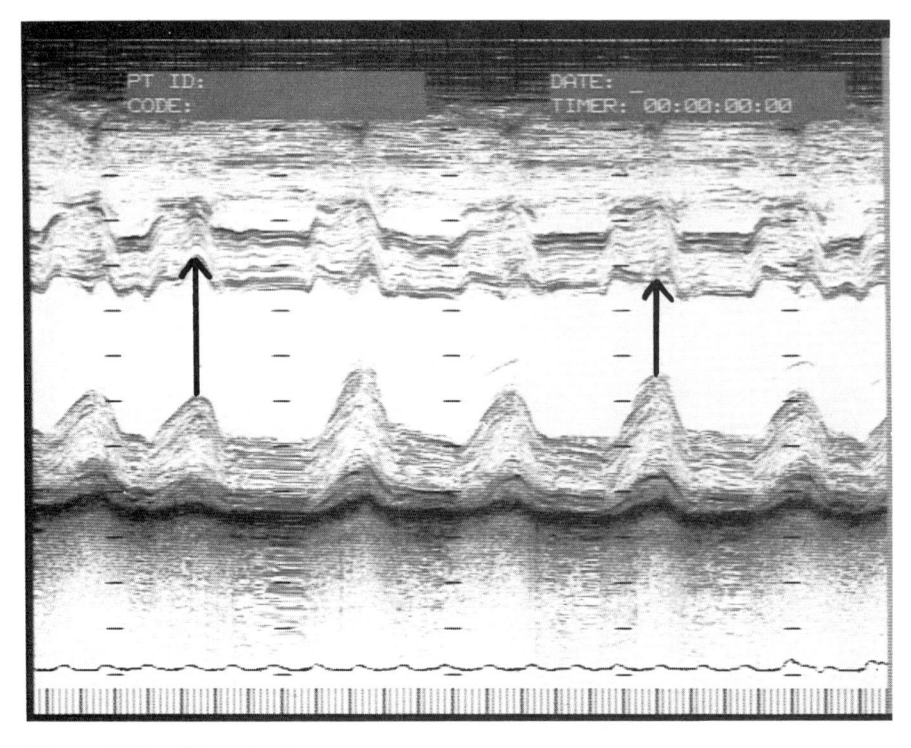

Figure 9-76 M-mode demonstrating paradoxical septal motion. Note the IVS moving in the same direction as the LVPW.

ity. The m-mode is sensitive and can easily detect paradoxical septal motion. The IVS and LVPW are moving in the same direction instead of in the opposite direction (Figure 9-76).

Mitral Stenosis

Mitral stenosis is a disease state in which there is a restriction of the mobility of the mitral valve leaflets, impairing the blood flow through the orifice. Rheumatic mitral stenosis is the type most commonly seen. It is the result of rheumatic fever, which causes a scarring on the valves. Mitral stenosis can also be acquired, the result of a slow, natural process of calcium buildup.

Mitral stenosis is classified by degrees of severity: mild, moderate, and severe. The degree is determined by evaluating the left atrial size and the actual pliability of the mitral valve leaflet, as well as by measuring the E-to-F slope on the m-mode.

When viewing an echo for mitral stenosis, it could be expected that a thickened mitral valve with restricted motion of the valve leaflet would be seen. An enlarged left atrium would also be a significant finding.

Rheumatic mitral stenosis on the two-dimensional exam would exhibit

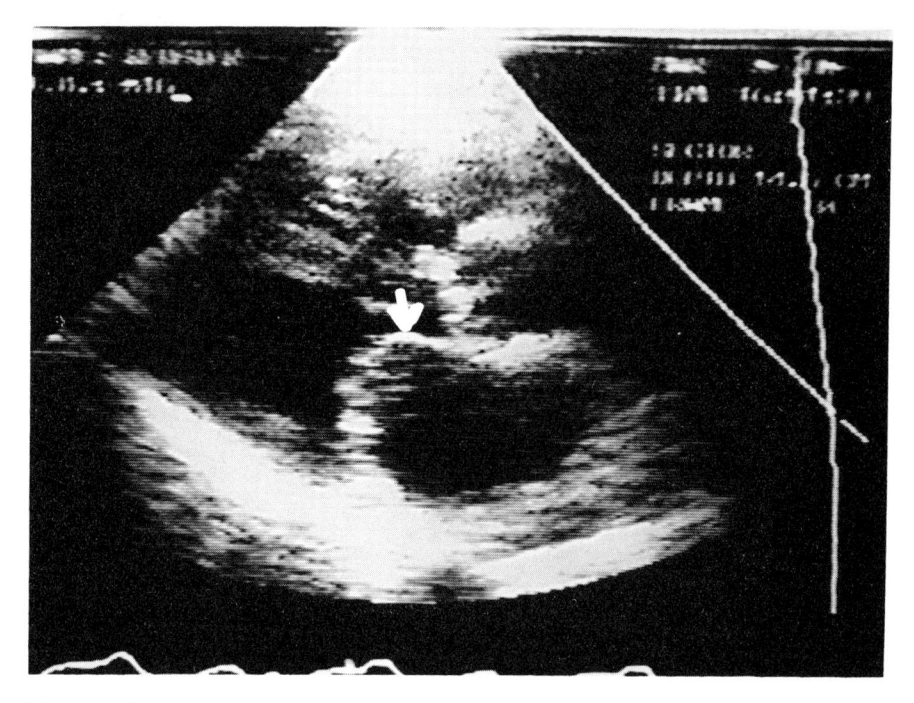

Figure 9-77 Parasternal long-axis view consistent with rheumatic mitral stenosis. The anterior mitral valve leaflet demonstrates the "diastolic bowing" (arrow).

a thickened valve with "diastolic bowing of the anterior mitral valve leaflet." It appears to have a hook-shaped configuration in diastole. The anterior and posterior mitral valve leaflets appear fused in diastole, at the maximum point of separation, in both the parasternal long-axis view and the apical four-chamber view (Figures 9-77 and 9-78). The left atrium would be enlarged as well. All views can be used to detect mitral stenosis. In long-standing mitral stenosis, atrial fibrillation could develop, due to the increase in left atrial size.

On two-dimensional exam, acquired mitral stenosis would show a highly thickened, calcific valve. This process usually starts in the annular region of the mitral valve and moves inward, toward the coapt point. Rocklike calcific lesions are seen on both leaflets, restricting orifice size and pliability. Once again, the left atrial size would be increased.

When evaluating rheumatic mitral valve stenosis on m-mode, a dilated left atrium would be noticed. The anterior mitral valve leaflet would flatten out, decreasing the E-to-F slope. The greater the decrease in the E-to-F slope, the more severe the mitral stenosis. The posterior leaflet is also flattened, moving anteriorly in diastole (Figure 9-79).

On m-mode, acquired mitral stenosis would appear as a thickened mitral valve with a heavily calcified mitral valve annulus. The E-to-F slope/D-to-E slope would be reduced, and an enlarged left atrium would also be seen.

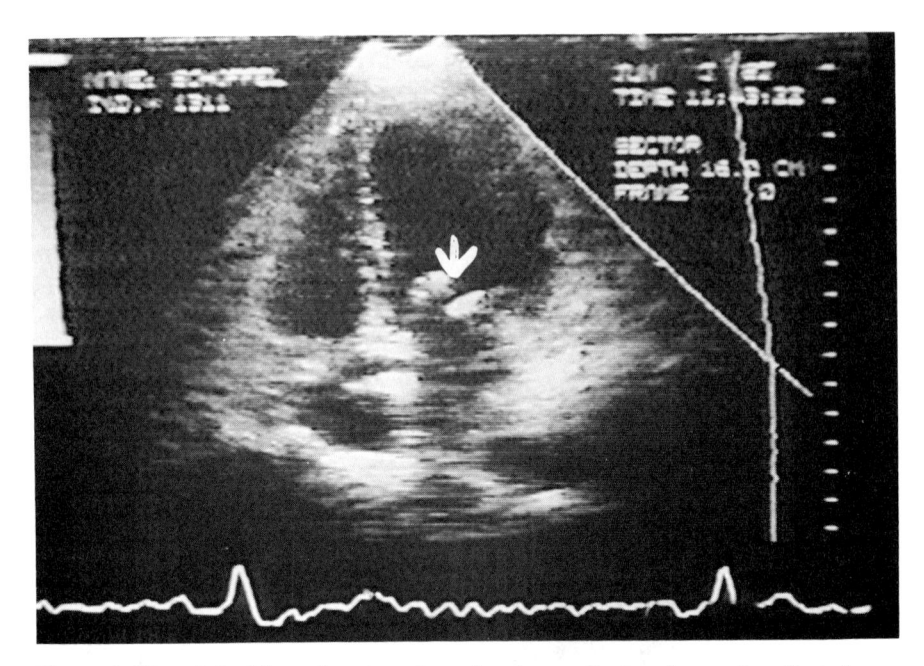

Figure 9-78 Apical four-chamber view also demonstrates rheumatic mitral stenosis (arrow).

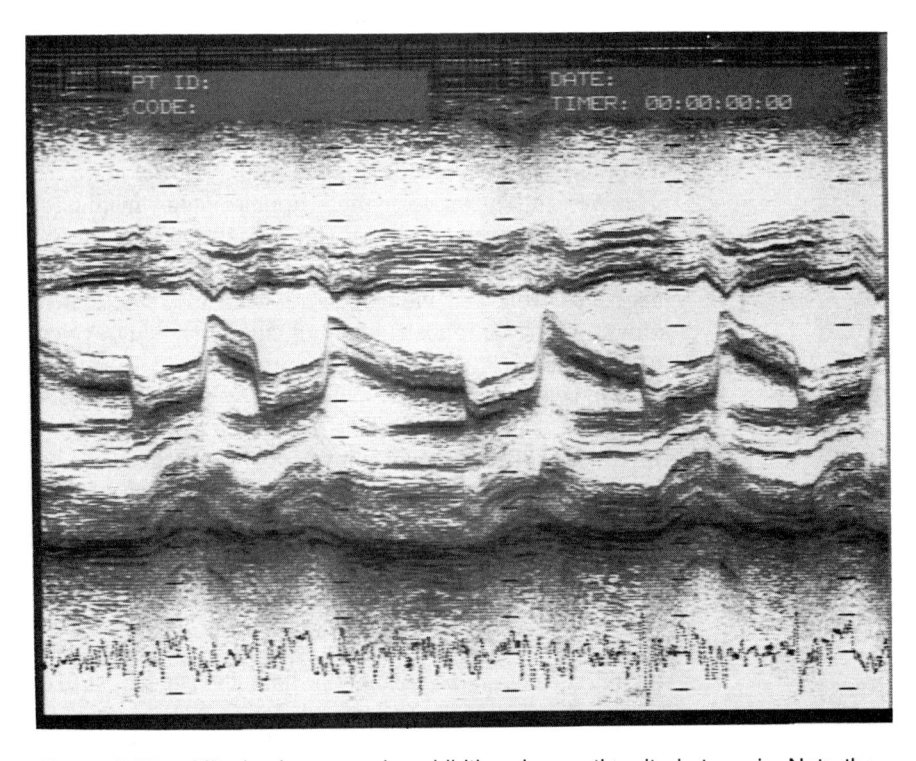

Figure 9-79 Mitral valve m-mode exhibiting rheumatic mitral stenosis. Note the decreased EF slope. The posterior mitral valve leaflet moves anteriorly in diastole.

Mitral Regurgitation

In mitral regurgitation, the mitral valve fails to close properly, allowing blood to flow backward into the left atrium in ventricular systole. Mitral regurgitation may not necessarily be seen directly on the echo examination, but its secondary results can be seen. Some findings include left atrial dilatation as well as left ventricular dilatation, exaggerated interventricular septal motion, and abnormal left atrial wall motion. Mitral regurgitation can result from mitral valve prolapse, damaged chordae, a calcified mitral valve annulus, bacterial endocarditis, or many other disease states. Doppler echocardiography is an excellent diagnostic tool used to detect and actually to quantitate the amount of regurgitant blood flow.

Left Ventricular Clots

Ventricular clots are generally seen at the apex of the heart. Clots are composed of fibrinous material as well as stagnated blood. Ventricular clots usually form because of a pooling of blood. Apical clots may be seen following a myocardial infarction. The area of the clot would be hypokinetic or akinetic and the surrounding muscle may thicken. At times, the apex may appear dyskinetic, where the clot has adhered to the wall. M-mode echocardiography cannot detect apical clots, because of the "ice-pick" effect; however, two-dimensional echocardiography is an excellent method of detecting these clots. The parasternal views are not routinely used for detecting clots because on cannot see the true apex. The apical four-chamber and apical two-chamber views are used when evaluating clots. A "bright" area would be seen in the apical region (Figures 9-80 and 9-81). Remember, the clot has adhered to the wall and a balllike image would be noted attached to the endocardial surface. The surrounding muscle would also be affected, showing an akinetic segment. An artifact should not be confused with an apical clot. An artifact is a product of artificial character caused by extraneous echoes, improper gain settings, or reverberations that may mimic intracardiac abnormalities. Angulation can create extra echoes which could be confused with a thrombus.

Cardiomyopathy (Congestive)

Congestive cardiomyopathy by echo would exhibit a dilated, poorly moving left ventricle. Diffuse hypokinesis is generally seen, and the left atrium is also dilated. The cardiac output in turn would be decreased, causing a poorly moving aortic root; at times, early closure of the aortic valve is noted. The mitral valve would appear free-floating within the left ventricle. An increased E point–septal separation, could also be seen, indicating low cardiac output. Normally, the anterior mitral valve leaflet (in diastole) reaches the intraventricular septum. However, in a congestive cardiomyopathy, there is a significant separation between the E point of the mitral valve and the

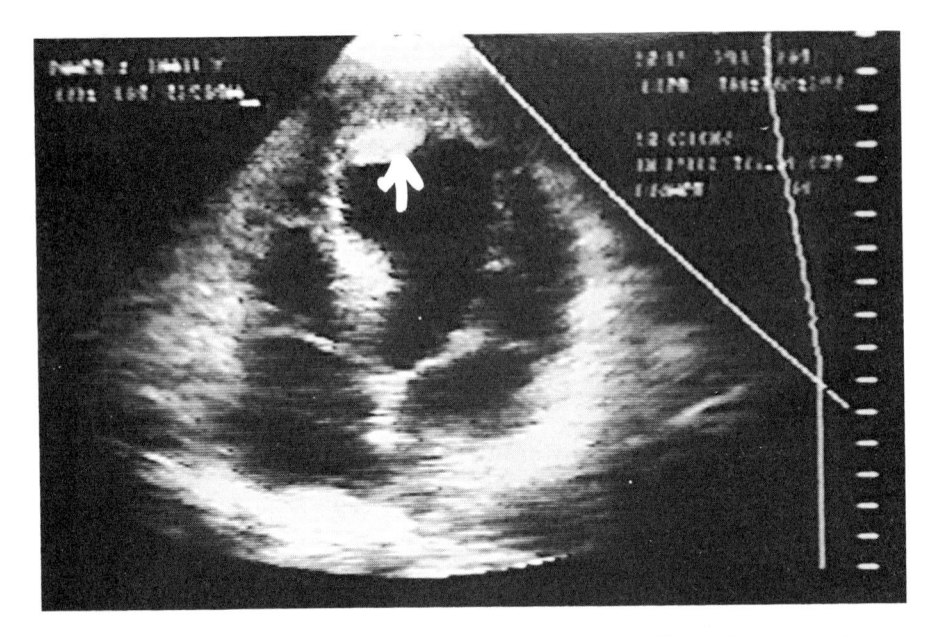

Figure 9-80 Apical four-chamber view exhibiting an apical thrombus (arrow).

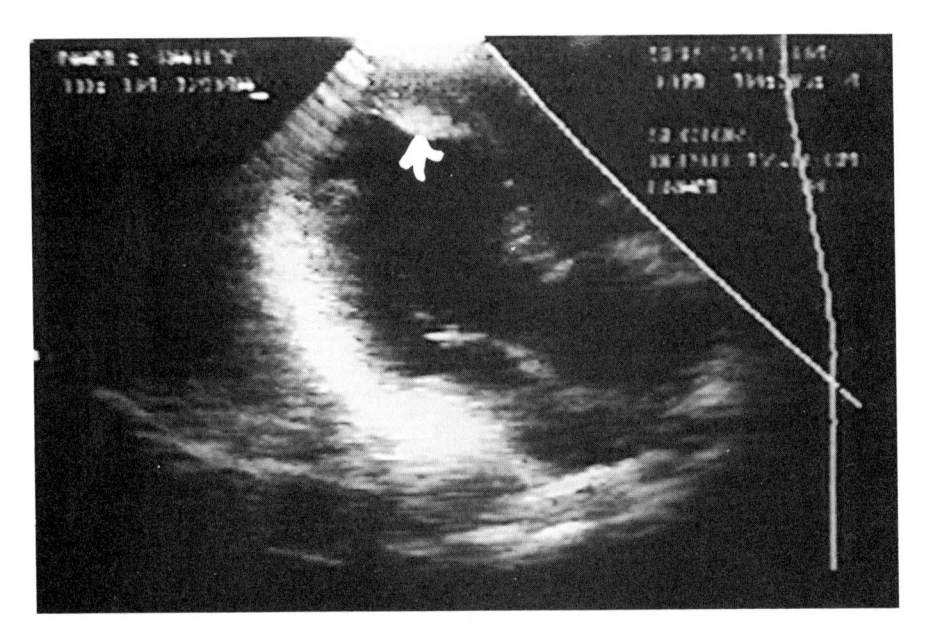

Figure 9-81 Apical two-chamber view is also useful when evaluating apical clots (arrow).

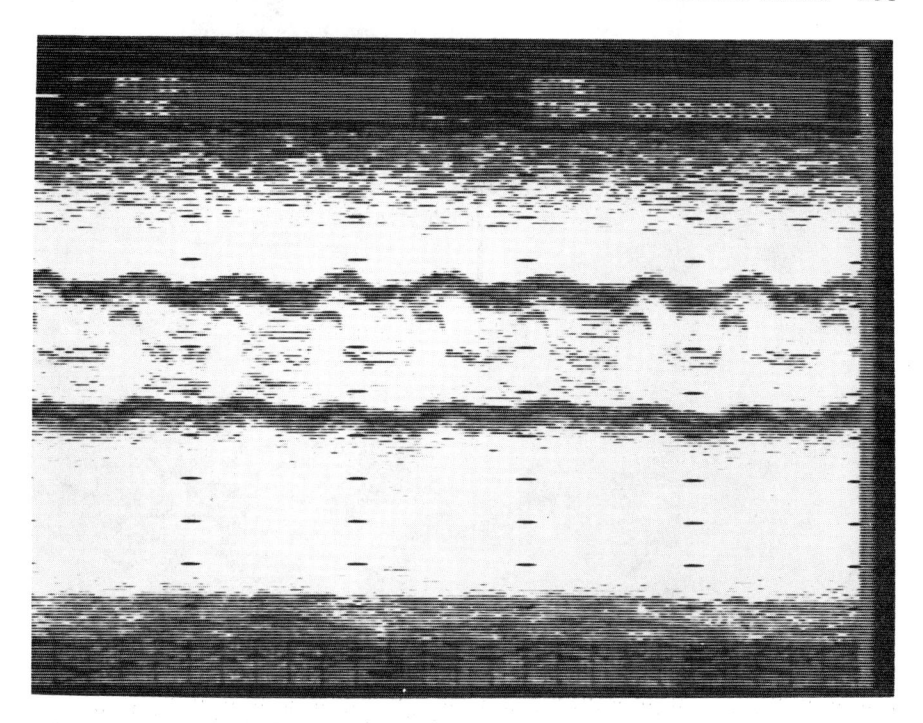

Figure 9-82 Aortic valve m-mode showing decreased aortic root motion with a slightly dilated left atrium.

intraventricular septum. Mitral regurgitation is another common finding in a patient with cardiomyopathy. The cardiac Doppler would confirm this finding. Both the m-mode and two-dimensional echo are accurate for diagnosing this disease state. There are several types of cardiomyopathies. As an echocardiographer, it is not to diagnosis for type, but to detect the abnormalties by the echo examination (Figures 9-82 through 9-84).

Flail Mitral Valve Leaflet

A flail mitral valve leaflet can affect either the anterior or posterior leaflet. A flail leaflet is usually the result of a ruptured chardae tendineae, causing the leaflets to close improperly. A ruptured chordae tendineae can be the result of an acute myocardial infarction, or simply result from wear and tear on the chordae from an abnormality such as mitral valve prolapse. A flail mitral valve leaflet usually requires a valve replacement.

The two-dimensional echo is more sensitive in detecting this abnormality, because visualization of the valve is much greater. All views are used to visualize a flail mitral valve leaflet. The parasternal short-axis view at the mitral valve is the least common view used. A leaflet that does not close

(Text continues on page 238)

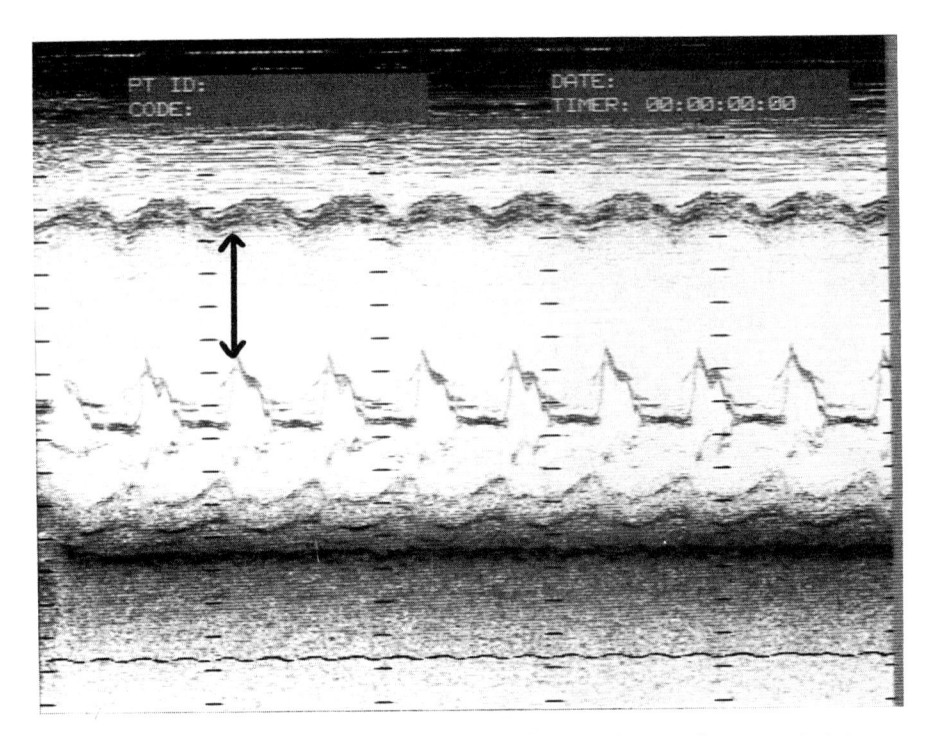

Figure 9-83 A "free-floating" mitral valve indicates a low cardiac output state, seen in patients with congestive cardiomyopathy.

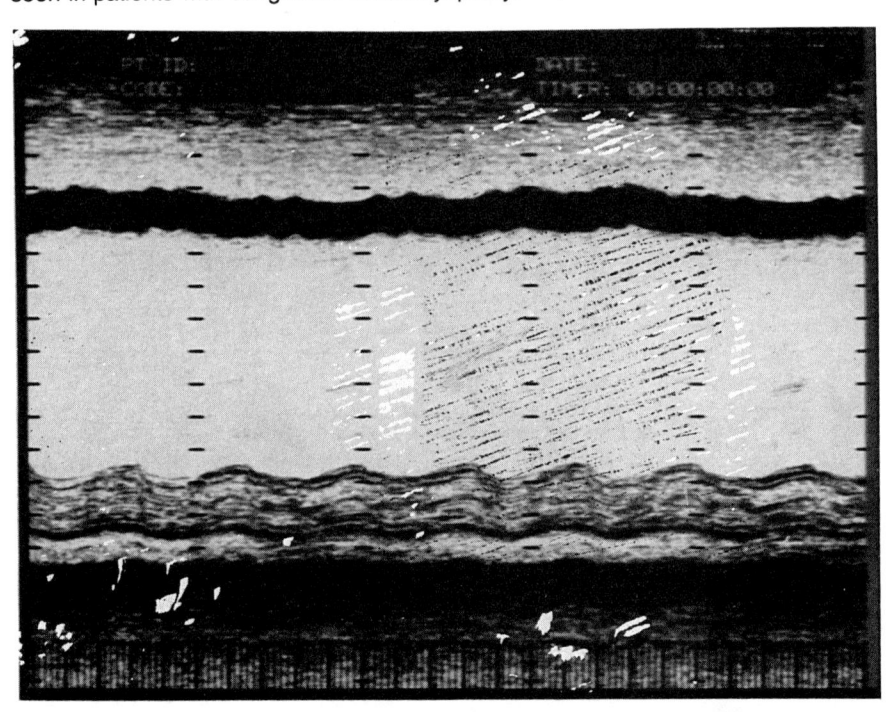

Figure 9-84 An LV m-mode demonstrating a dilated, poorly moving left ventricle. Patient also demonstrates a small posterior pericardial effusion.

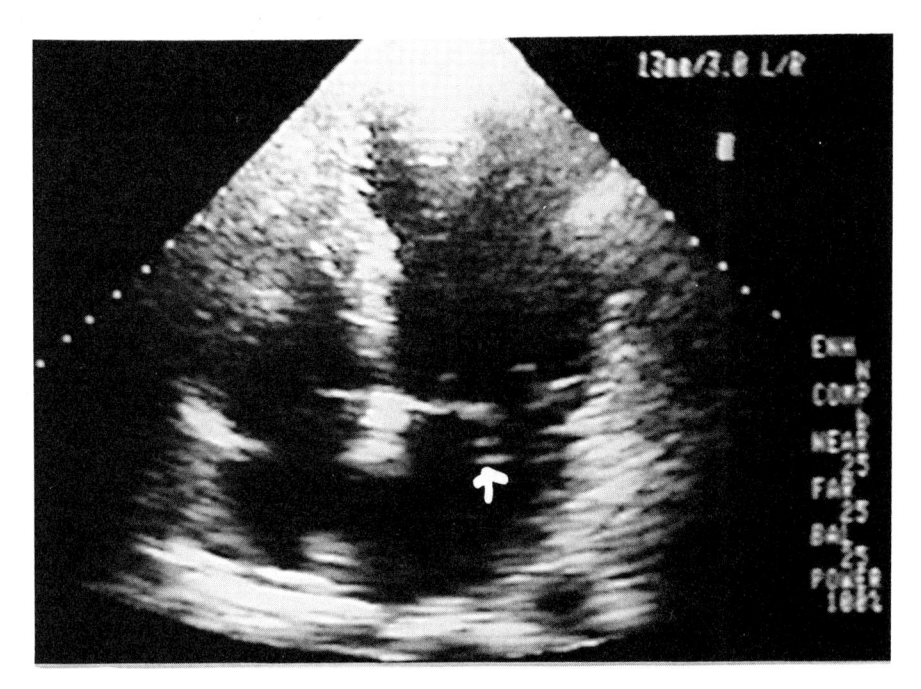

Figure 9-85 An apical four-chamber view demonstrating a flail mitral valve leaflet. Notice that a portion of the MV leaflet is freely moving into the left atrium, detached from the normal valve apparatus.

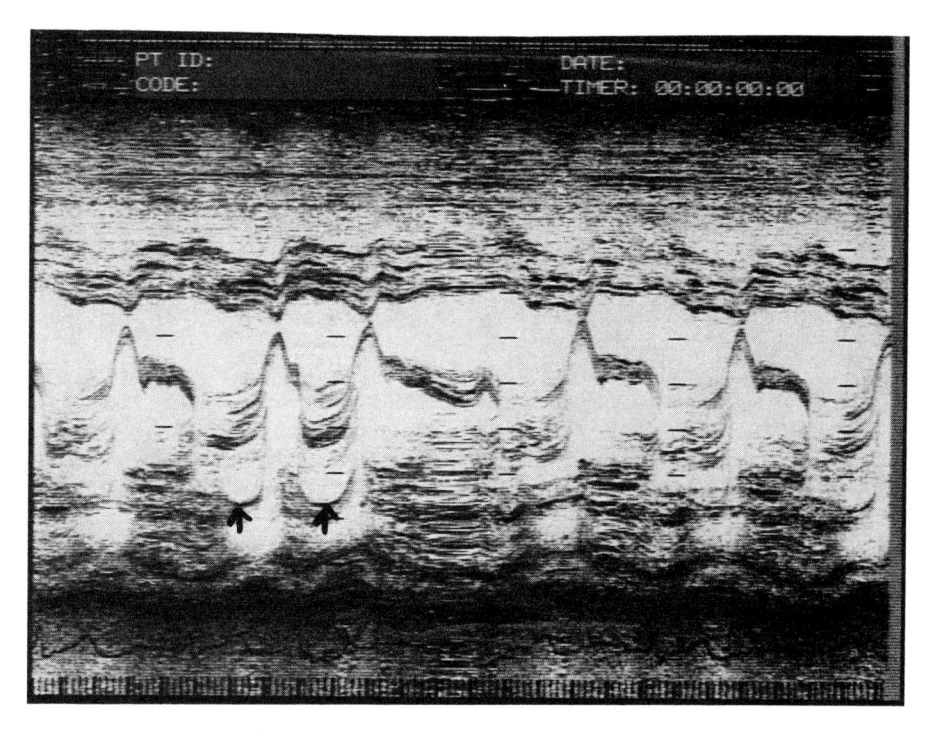

Figure 9-86 A mitral valve m-mode exhibiting a flail mitral valve leaflet. This resembles MVP, but to a much more exaggerated degree.

tightly in ventricular systole can be seen. The leaflet affected would be moving about freely, due to the inability of the valve leaflet to close properly from the ruptured chordae tendineae (Figure 9-85). Unlike MVP, which causes a sagging into the left atrium when the leaflets are closed, a flail mitral valve leaflet would not close at all, seeing an erratic moving leaflet. Severe mitral regurgitation is the effect of a flail mitral valve leaflet. Once again, a valve replacement is usually the prognosis.

The m-mode is not a precise way to diagnose a flail mitral valve leaflet. The m-mode recording of the posterior flail leaflet can mimic those of atrial myxomas, mitral valve prolapse, or infective endocarditis. Detection of an anterior flail leaflet by m-mode is even less satisfactory. An exaggerated excursion of the anterior leaflet could be seen and, possibly, diastolic fluttering that could mimic aortic insufficiency or atrial fibrillation (Figure 9-86).

Bibliography

Brown WT, Devereaux RB, Kramerfox R, Sachs I: Evolution of echocardiographic findings in patients with mitral valve prolapse. J Cardiovasc Ultrasonography 2(1):29, 1983

Burke JF, Pauletto FJ, Weinreich DJ: Left ventricular mural thrombi in patients with remote myocardial infarction: Long term follow-up with serial echocardiography. J Cardiovasc Ultrasonography 3(4):375, 1984

Chung EK, Joyer: Non-Invasive Cardiac Diagnosis. Philadelphia, Lea & Febiger, 1976

Feigenbaum: Echocardiography, 3rd ed, p 137. Philadelphia, Lea & Febiger, 1981

Goldberg SJ, Allen H, Sohn D: Pediatric and Adolescent "Echocardiography"—A Handbook, pp 13–15. Chicago, Year Book Medical Pub, 1975

Hurst JW, Logue RD, Schlant RC, Wenger NK: The Heart, pp 449–458. New York, McGraw-Hill, 1978

Kerin NZ, Matsuo M, O'Donnell L, Rubenfire M: Mitral valve fluttering in aortic insufficiency: Echocardiography and angiographic correlation. J Cardiovasc Ultrasonography 3(1):65, 1984

Phillips BJ, Friedwald VE: Manual of Echocardiography Techniques, p 64. Philadelphia, WB Saunders, 1980

Rahimtoola SH: Infective Endocarditis, p 138. Orlando, Grune & Stratton, 1978

Takamoto T, Popp RC: Conduction disturbances related to the site and severity of mitral annular calcification. A J Cardiol 51(10):1573–1855, 1983

Talano JV: Cardiac Ultrasound Workbook, p 5. Orlando, Grune & Stratton, 1982

Termini BA, Yu-Chen L: Essentials of Echocardiography, pp 67–69. Litten Industries, 1976

Weisslerr AM: Noninvasive Cardiology, p 184. Orlando, Grune & Stratton, 1974

Chapter 10

Basic Doppler Echocardiography

Linda Martin

The cardiac Doppler is a new addition to the cardiac ultrasound examination. The Doppler principle examines alteration in sound wave frequency reflected from moving objects. This change in frequency is called *the Doppler frequency shift*, which is directly proportional to the velocity of the sound waves and moving objects. Velocity is measured in meters per second. Some machines calculate m/sec automatically; however, other instruments give the Doppler shift in kiloHertz (kHz), which then has to be changed by the operator to m/sec (Figures 10-1*A*, *B* and *C*). Currently available instruments display this information graphically, placing velocity on the "Y" axis and time on the "X" axis. This representation is called the *spectral display* (Figure 10-2).

An audible signal is also generated with high pitch signals representing high velocity. The cardiac Doppler is capable of detecting valvular regurgitations, quantitating valvular stenosis (gradients in mm Hg), calculating valve areas (cm^2), quantitating cardiac outputs, and determining intracardiac shunts (such as ventricular septal defects (VSD's), atrial septal defects (ASD's), and *patent ductus* arteriosus (PDA's). All cardiac valves and structures can be examined for either regurgitant lesions, valvular stenosis, or structural defects.

Specific views and echo approaches must be used, because the ultrasound beam must be *parallel* to blood flow. The correct angle between the ultrasound jet and the moving target must be used to assure accurate calculations. Blood flow must be 0° or 180° ± 20° to the ultrasound beam. The direction of blood flow from the transducer indicates the Doppler shift. A

(Text continues on page 243)

240 Basic Doppler Echocardiography

Doppler Shift Conversion
2.25 MHz

Frequency Shift	Velocity Conversion
1.0 kHz	.34 m/sec
1.5 kHz	.54 m/sec
2.0 kHz	.68 m/sec
2.5 kHz	.86 m/sec
3.0 kHz	1.03 m/sec
3.5 kHz	1.20 m/sec
4.0 kHz	1.37 m/sec
4.5 kHz	1.55 m/sec
5.0 kHz	1.72 m/sec
5.5 kHz	1.89 m/sec
6.0 kHz	2.06 m/sec
6.5 kHz	2.24 m/sec
7.0 kHz	2.41 m/sec
7.5 kHz	2.58 m/sec
8.0 kHz	2.75 m/sec
8.5 kHz	2.93 m/sec
9.0 kHz	3.10 m/sec
9.5 kHz	3.27 m/sec
10.0 kHz	3.44 m/sec
10.5 kHz	3.62 m/sec
11.0 kHz	3.79 m/sec
11.5 kHz	3.96 m/sec
12.0 kHz	4.13 m/sec
12.5 kHz	4.30 m/sec
13.0 kHz	4.48 m/sec
13.5 kHz	4.65 m/sec
14.0 kHz	4.82 m/sec
14.5 kHz	5.00 m/sec
15.0 kHz	5.17 m/sec
15.5 kHz	5.34 m/sec
16.0 kHz	5.51 m/sec
16.5 kHz	5.68 m/sec
17.0 kHz	5.86 m/sec
17.5 kHz	6.03 m/sec
18.0 kHz	6.20 m/sec
18.5 kHz	6.37 m/sec
19.0 kHz	6.55 m/sec
19.5 kHz	6.70 m/sec
20.0 kHz	6.89 m/sec

Figure 10-1 (*A*) If a 2.25 megaHertz (MHz) transducer is being used, the above chart can be utilized to convert kiloHertz (kHz) shift to a velocity reading in milliseconds.

Doppler Shift Conversion
3 MHz

Frequency Shift	Velocity Conversion
1.3 kHz	.25 m/sec
1.5 kHz	.38 m/sec
2.0 kHz	.51 m/sec
2.5 kHz	.64 m/sec
3.0 kHz	.76 m/sec
3.5 kHz	.89 m/sec
4.0 kHz	1.02 m/sec
4.5 kHz	1.15 m/sec
5.0 kHz	1.28 m/sec
5.5 kHz	1.41 m/sec
6.0 kHz	1.53 m/sec
6.5 kHz	1.66 m/sec
7.0 kHz	1.79 m/sec
7.5 kHz	1.92 m/sec
8.0 kHz	2.05 m/sec
8.5 kHz	2.17 m/sec
9.0 kHz	2.30 m/sec
9.5 kHz	2.43 m/sec
10.0 kHz	2.50 m/sec
10.5 kHz	2.69 m/sec
11.0 kHz	2.82 m/sec
11.5 kHz	2.94 m/sec
12.0 kHz	3.07 m/sec
12.5 kHz	3.20 m/sec
13.0 kHz	3.33 m/sec
13.5 kHz	3.46 m/sec
14.0 kHz	3.58 m/sec
14.5 kHz	3.71 m/sec
15.0 kHz	3.84 m/sec
15.5 kHz	3.97 m/sec
16.0 kHz	4.10 m/sec
16.5 kHz	4.25 m/sec
17.0 kHz	4.35 m/sec
17.5 kHz	4.48 m/sec
18.0 kHz	4.61 m/sec
18.5 kHz	4.75 m/sec
19.0 kHz	4.87 m/sec
19.5 kHz	5.00 m/sec
20.0 kHz	5.12 m/sec

Figure 10-1 (*B*) A 3MHz transducer would use these figures for the Doppler shift conversion.

(*Continued*)

242   Basic Doppler Echocardiography

Doppler Shift Conversion
5 MHz

Frequency Shift	Velocity Conversion
1.0 kHz	.15 m/sec
1.5 kHz	.23 m/sec
2.0 kHz	.30 m/sec
2.5 kHz	.38 m/sec
3.0 kHz	.46 m/sec
3.5 kHz	.53 m/sec
4.0 kHz	.61 m/sec
4.5 kHz	.69 m/sec
5.0 kHz	.76 m/sec
5.5 kHz	.84 m/sec
6.0 kHz	.91 m/sec
6.5 kHz	1.00 m/sec
7.0 kHz	1.07 m/sec
7.5 kHz	1.15 m/sec
8.0 kHz	1.23 m/sec
8.5 kHz	1.30 m/sec
9.0 kHz	1.38 m/sec
9.5 kHz	1.46 m/sec
10.0 kHz	1.53 m/sec
10.5 kHz	1.61 m/sec
11.0 kHz	1.69 m/sec
11.5 kHz	1.76 m/sec
12.0 kHz	1.84 m/sec
12.5 kHz	1.92 m/sec
13.0 kHz	2.00 m/sec
13.5 kHz	2.07 m/sec
14.0 kHz	2.15 m/sec
14.5 kHz	2.23 m/sec
15.0 kHz	2.30 m/sec
15.5 kHz	2.38 m/sec
16.0 kHz	2.46 m/sec
16.5 kHz	2.53 m/sec
17.0 kHz	2.61 m/sec
17.5 kHz	2.69 m/sec
18.0 kHz	2.76 m/sec
18.5 kHz	2.84 m/sec
19.0 kHz	2.92 m/sec
19.5 kHz	3.00 m/sec
20.0 kHz	3.07 m/sec

Figure 10-1   (C) The 5MHz transducer is used primarily when dealing with pediatric echo examinations, and the appropriate conversion table should be used.

Basic Doppler Echocardiography 243

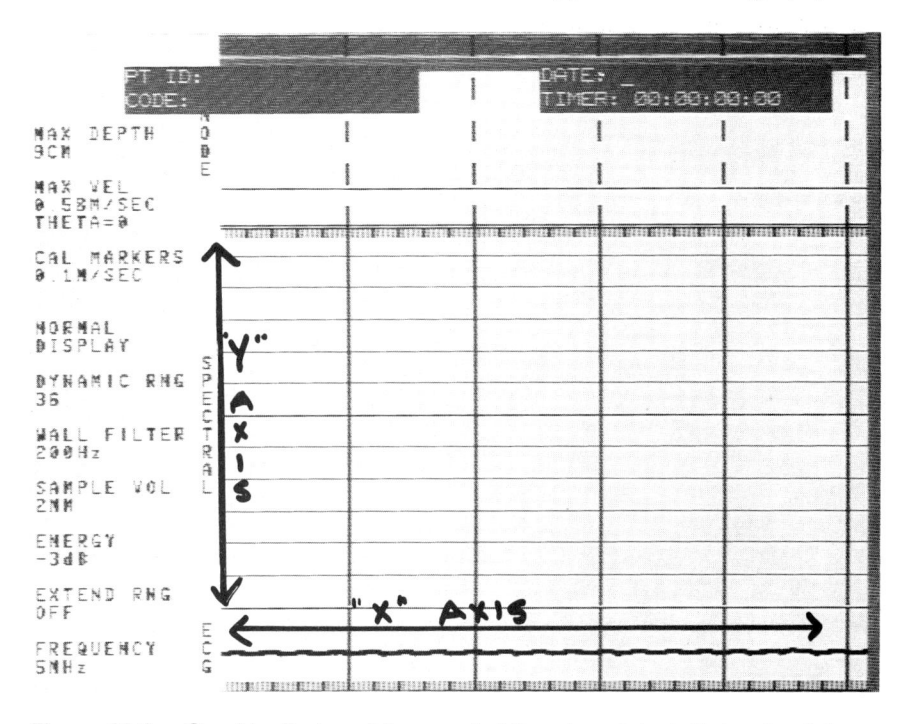

Figure 10-2 Graphic display of the spectral Doppler printout. Note other information given on the spectral display.

positive deflection indicates blood flow *toward* the transducer and negative deflection indicates blood flow *away* from the transducer (Figure 10-3).

There are three types of Dopplers: the *pulse wave Doppler* (PW); its variation called *pulsed repetition frequency Doppler* (PRF) and the *continuous wave Doppler* (CW). The pulsed Doppler sends a burst of ultrasound to a specific area at a specific depth. Only one burst of ultrasound is sent at a time and another signal can not be sent until the first has been returned. The major difference between the PRF Doppler and the standard pulsed Doppler is that the PRF system allows several pulsed signals in the body simultaneously. Higher velocities may be obtained with the PRF system compared to the standard pulsed Doppler. The two-dimensional image is used to locate cardiac structures. Interrogation of an exact location can be accomplished by a feature known as *"range gating."* A sample volume is used as an indicator to guide the ultrasound signal to the exact location (Figure 10-4).

The range gated signal can vary from 2 to 20 millimeters in depth. Pulsed Doppler has high-velocity measurement limitations that may hinder stenotic valve calculations. The PRF system helps eliminate this limitation of the standard pulsed Doppler.

244 Basic Doppler Echocardiography

	Blood flow above the zero line indicates positive flow towards the transducer.
ZERO LINE	The zero line represents the location of the sample volume as a reference point for determining blood flow direction.
	Blood flow below the zero line indicates negative flow away from the transducer.

Figure 10-3 Doppler graph in schematic representation. The dark center line represents the location of the sample volume used as a reference point to blood flow from the transducer.

The continuous wave Doppler uses two crystals (the pulsed wave unit uses only one). One crystal continuously sends bursts of ultrasound to the desired location, and one crystal constantly receives the transmitted information after the ultrasound has reached its desired locale. Range gating is not possible with the CW Doppler unit, because it receives information all along the Doppler beam. One can not determine the exact depth at which the frequency shift has occurred. High-velocity tracings, however, are easily obtainable with the CW Doppler.

The Examination

The Doppler exam is usually combined with two-dimensional examination, and can be quite lengthy, averaging approximately 45 to 60 minutes. The patient must be extremely comfortable and cooperative while the exam is being performed in order to obtain accurate results. Some laboratories perform a Doppler exam routinely with each two-dimensional study. Other

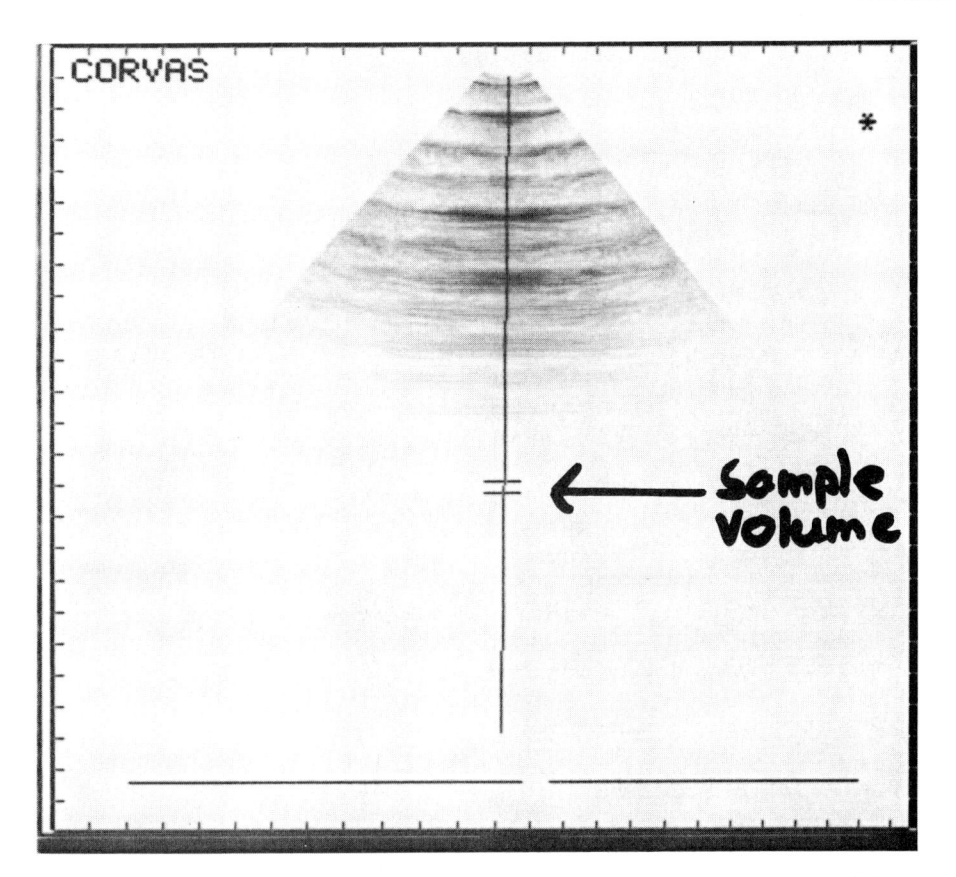

Figure 10-4 The sample volume is set along the cursor. Both the cursor and the sample volume can be moved to various locations in the two-dimensional field for exact interrogation.

laboratories perform Dopplers when specifically indicated. A three lead ECG is always hooked up to the patient for differentiating cardiac cycles.

Various echocardiographic views are taken when performing the Doppler examination. Standard parasternal and apical views are used; positioning the patient in the left lateral decubitus position will help achieve the best results. Suprasternal and subcostal views are also used, positioning the patient in the supine position. Another view, termed the *high right parasternal view*, in which the transducer is placed in the upper right sternal border, is helpful when searching for aortic root velocities. As previously mentioned, the patient must be completely cooperative, because of constant repositioning. Numerous views are used, depending on the specific disease state being evaluated (Table 10-1). Diagnosing abnormalities is determined by spectral and audible signals. Calculations may need to be made, depending on the specific diagnosis.

246 Basic Doppler Echocardiography

Table 10-1   Views in Evaluating Disease States

Diseases Evaluated by the Cardiac Doppler	Imaging Planes Used
Mitral Stenosis	Apical/2 Chamber—4 Chamber
Mitral Regurgitation	Apical or Parasternal
Aortic Stenosis	Apical/Suprasternal/High Right Parasternal
Aortic Regurgitation	Apical/Parasternal
Pulmonic Stenosis	Parasternal Short Axis View
	Subcostal/Parasternal Long Axis View
Pulmonic Regurgitation	Parasternal Short Axis/Subcostal/Parasternal Long Axis View
Tricuspid Stenosis	Apical/Parasternal Short Axis View
Tricuspid Regurgitation	Parasternal Short Axis View
	Parasternal RV Inflow/Apical
VSD	Parasternal Long Axis View
	Subcostal
ASD	Parasternal Short Axis View
	Apical
PDA	Parasternal Short Axis View
	Suprasternal Short Axis
IHSS or Subvalvular AS	Apical/Parasternal

Normal Mitral Blood Flow

Mitral valve blood flow is examined by sampling the actual mitral valve orifice near the left ventricular inflow tract, slightly distal to the mitral valve leaflets. Both the apical four-chamber and apical two-chamber view are used (Figure 10-5).

This tracing is important when evaluating mitral stenosis. Normal mitral valve flow is displayed in a shape resembling that of an "M." From the baseline reference point, a positive deflection is obtained in diastole, representing blood flow towards the transducer. In systole, there is no blood flow turbulance because the valve is tightly closed (Figure 10-6).

Figure 10-5   (A) The apical four-chamber view can be used for mitral flow tracings. The sample volume is situated on the mitral valve orifice near the left ventricular inflow tract. (B) The apical two-chamber view can also be used to obtain mitral flows. Again, the sample volume is placed slightly in the left ventricular inflow tract.

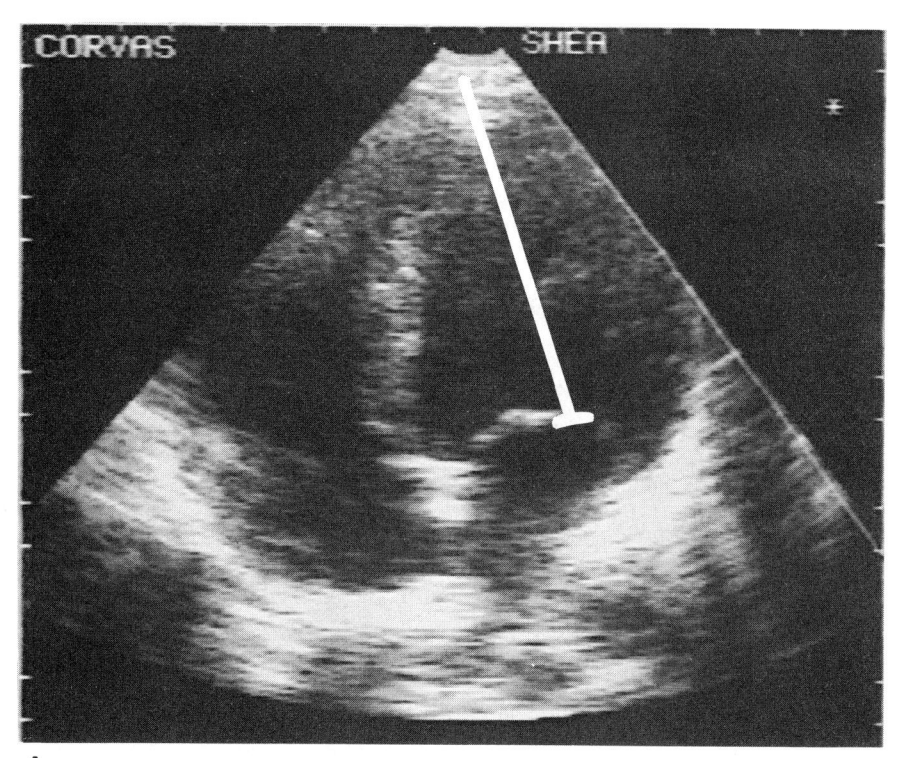

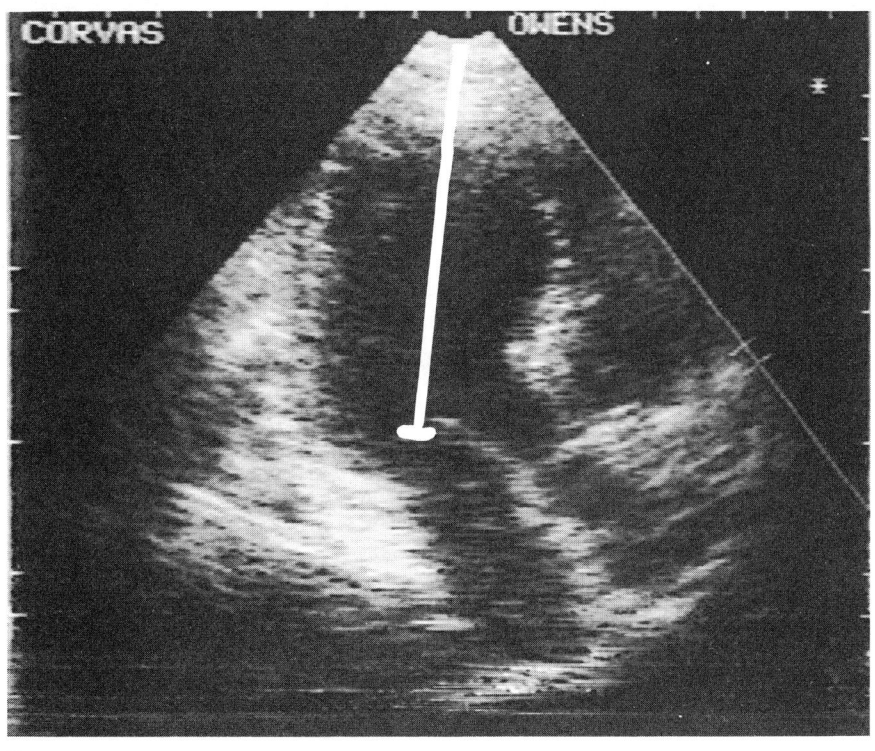

A

B

247

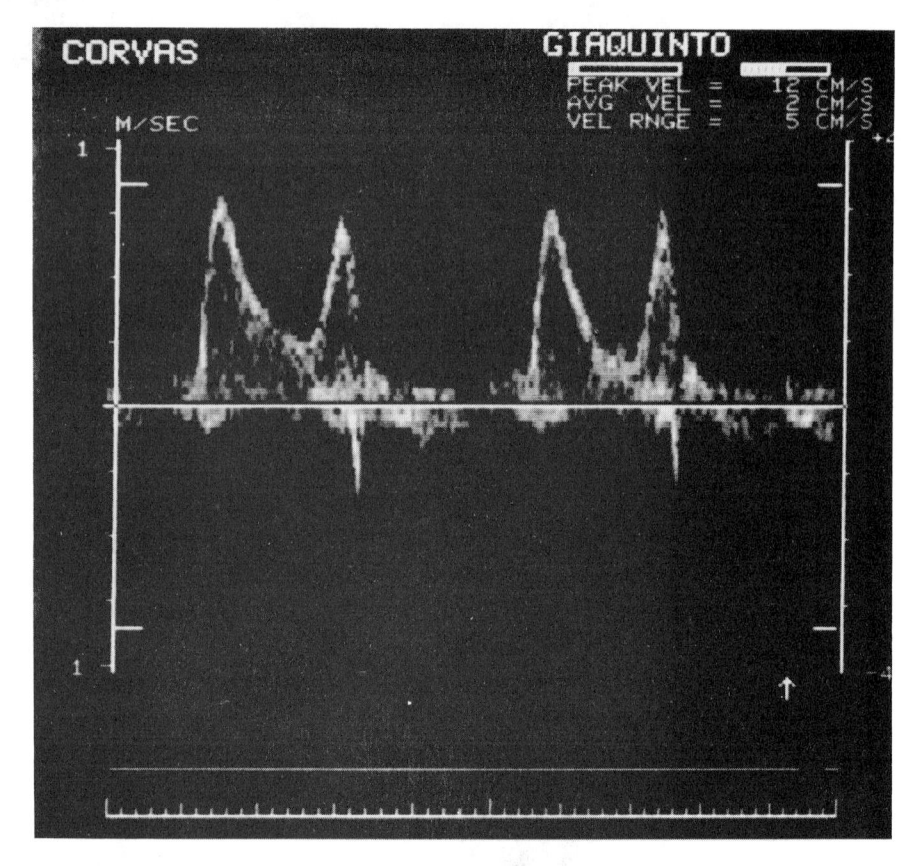

Figure 10-6 Normal mitral valve spectral display.

Normal Aortic Valve Flow

Apical, suprasternal, and high right parasternal views are used when evaluating aortic blood flow. The apical five-chamber or the apical two-chamber view can be used, with the sampling site slightly distal to the valve orifice, towards the ascending aorta (Figure 10-7). The spectral display depicts a negative deflection in ventricular systole because blood flow is away from the transducer as the aortic valve is open for the ventricular ejection of blood. In diastole, flow is even with the baseline, indicating the closing of the aortic valve (Figure 10-8).

Figure 10-7 (*A*) The apical five-chamber view can be used to record aortic flow. (*B*) The apical two-chamber view is also used in the evaluation of aortic valve flow.

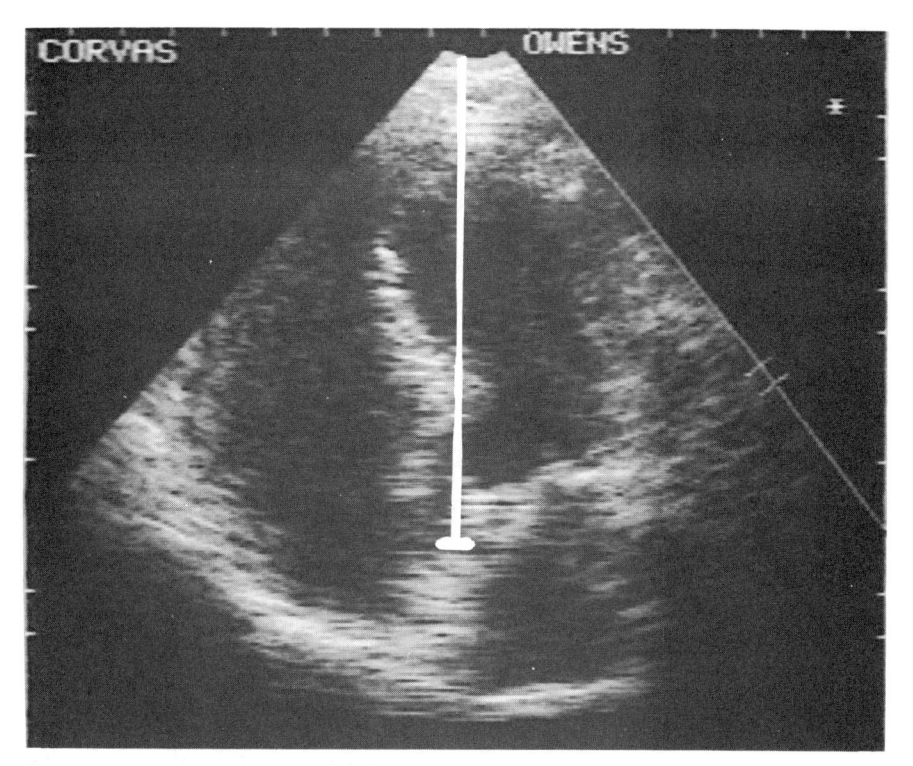

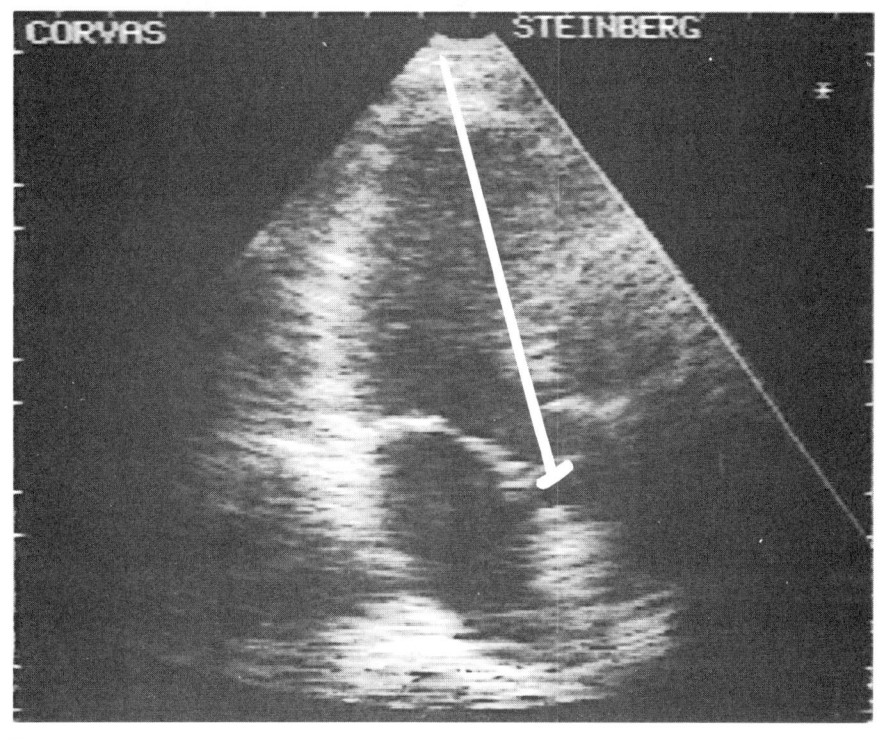

A

B

249

250 Basic Doppler Echocardiography

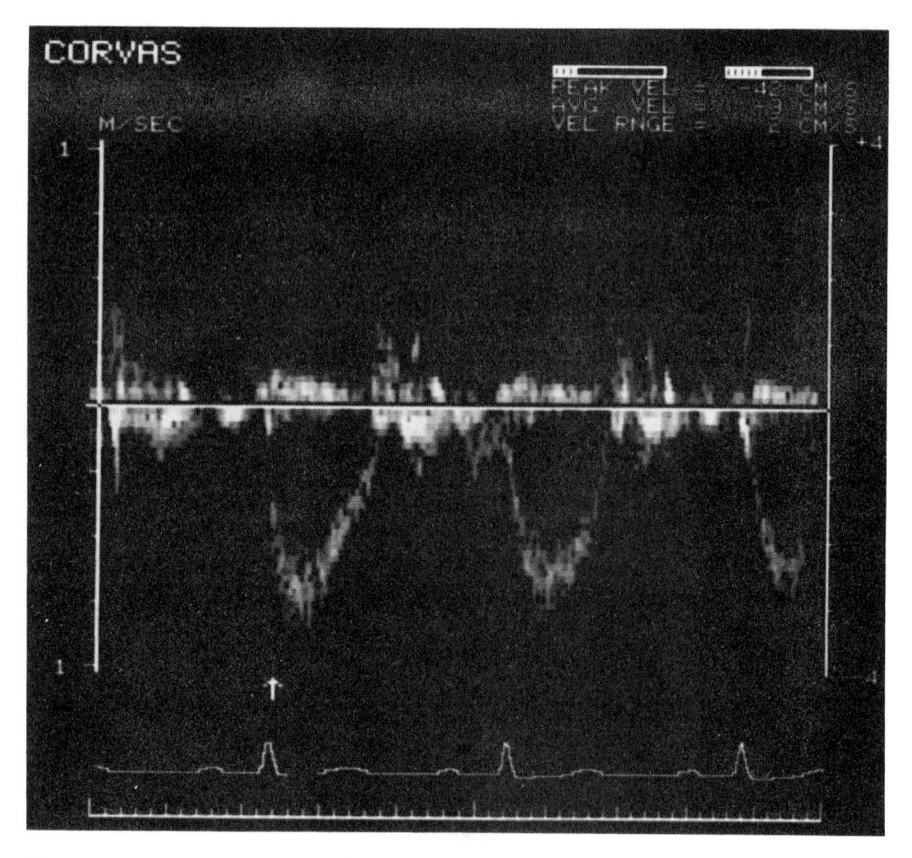

Figure 10-8 Normal aortic flow.

The suprasternal view is another view commonly used for aortic valve flow studies. The sampling site used is in the ascending aorta. When visualizing the suprasternal image, one can actually see the ascending aorta, arch, and descending aorta (Figure 10-9). Blood flow will be positive because blood normally flows from the aortic valve to the ascending aorta towards the transducer. In systole, a positive spectral image is seen above the baseline, whereas in diastole, the signal should stay at the central baseline (Figure 10-10).

The high right parasternal view is another view commonly used. As mentioned earlier, the transducer is placed in the high right sternal border. Audible and visible techniques must be demonstrated because an image is often difficult to obtain. The spectral display is positive above the zero baseline, as seen when using the suprasternal approach. A clear, crisp high-pitched signal is heard in systole, in an aortic valve study.

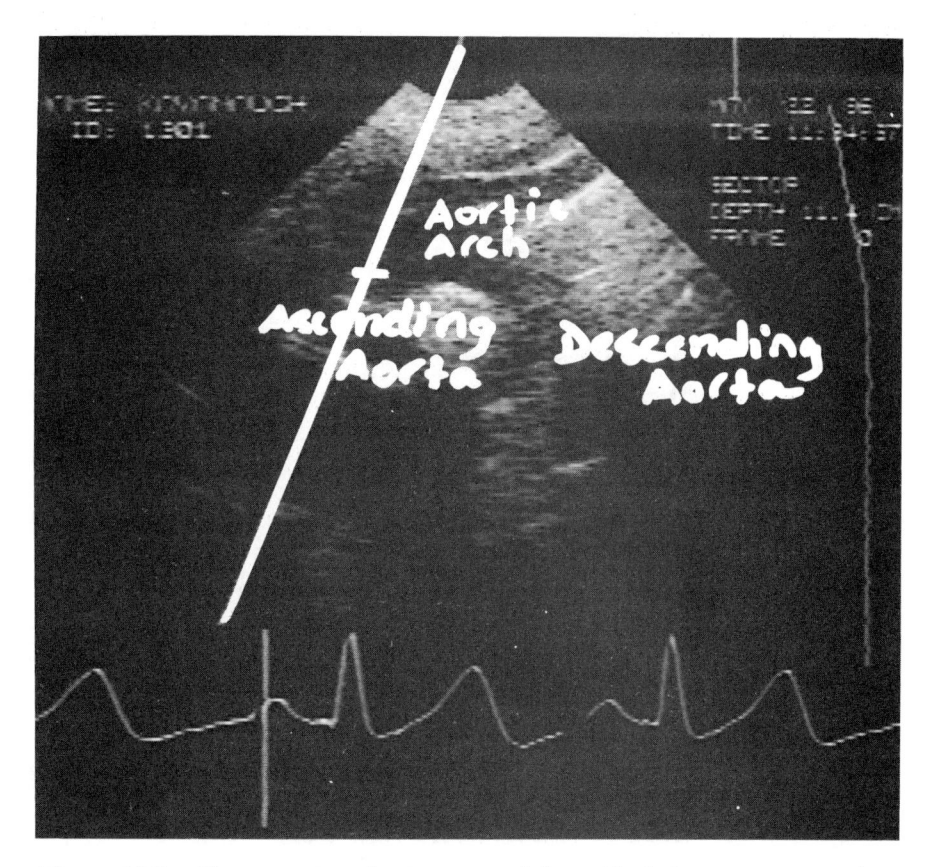

Figure 10-9 The suprasternal echo approach is an ideal view to access aortic valve flow. Sampling in the ascending aorta provides an accurate flow recording.

252 Basic Doppler Echocardiography

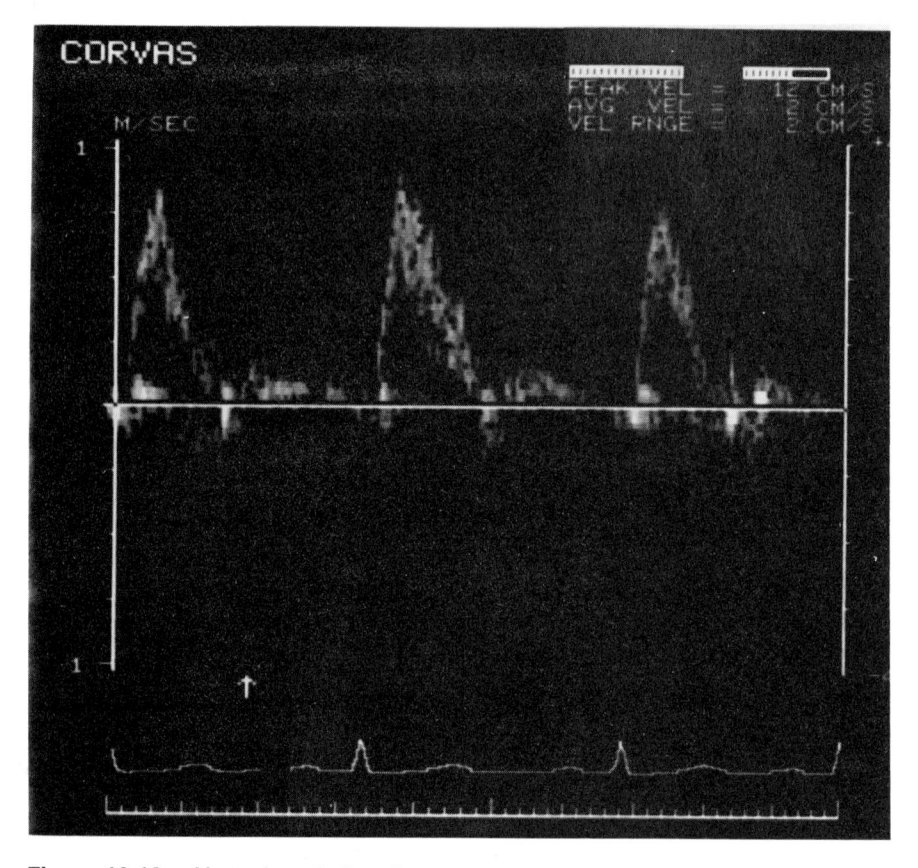

Figure 10-10 Normal aortic flow from the suprasternal approach.

Normal Pulmonic Flow

To obtain pulmonic blood flow tracings, the exam can be performed from the parasternal long-axis view, the parasternal short-axis view at the level of the aortic valve (Figure 10-11), or from the subcostal approach. The sampling site is slightly distal to the pulmonic valve near the pulmonary artery inflow tract. When the long-axis approach is being used, the transducer must be tipped anteriorly towards the patient's left shoulder. The right ventricle, pulmonary artery, and pulmonic valve can be visualized (Figure 10-12). The subcostal approach often is used when dealing with pediatric patients (Figure 10-13). A negative deflection is seen in systole as the pulmonic valve opens. Diastolic flow should be at the baseline as the valve closes. Blood flow is negative because flow is away from the transducer. The pattern of flow resembles that of the aortic flow spectral display (Figure 10-14).

The Examination 253

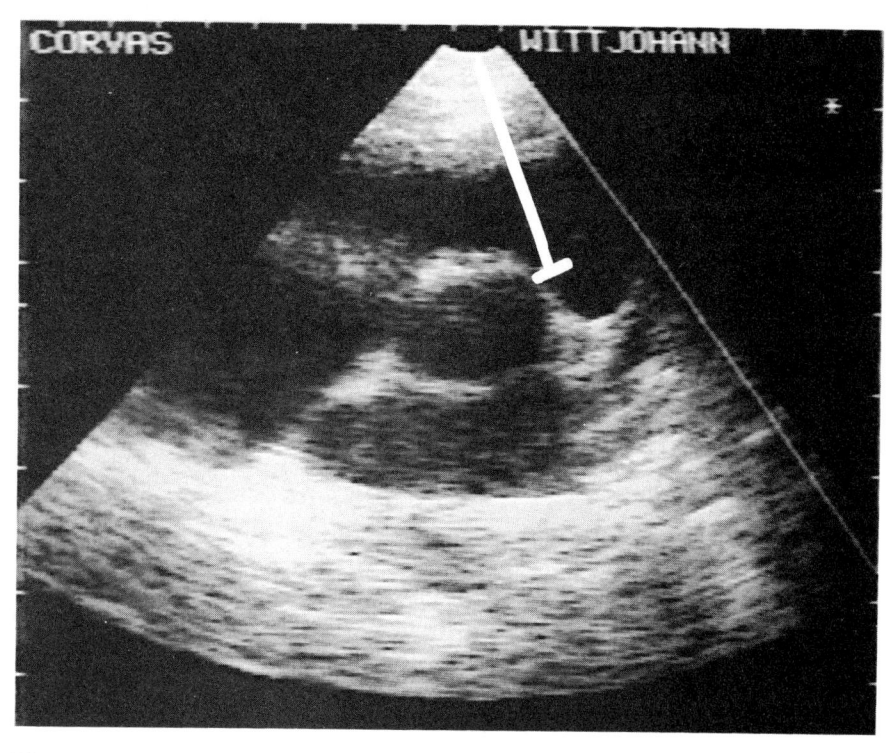

Figure 10-11 The parasternal short-axis view is often used for the evaluation of pulmonic blood flow.

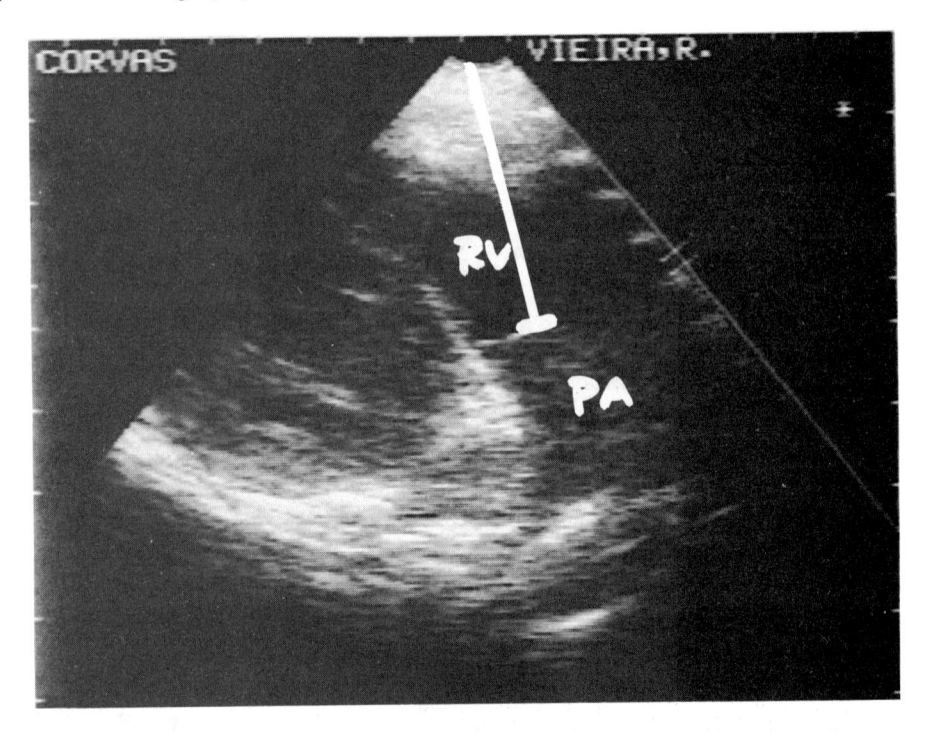

Figure 10-12 The parasternal long-axis approach is often used in echogenic patients or in pediatric patients because, in these cases, blood flow tracings are often hard to obtain. The sampling site is in the pulmonic valve orifice near the pulmonary artery inflow tract.

Normal Tricuspid Flow

Tricuspid flow is measured in the same manner as mitral flow. The apical four-chamber view, the parasternal short-axis view at the level of the aortic valve, and the parasternal long-axis view can be used (Figures 10-15 and 10-16). The long-axis approach can be altered to visualize the tricuspid valve. The transducer is angled inferiorly from the standard parasternal long-axis approach. The right atrium, tricuspid valve, and right ventricle are visualized with blood flow parallel to the ultrasound beam (Figure 10-17). The sampling site is slightly distal to the tricuspid valve orifice near the right ventricular inflow tract. Normal tricuspid flow display resembles that of a mitral flow display since both are atrioventricular valves. Diastolic flow will be positive, indicating blood flow towards the transducer as the ventricle is filling. Systolic flow remains at the baseline as the valve closes (Figure 10-18).

(Text continues on page 259)

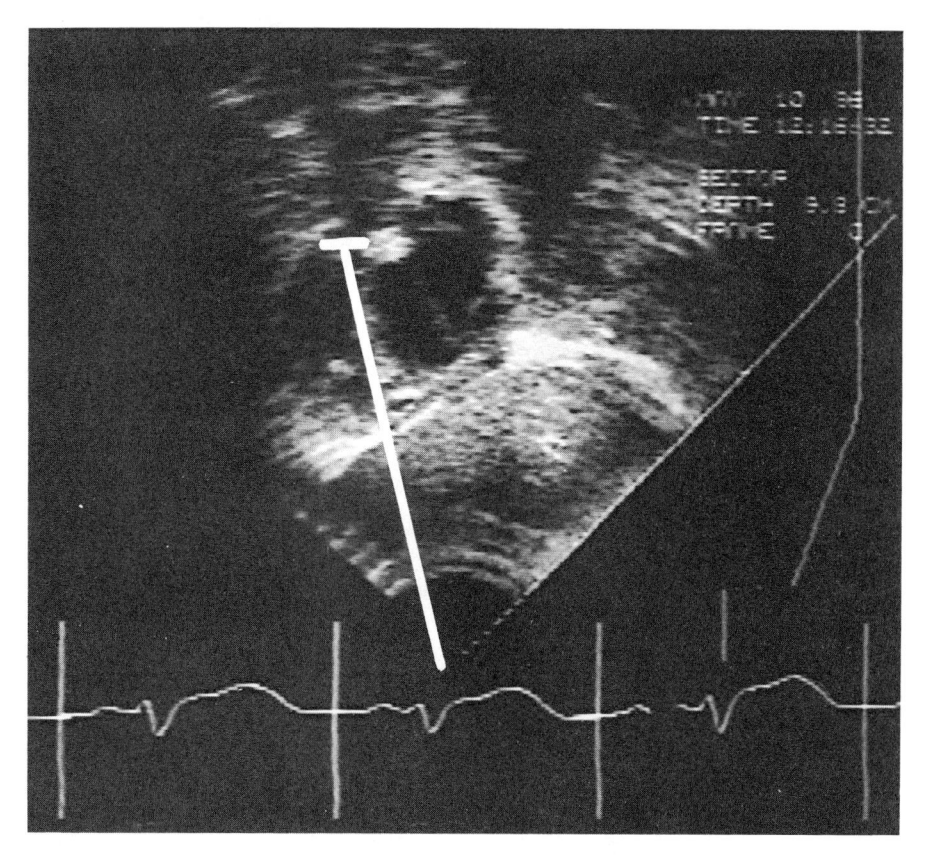

Figure 10-13 Subcostal approaches are often used when dealing with pediatric patients. If obtainable, evaluation from this approach helps supplement the pulmonic blood flow exam.

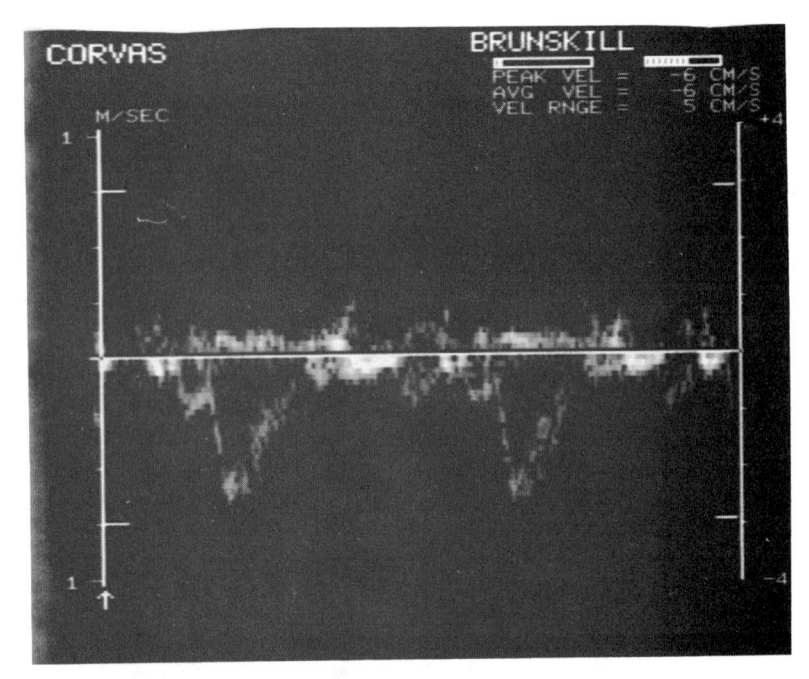

Figure 10-14 Normal pulmonic flow.

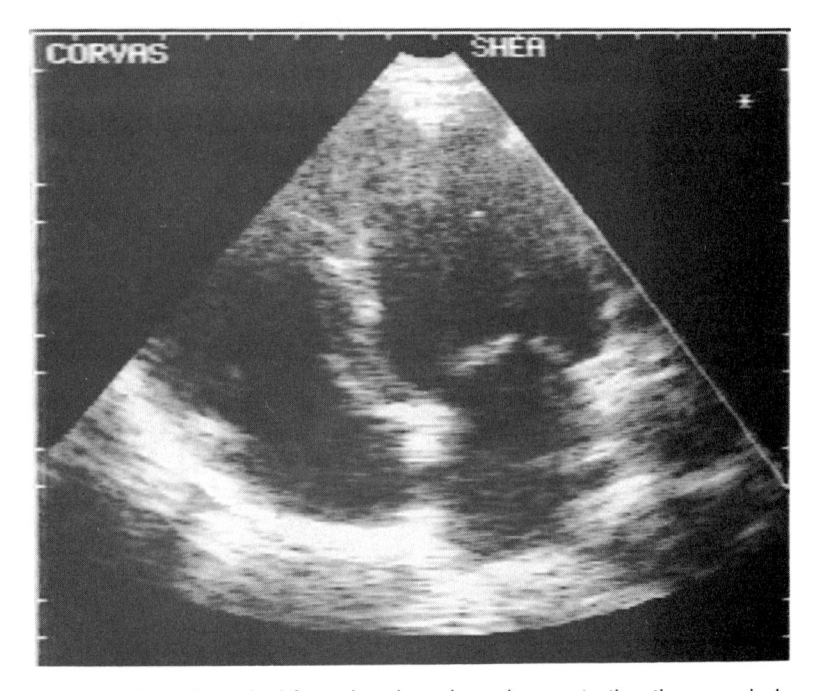

Figure 10-15 An apical four-chamber view, demonstrating the sampled area for the evaluation of tricuspid flow.

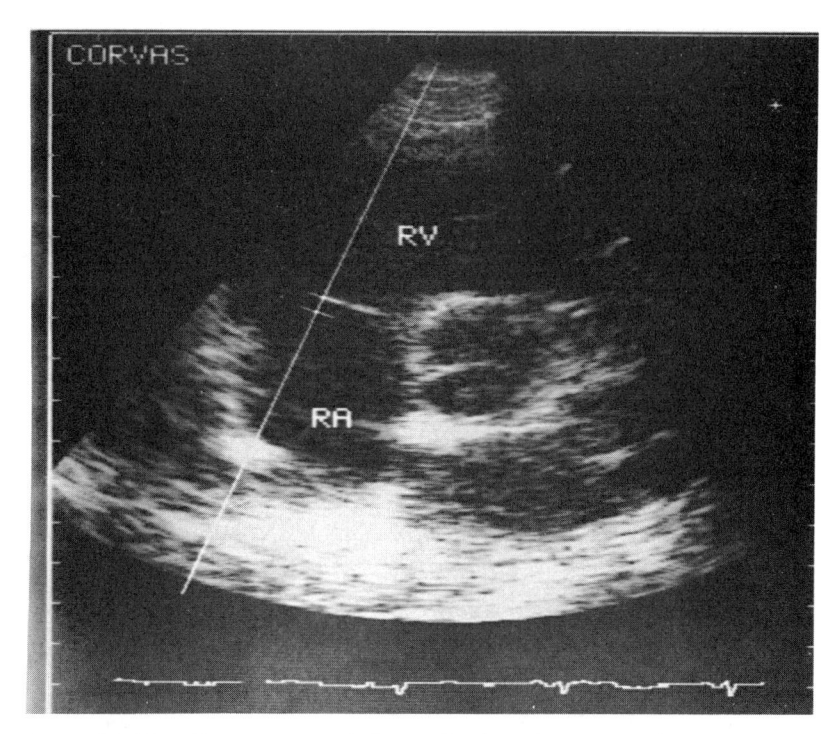

Figure 10-16 The parasternal short-axis view also is used for obtaining tricuspid flow.

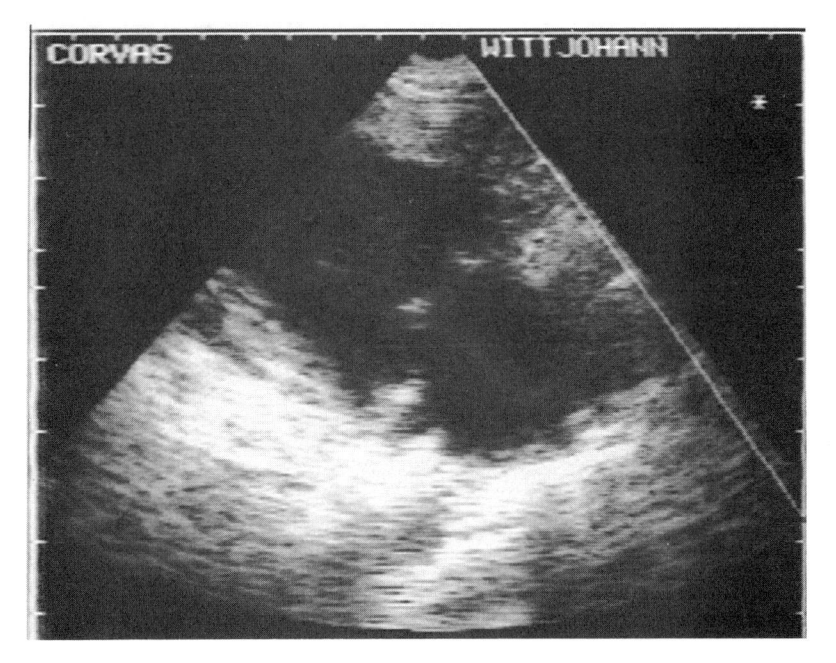

Figure 10-17 The parasternal long-axis approach is often hard to visualize, but is extremely useful when evaluating tricuspid flow.

258 Basic Doppler Echocardiography

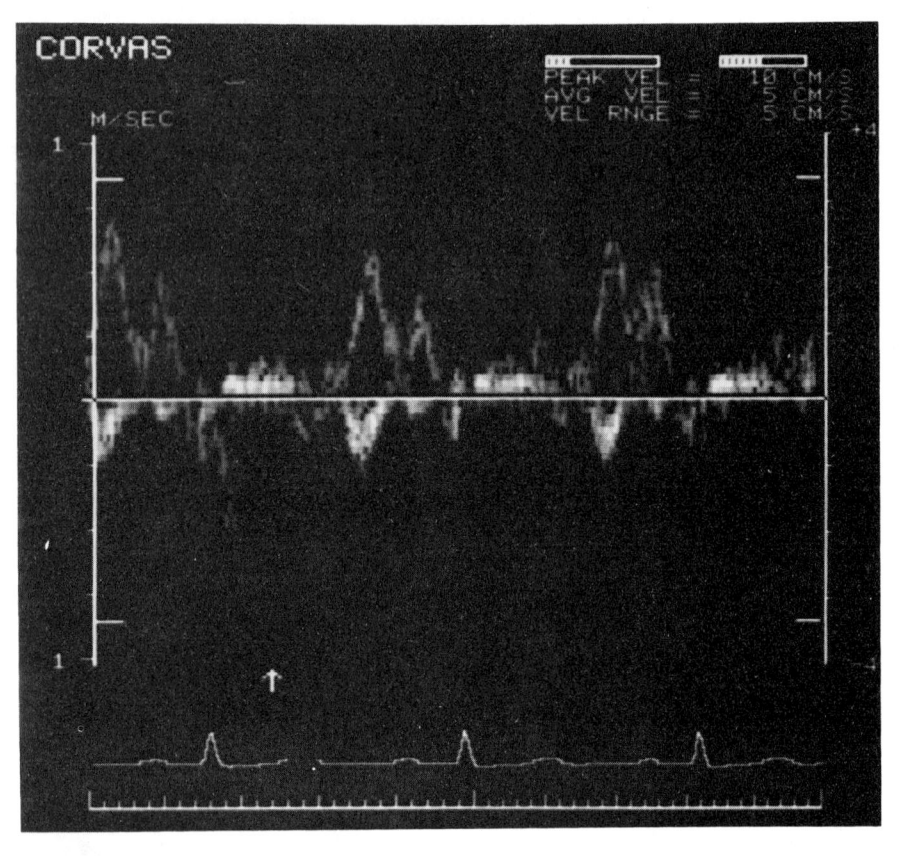

Figure 10-18 Normal tricuspid flow display.

Regurgitant Lesions

Regurgitant lesions and valvular areas/gradients can be detected by the Doppler principle. Using the previously described views and techniques, actual quantitation can be calculated. Regurgitant flow can be detected by placing the sample volume slightly beneath the valvular coaptation point. All cardiac valves can be evaluated for valvular regurgitations. The sampling sites for valvular regurgitations are described below.

Disease	Sampling Site	Views Used
Mitral regurgitation	Left atrium	Parasternal long-axis, apical four-chamber, apical 2-chamber
Tricuspid regurgitation	Right atrium	Parasternal short-axis, apical four-chamber, parasternal long-axis
Aortic insufficiency	Left ventricular outflow tract	Apical four-chamber, apical two-chamber
Pulmonic insufficiency	Right ventricle	Parasternal short-axis, parasternal long-axis

When evaluating for mitral regurgitation, the apical four-chamber and the apical two-chamber views are used. The sample volume is placed directly behind the mitral valve in the left atrium (Figures 10-19 and 10-20). The normal mitral flow was previously described, noting positive blood flow towards the transducer in diastole. If mitral regurgitation is present, a negative deflection in systole will result (Figure 10-21).

There may be aliasing if excessive flow is present. (See Basic Doppler Terminology, page 278). After locating a regurgitant jet, the sample volume is moved carefully around the valve leaflets and the orifice, then dropped back into the left atrium to see how far the jet is still detectable, thus quantitating the severity of aliasing. If the jet is detected deep into the atrium, this could signify moderate mitral regurgitation. The regurgitant jet may be only behind the anterior or the posterior leaflet, so thorough Doppler techniques must be applied. Careful evaluation of the valve must be made because small regurgitant jets can be missed easily. The audible detection of mitral regurgitation would sound like hands clapping, coinciding with the regurgitant jet in systole.

Tricuspid regurgitation can be detected in the same manner as mitral regurgitation. The apical four-chamber view, the parasternal short-axis view at the level of the aortic valve, and the parasternal long axis view can all be used (Figures 10-22 through 10-24). The sample volume is placed in the right atrium and the same techniques are applied. Once again, if tricuspid

(Text continues on page 263)

260 Basic Doppler Echocardiography

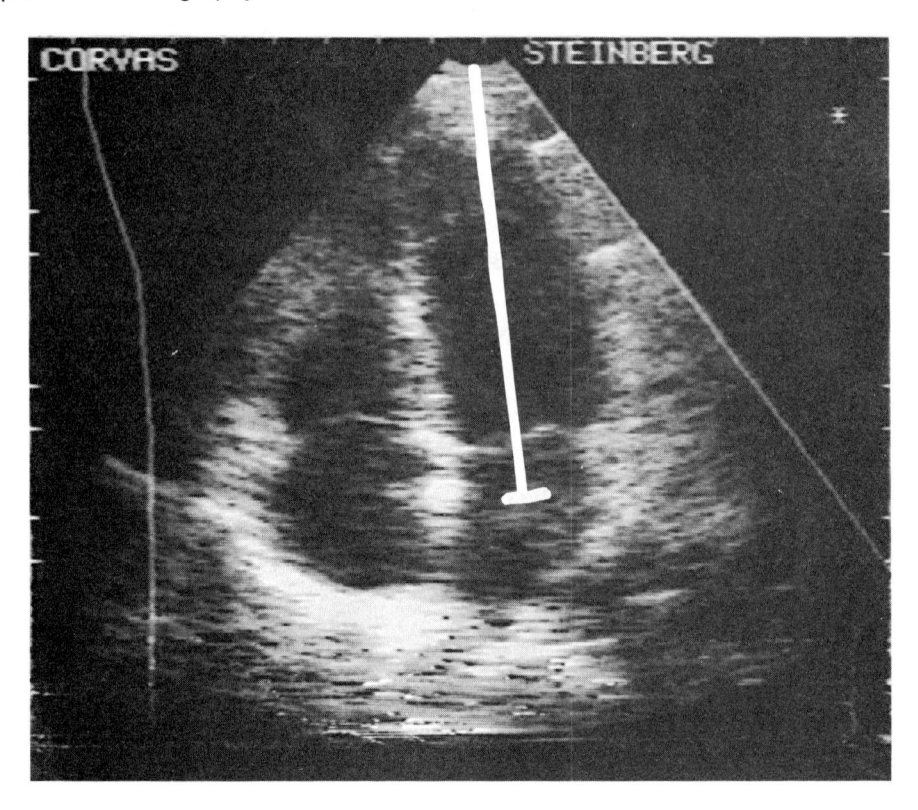

Figure 10-19 Apical four-chamber view demonstrating placement of the sample volume for mitral regurgitation.

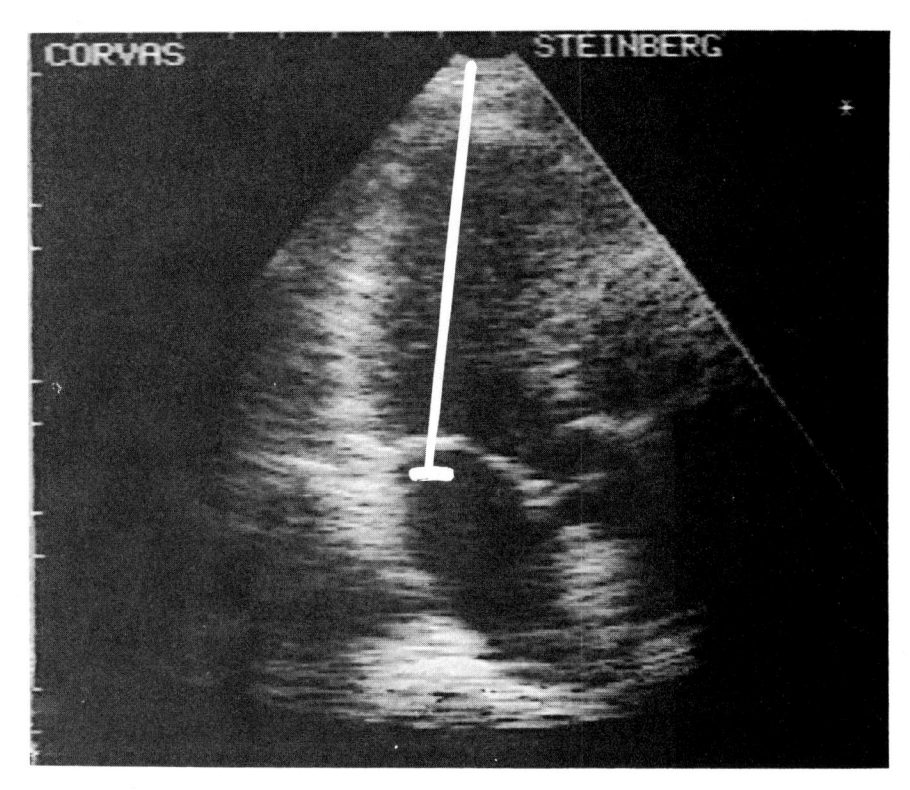

Figure 10-20 An apical two-chamber view for evaluation of mitral regurgitation.

normal mitral flow in diastole

regurgitant jet in systole

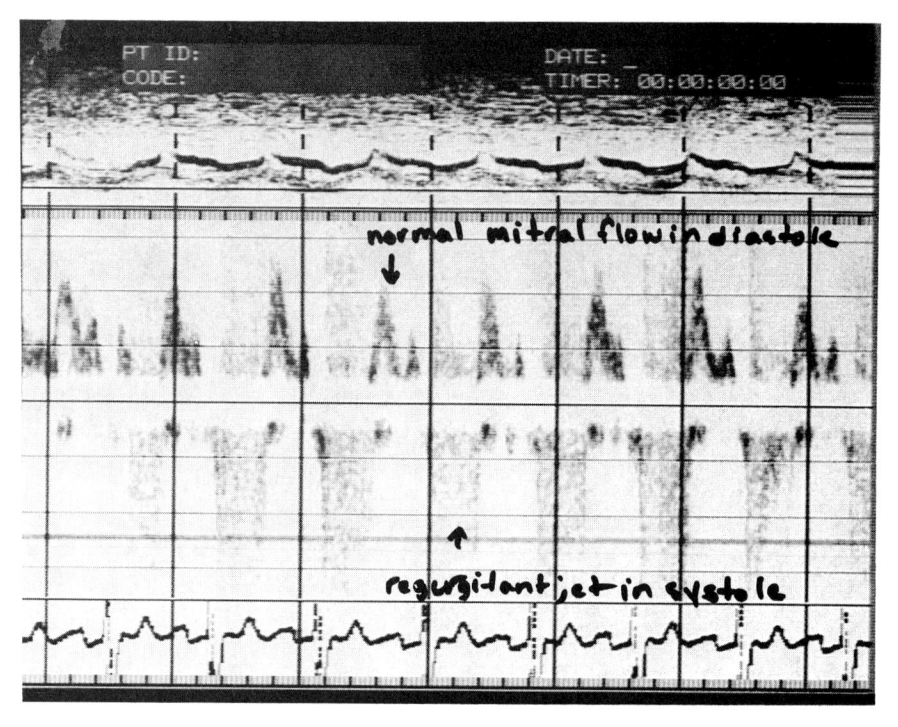

Figure 10-21 Spectral display of mitral regurgitation.

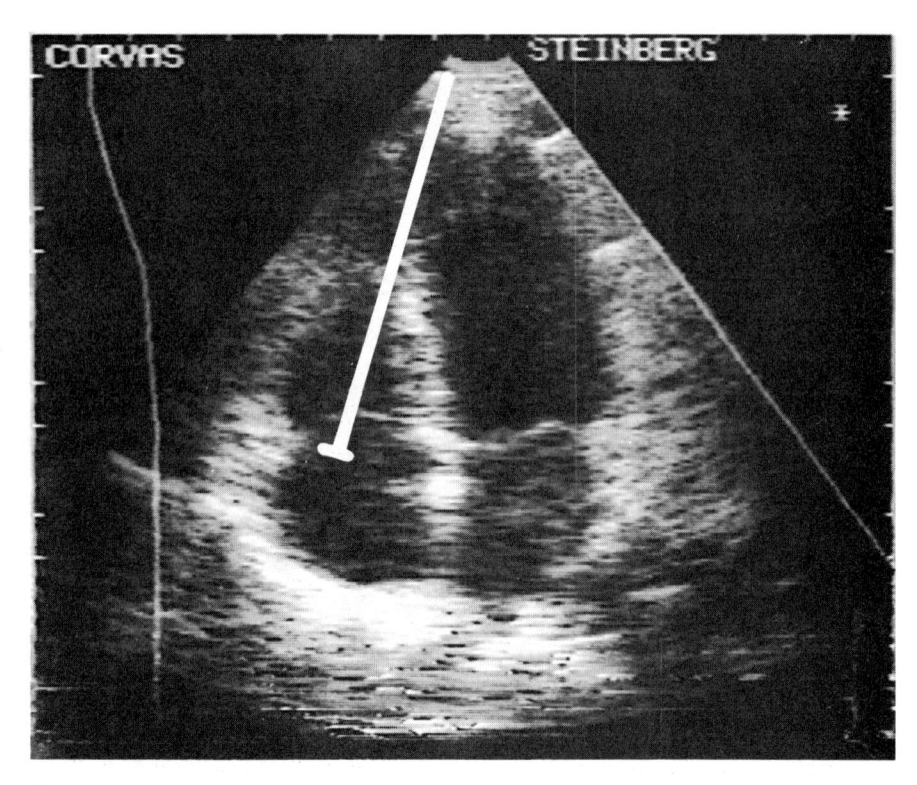

Figure 10-22 Apical four-chamber view for evaluating tricuspid regurgitation.

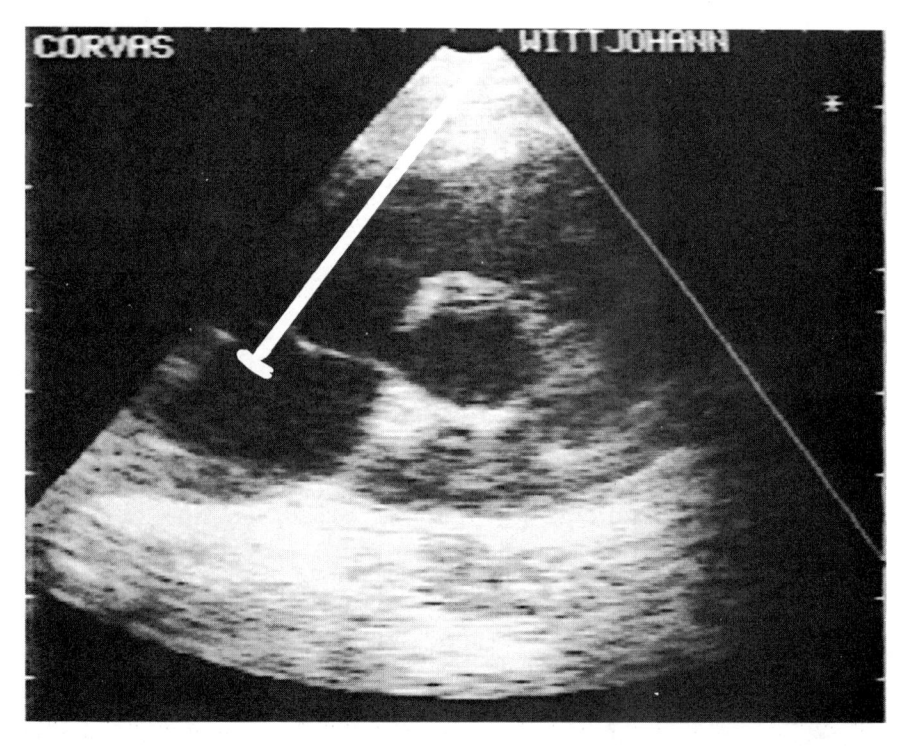

Figure 10-23 Parasternal short-axis view for the evaluation of tricuspid regurgitation.

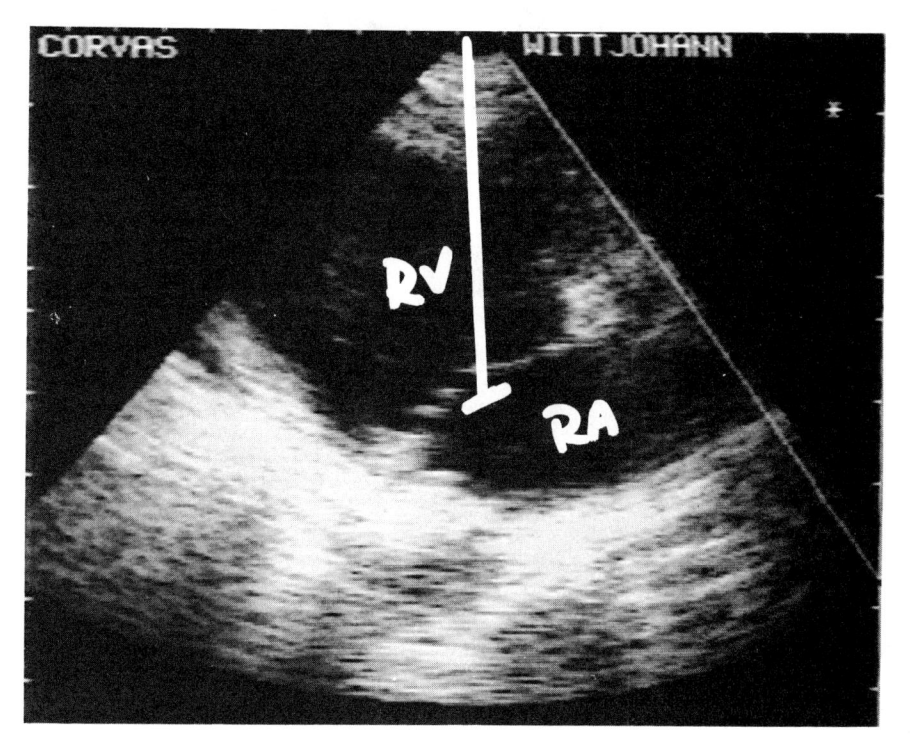

Figure 10-24 A variated parasternal long-axis view for the detection of tricuspid regurgitation.

regurgitation is present, the spectral display will depict normal positive diastolic flow with negative flow away from the transducer in systole, indicating a regurgitant jet (Figure 10-25).

When evaluating for aortic insufficiency, the apical five-chamber, or apical two-chamber view is used, placing the sample volume in the left ventricular outflow tract. Flow is normally from the left ventricle to the aortic valve, resulting in a negative deflection away from the transducer. If aortic insufficiency is present, the normal negative systolic aortic flow is present, with a positive diastolic display indicating a back flow of blood into the left ventricle towards the transducer (Figures 10-26 through 10-28).

The audible sound resulting from aortic regurgitation can be described as a low, harsh "wooshing" sound. Tracking the regurgitant lesion along the intraventricular septum can help quantitate the severity. If diastolic flow is seen far down along the septum, this could indicate severe aortic insufficiency.

Pulmonic insufficiency uses the parasternal short-axis view at the level of the aortic valve, or the parasternal long-axis view, placing the sample volume behind the pulmonic valve in the right ventricle. Blood flows nor-

(Text continues on page 266)

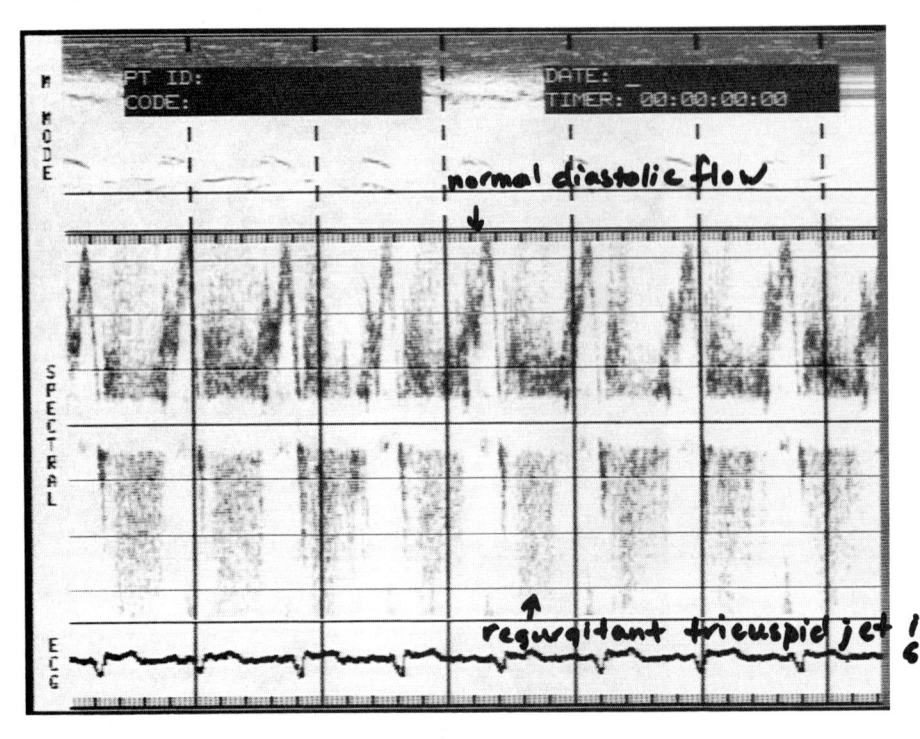

Figure 10-25 A spectral display of tricuspid regurgitation.

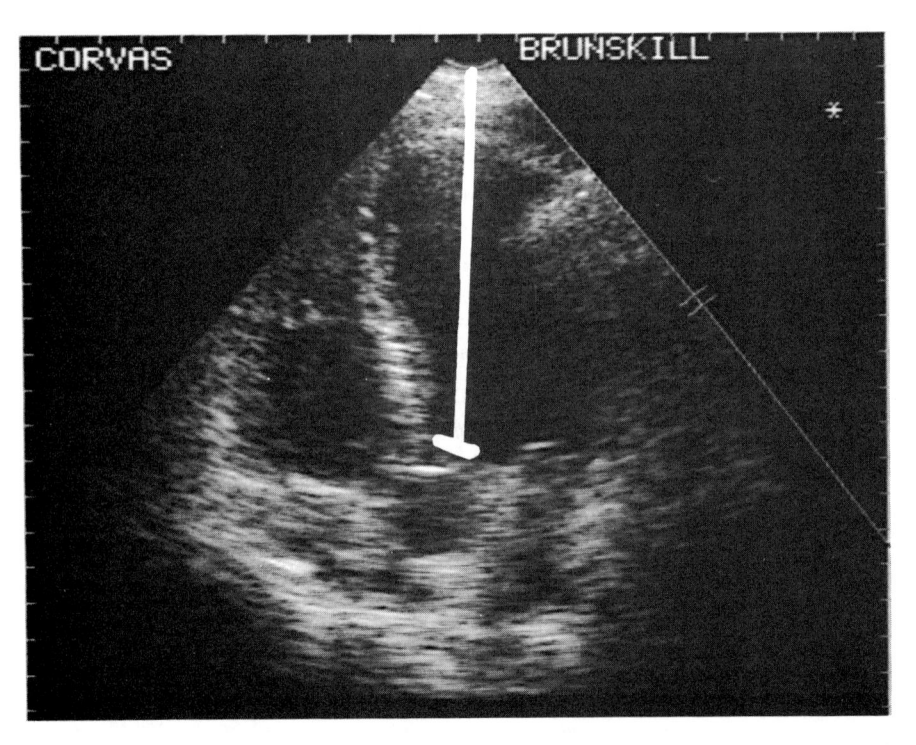

Figure 10-26 Apical four-chamber view with the left ventricular outflow tract used as the sampling site.

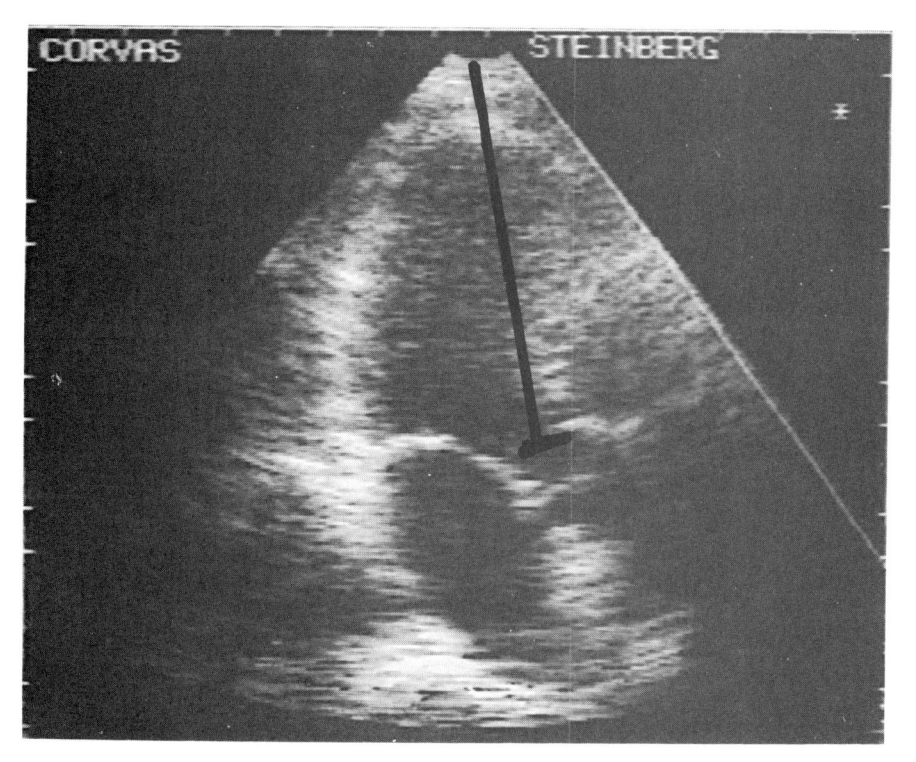

Figure 10-27 Apical two-chamber view with the sample volume placed in the left ventricular outflow tract.

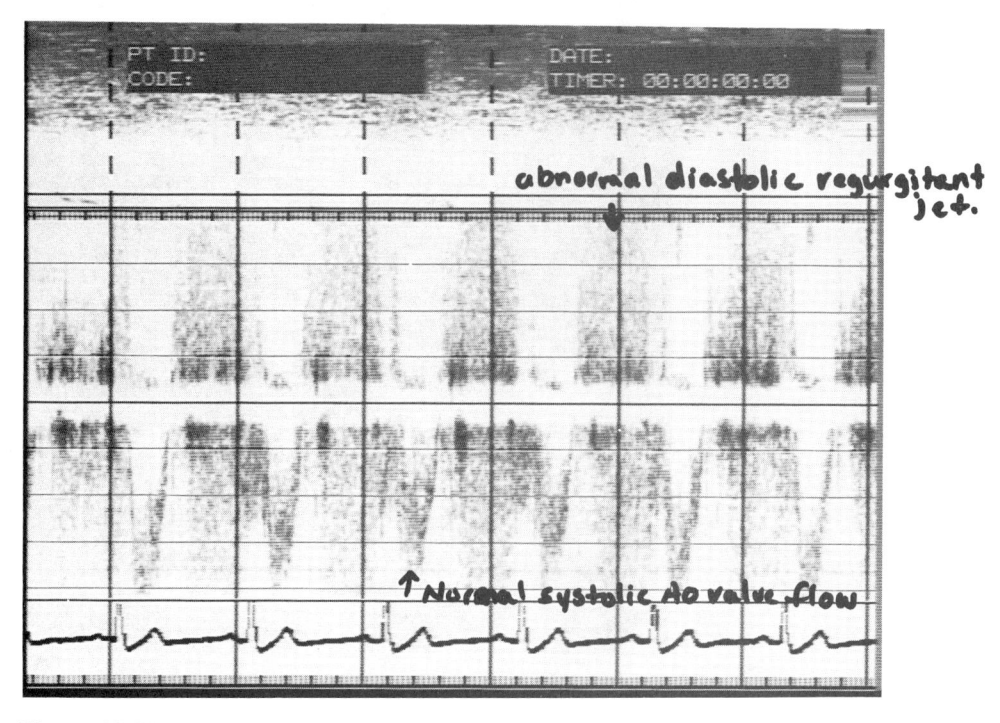

Figure 10-28 A spectral display of aortic insufficiency.

265

266 Basic Doppler Echocardiography

mally from the right ventricle to the pulmonary artery, resulting in a negative deflection in systole. If pulmonic insufficiency is present, one will see a positive spectral display in ventricular diastole, which would indicate valvular regurgitation, similar to that of aortic insufficiency (Figures 10-29 through 10-31).

Thorough searching and various views must be applied, in order to detect and quantitate regurgitant jets. Time and patience are the key factors when performing a Doppler exam.

Evaluating Valvular Stenosis

The cardiac Doppler can be used to evaluate and quantitate any valvular stenosis. The sampling site used for any valvular lesion is slightly distal to the actual valve, as previously described for the normal blood flow tracings. Various views and echo approaches must be applied for accurate results. Obtaining correct maximum velocities can be time consuming especially when dealing with severely stenotic valves, because of the narrowed orifice. As a result, high velocity flow tracings are displayed on the spectral image. The continuous wave or PRF Doppler systems help obtain peak maximum velocities. The standard pulsed Doppler systems have difficulties displaying

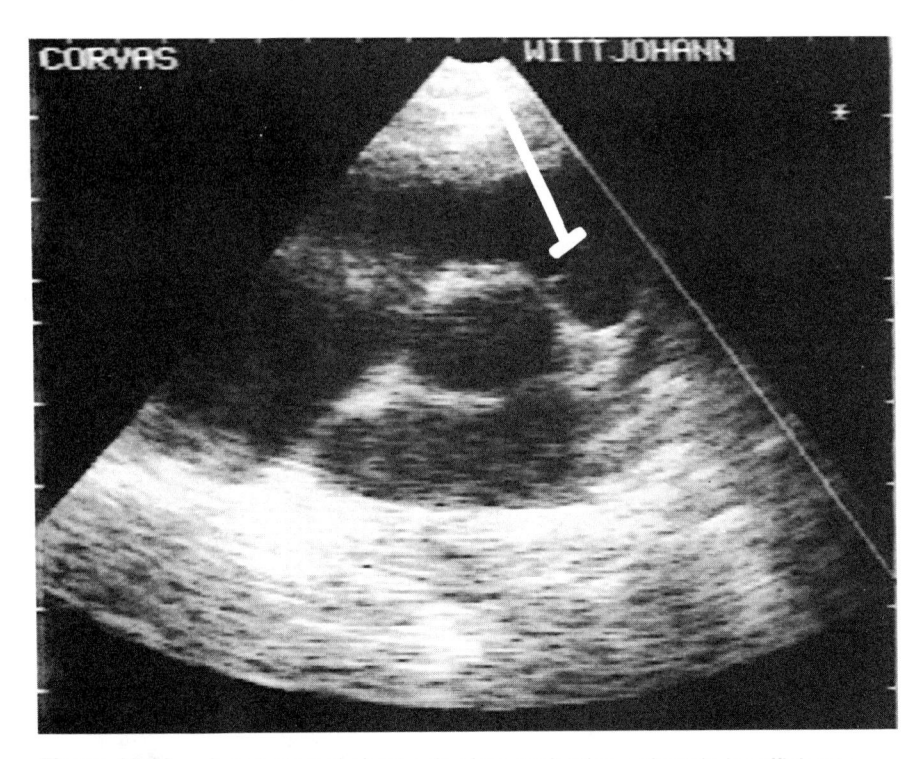

Figure 10-29 A parasternal short-axis view evaluating pulmonic insufficiency.

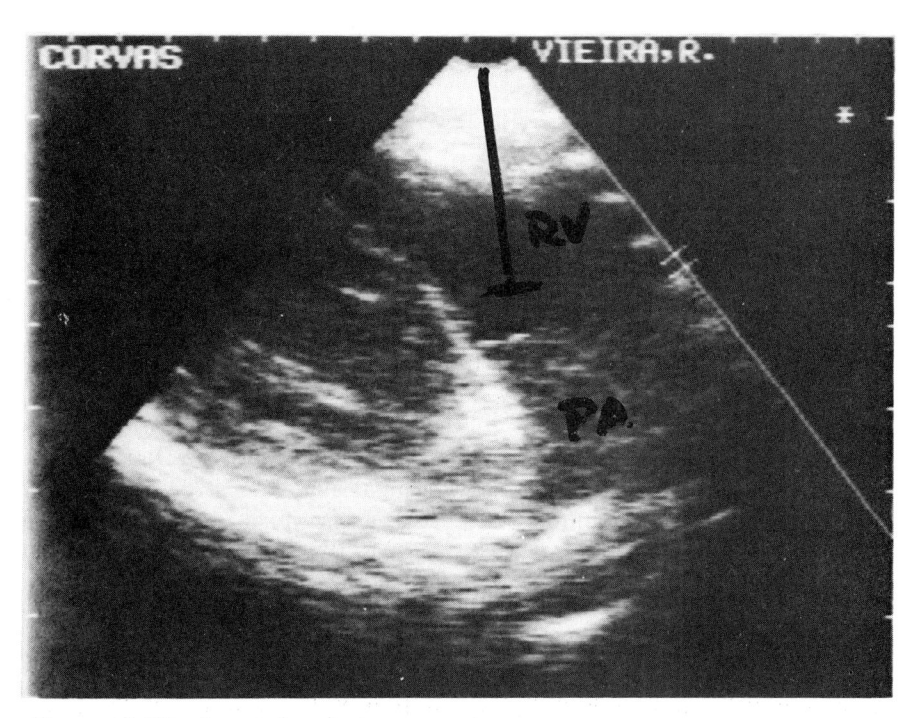

Figure 10-30 A variation of the parasternal long-axis view is used when evaluating pulmonic insufficiency.

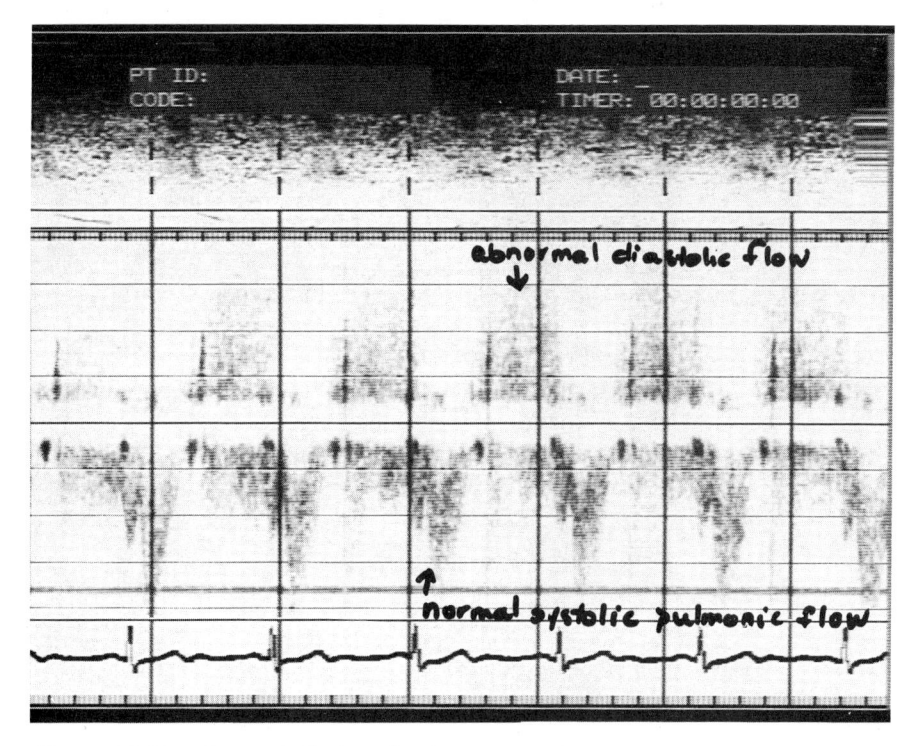

Figure 10-31 Spectral display of pulmonic insufficiency.

high velocity flow recordings. Aliasing may occur with the pulsed Doppler system.

Evaluating Aortic Stenosis

When evaluating aortic stenosis, the following views can be used: the apical five-chamber view, the apical two-chamber view, the suprasternal approach, or the high right parasternal approach. The sampling site is slightly distal to the valve orifice, almost in the ascending aorta. At times the aortic valve and ascending aorta are hard to visualize, making audible and visible display extremely important. The direction of blood flow will be reflected on the spectral display, which can help identify the vessel. All views should be used when trying to obtain the maximum "Doppler shift" in an aortic stenosis exam. Because of the narrowed orifice, the Doppler shift will be of a higher velocity. Various views and angles must be tried in a search for the maximum shift. An aortic stenosis signal is of high pitch intensity, in systole.

When apical views are used, the sampling site is just slightly distal to the valve, almost in the ascending aorta. The flow pattern will be negative, because blood flow is away from the transducer. The velocity will be much higher than a normal aortic valve flow tracing. Thorough searching for maximum Doppler shifts is essential for accurate calculations. The degree of stenosis is directly determined by the frequency of the Doppler shift. The more severe the stenosis, the higher the Doppler shift.

The suprasternal approach and the high right parasternal view are excellent for quantitating aortic valve gradients. When using the suprasternal view, the sampling site is distal to the valve, in the ascending aorta. A positive deflection will be displayed because blood flow is moving towards the transducer. Although this particular view is extremely accurate in obtaining a peak velocity (because blood flow is almost exactly parallel with the ultrasound Doppler beam), it is often hard to get good Doppler signals from this approach.

The high right parasternal approach is another view that is extremely accurate when searching for peak velocity flows. Visualization of the aortic valve and ascending aorta in this view are not always seen, so audible and spectral analysis must be evaluated. A positive deflection is seen on the spectral tracing, because blood flow is moving toward the transducer.

Maximum peak velocities are used when calculating gradients. As previously mentioned, all views should be used and thorough Doppler techniques should be taken. A heavily calcified or stenotic valve makes obtaining peak velocities difficult.

Evaluating Mitral Stenosis

Mitral stenosis can be calculated in the same manner as aortic stenosis; however, the sampling site is in the mitral valve orifice, slightly in the left ventricular cavity. The sample volume is placed within the opening excursion in diastole. Valve areas are quantitated in cm². The apical four-chamber or apical two-chamber view is used to obtain these tracings. When mitral stenosis is present, the tracing obtained resembles that of an m-mode of mitral stenosis. The paper speed is usually switched to 100 m/sec for ease of measurements. The zero baseline is generally moved to the bottom of the spectral display, so full tracings can be recorded. Thorough searching is essential for clear tracings with the highest velocity peaks (Figure 10-32). The formula shown in Figure 10-33 can be utilized to obtain a mitral valve area.

Evaluating Pulmonic and Tricuspid Stenosis

Pulmonic valve gradients are calculated in the same manner as the aortic valve gradients. The gradient obtained is measured in mm Hg. Three views are generally used when evaluating pulmonic stenosis: the parasternal long-axis view, parasternal short-axis view, and the subcostal approach. The sample volume is located in the pulmonary artery inflow tract, in the pulmonic valve leaflet orifice (in systole).

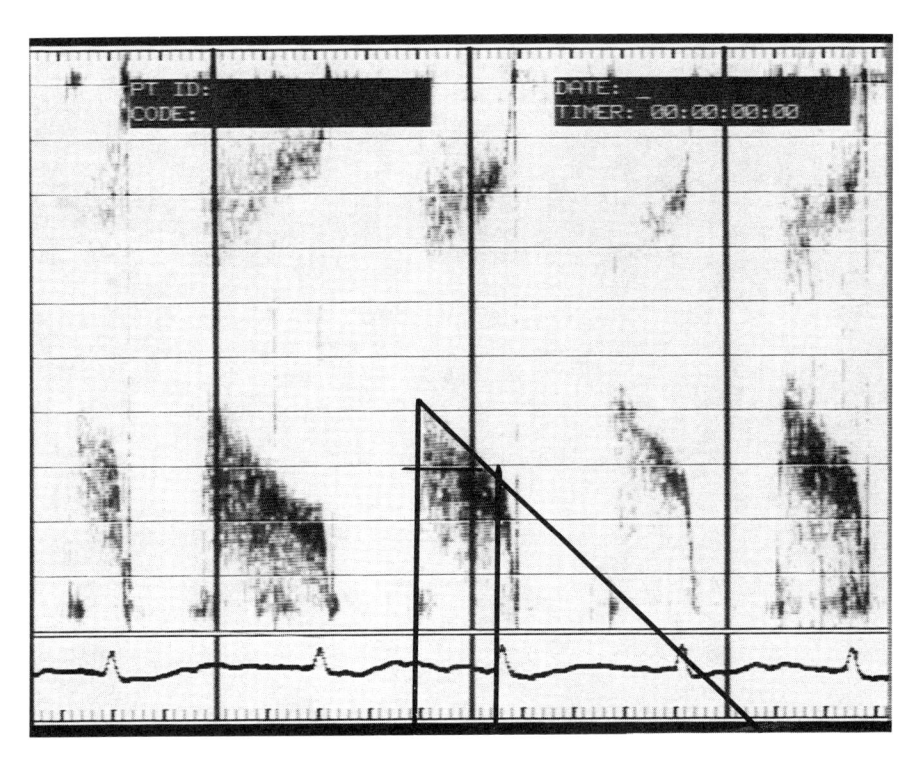

Figure 10-32 An example of a mitral stenosis tracing with the zero baseline shifted to the bottom of the spectral display and the paper speed at 100 m/sec. By following the pressure half-time formula, mitral valve areas can be calculated.

270 Basic Doppler Echocardiography

MITRAL VALVE AREA
Pressure Half-Time

$$\text{MVA (cm}^2) = \frac{220}{\text{pressure half-time}}$$

Pressure half time = Time (milliseconds) from peak pressure to one-half peak pressure.

Once an image representing blood flow through the mitral valve orifice has been obtained, the following formula can be applied. This tracing should be recorded at a paper speed of 50 and, even more preferable, at a speed of 100. The image should also arise from the bottom of the strip chart for easier calculations.

Simplified Formula

1. Draw a vertical line from the peak of the curve down to the time markers.
2. Next, draw a line from the peak of the curve to the initial downslope, again reaching the time markers.
3. Measure the distance (in mm) of the vertical line first drawn. Once this number has been obtained, divide this number by $\sqrt{2}$ or 1.4 (a constant)

$$\frac{52 \text{ mm}}{1.4} = 37.1$$

4. Mark this distance in mm on the first vertical line drawn. Measure up from the time markers.
5. Draw a horizontal line from the mark made in Step 4 across to the slope drawn in Step 2.
6. Drop a vertical line down to the time markers from the horizontal line drawn in Step 5.
7. Measure the distance from the line drawn in Step one to the vertical line drawn in Step 6. (Use the time markers.) Each small mark represents 40 milliseconds. Multiply the distance × 40

$$8 \times 40 = 320$$

8. Divide this number into 220

$$\frac{220}{320} = .68 \text{ cm}^2$$

Figure 10-33   Mitral valve pressure half-time calculates mitral valve areas in cm^2.

Calculating tricuspid stenosis has not been fully studied. Sampling the right ventricular inflow tract, slightly distal to the tricuspid valve, will give a tricuspid flow display. Evaluation of the maximum velocity can indicate the severity of the stenosis. The apical four-chamber view, parasternal short-axis view at the level of the aortic valve, and the modified parasternal long-axis view can all be used. The pressure half-time formula is not ideally used for tricuspid stenosis. Merely obtaining the maximum peak velocity has been the method used to evaluate tricuspid stenosis.

Stenotic valves can be evaluated in terms of the degree of severity. The numbers obtained by the cardiac Doppler (velocity or pressure gradients) can be utilized to detect the actual degree of obstruction or severity of the disease (Table 10-2).

Calculating Gradients

Pressure gradients are calculated for valvular stenosis, in particular for pulmonic and aortic stenosis. An actual pressure gradient in mm Hg is derived. First, a peak maximum velocity must be obtained. Thorough searching and scanning from different windows should be attempted before

Table 10-2

Stenotic Valve Obstruction (Severity of Disease)

Disease State	Mild	Moderate	Severe
Aortic Stenosis			
Peak Systolic:			
Velocity (m/sec)	1.0–2.7	2.7–4.0	>4.0
Pressure Gradient			
(mm Hg)	0–30	30–60	>60
Mitral Stenosis			
Mean Diastolic:			
Velocity (m/sec)	1.0–1.6	1.7–2.3	>2.3
Pressure Gradient			
(mm Hg)	4–10	11–20	>20
Pulmonic Stenosis			
Peak Systolic:			
Velocity (m/sec)	1.0–2.7	2.7–4.0	>4.0
Pressure Gradient			
(mm Hg)	5–30	30–60	>60
Tricuspid Stenosis			
Mean Diastolic:			
Velocity (m/sec)	.7–1.2	1.3–1.7	>1.7
Pressure Gradient			
(mm Hg)	2–6	7–12	>1.7

a maximum velocity is determined. Post arrhythmias and extra heart beats produce higher velocities and should not be used.

The formula used to calculate pressure gradients is: pressure gradient $= 4V^2$. Velocity is derived directly off the spectral display and is measured in m/sec. As mentioned, some Doppler instruments measure Doppler shifts in kHz, which have to be converted to m/sec. Once velocity has been determined, in m/sec, the above formula can now be applied (Figures 10-34A and 10-34B).

The corrected angle must be applied if blood flow is not parallel with the ultrasound beam. Most machines have the capability of correcting the angle by means of a software package within the system.

Evaluating Ventricular Septal Defects

Large ventricular septal defects (VSD's) can be detected by the two-dimensional echocardiogram, but small VSD's or pinhole VSD's are not easily seen. The cardiac Doppler not only can detect a VSD but actually

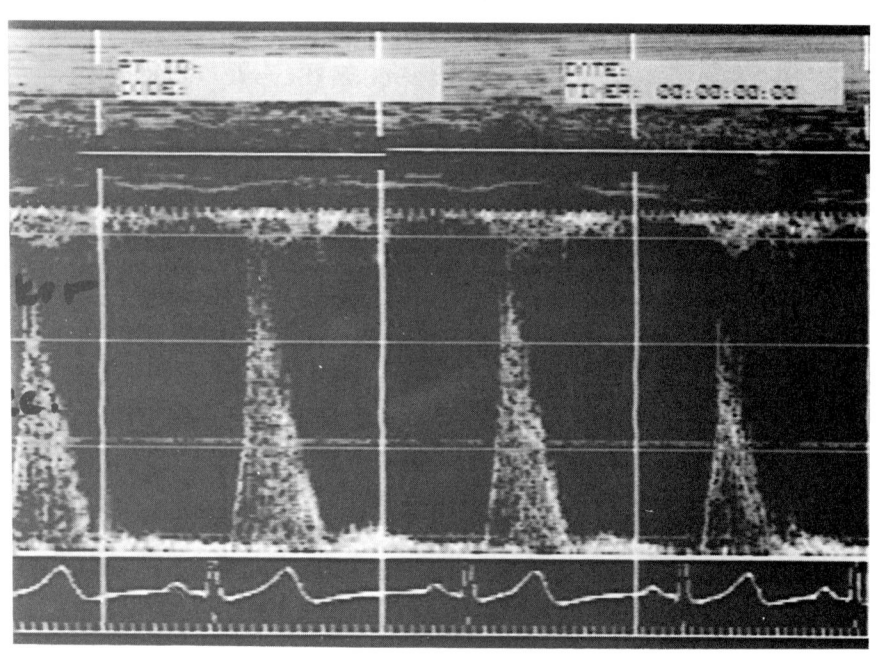

Aortic valve flow tracing consistent with mild aortic stenosis

Each cal marker is $= 4(V^2)$ to 1 m/sec

1. Peak flow velocity $= 2.5$ m/sec
2. $(2.5)^2 = 6.25$
3. $4(6.25) = 2.5$ mmHg

Figure 10-34a Pressure gradients in mm Hg use the following formula: $4V^2$.

Velocity (m/sec)	Pressure mmHg
1.5	9
1.6	10
1.7	11.5
1.8	13
1.9	14.5
2.0	16
2.1	18
2.2	19.5
2.3	21
2.4	23
2.5	25
2.6	27
2.7	29
2.8	31
2.9	34
3.0	36
3.1	38
3.2	41
3.3	44
3.4	46
3.5	49
3.6	51
3.7	55
3.8	58
3.9	61
4.0	64
4.1	67
4.2	72
4.3	74
4.4	77
4.5	81
4.6	85
4.7	88
4.8	92
4.9	96
5.0	100

Figure 10-34b Velocity conversions from mm/sec and actual pressure gradients are calculated.

274 Basic Doppler Echocardiography

locates the area of the defect. An isolated, noncomplicated VSD produces a left-to-right shunt, because of the higher pressure system of the left heart. When evaluating for a VSD, the sample volume is placed in the right ventricle and thorough sampling along the intraventricular septum and around the aortic valve is performed. The parasternal long-axis view, the apical four- and apical five-chamber views, and the subcostal four-chamber approach can all be used for the detection of a VSD (Figures 10-35 through 10-37). When Dopplering from the apical approach, detection of a VSD may be somewhat more difficult because the transducer is almost perpendicular to the jet, but flow disturbance can be found. The Doppler views used to detect a VSD are basically the same as a two-dimensional exam for a VSD. The spectal and audible signal that occurs when a VSD has been located is a high-pitched, high-velocity signal in systole. Small VSD's will create high-velocity flow, because of the greater pressure differences between the right and left ventricle. Large VSD's will create smaller velocity flows. Small and pinhole VSD's are often harder to detect, so thorough searching is necessary.

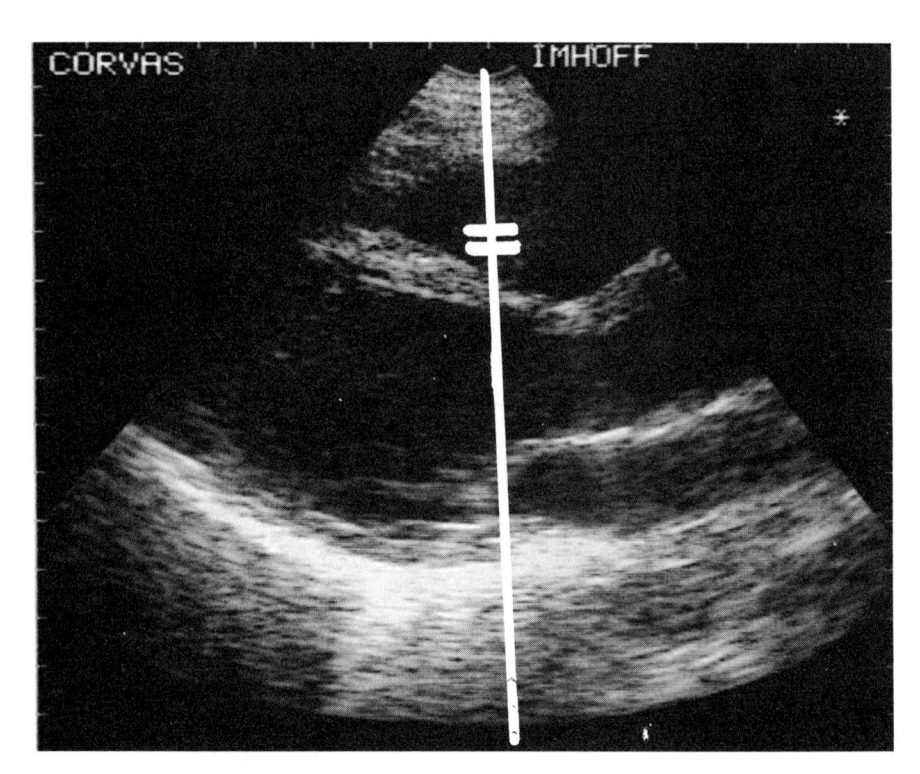

Figure 10-35   A parasternal long-axis view is used to detect VSD's. The sample volume is placed in the right ventricle.

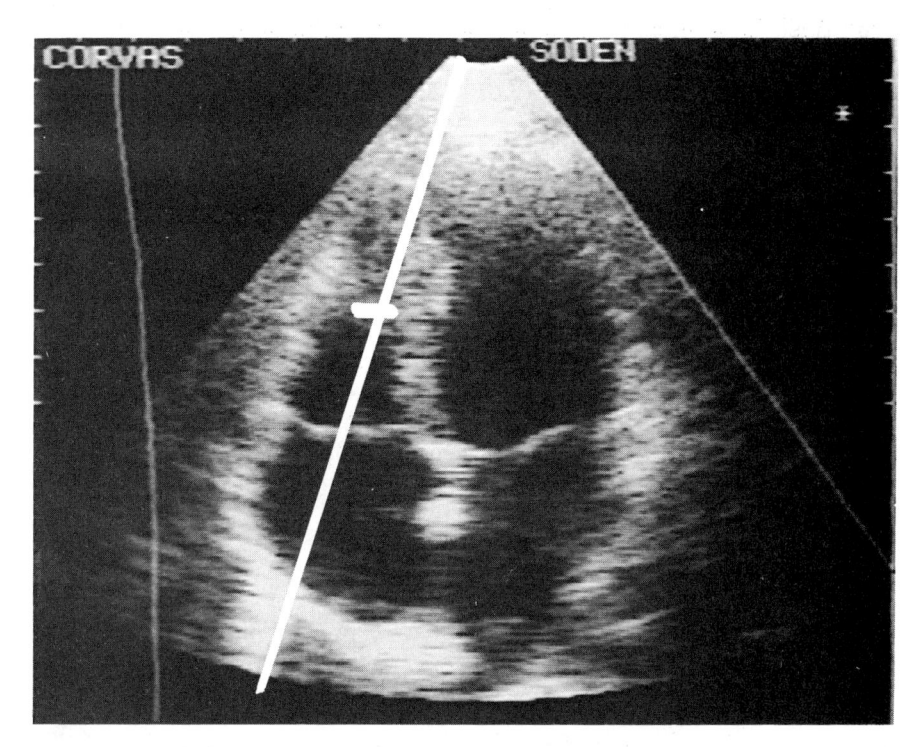

Figure 10-36 Apical four-chamber view for the evaluation of a VSD.

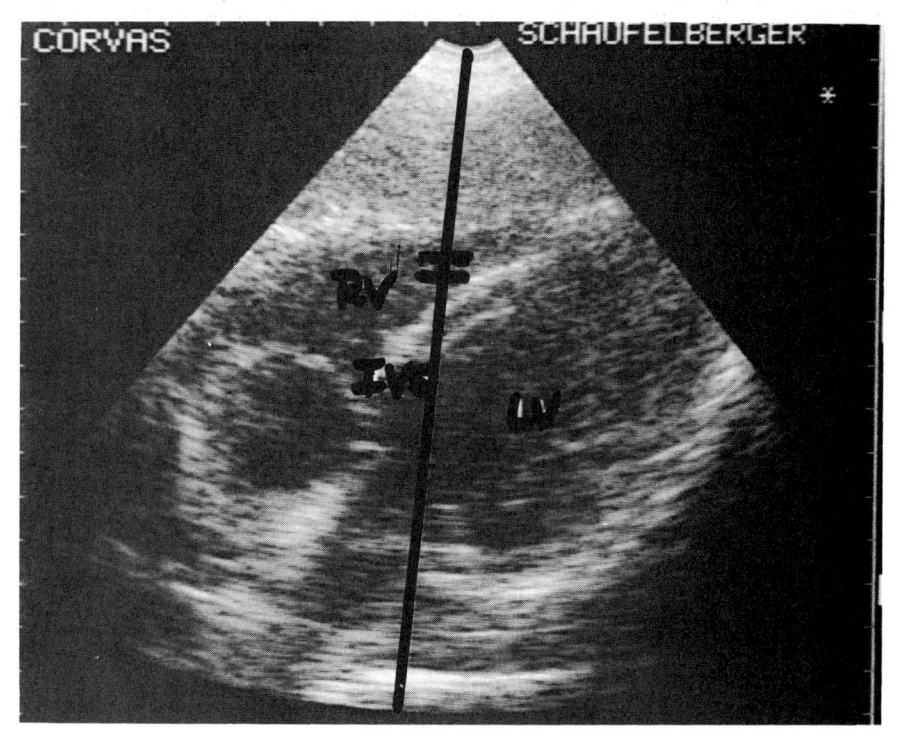

Figure 10-37 Subcostal approach demonstrating the sampled area for evaluating VSD.

Evaluating Atrial Septal Defects

Noncomplicated atrial septal defects (ASD's) can be evaluated with the cardiac Doppler. The technique used when examining for an ASD is the same as for a VSD. The intra-atrial septum is Dopplered, placing the sample volume in the right atrium, scanning the entire intra-atrial septum. The apical four-chamber view, the parasternal short-axis view at the level of the aortic valve, and, most ideally, the subcostal four-chamber view can all be used (Figures 10-38 through 10-40).

It is often difficult to obtain a subcostal four-chamber view in adults, so subsequent views must be used. The sample volume should be as perpendicular to the atrial septum as possible. Generally, the Doppler findings associated with ASD's are high-pitched audible signals with several spectral peaks (usually two or three). The largest occurs in systole, which is usually followed by a smaller one, with a broad peak, in systole.

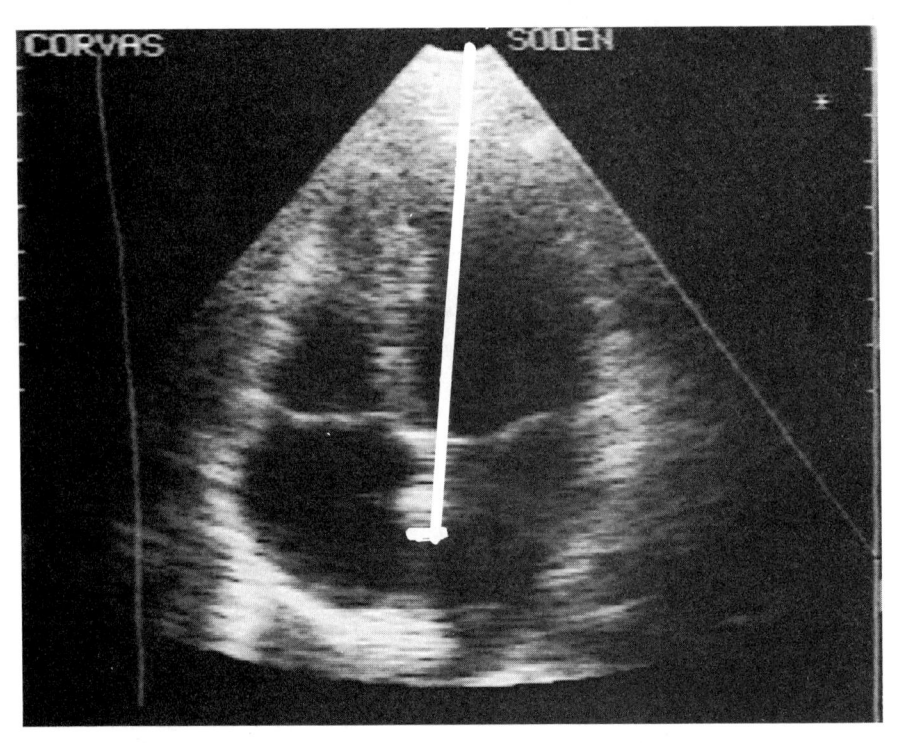

Figure 10-38 Apical four-chamber view demonstrates the sample volume placed in the right atrium.

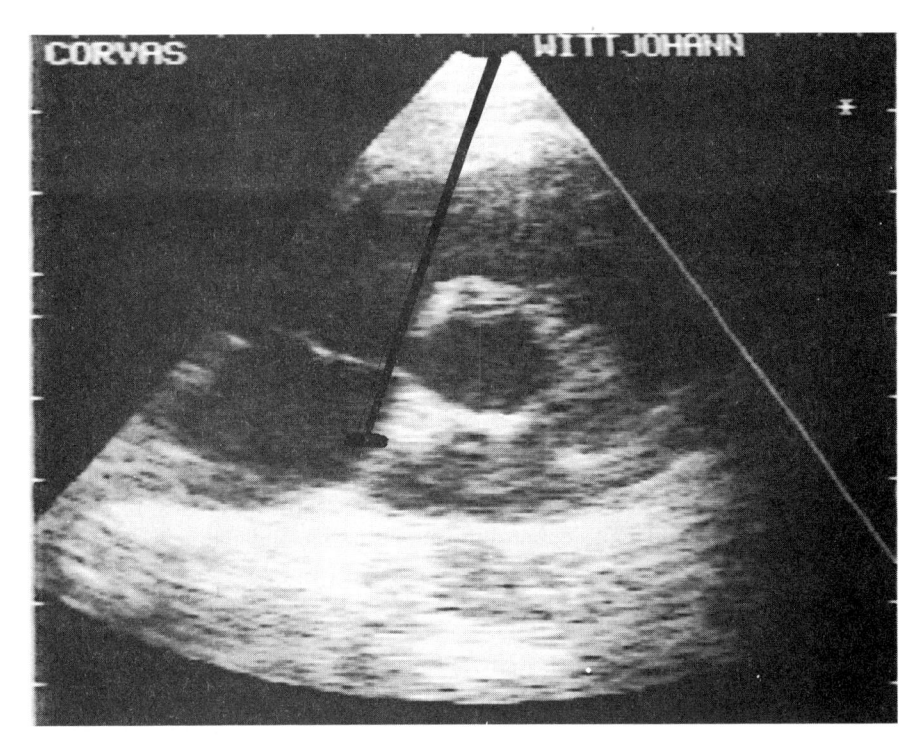

Figure 10-39 Parasternal short-axis view can be used to evaluate an ASD.

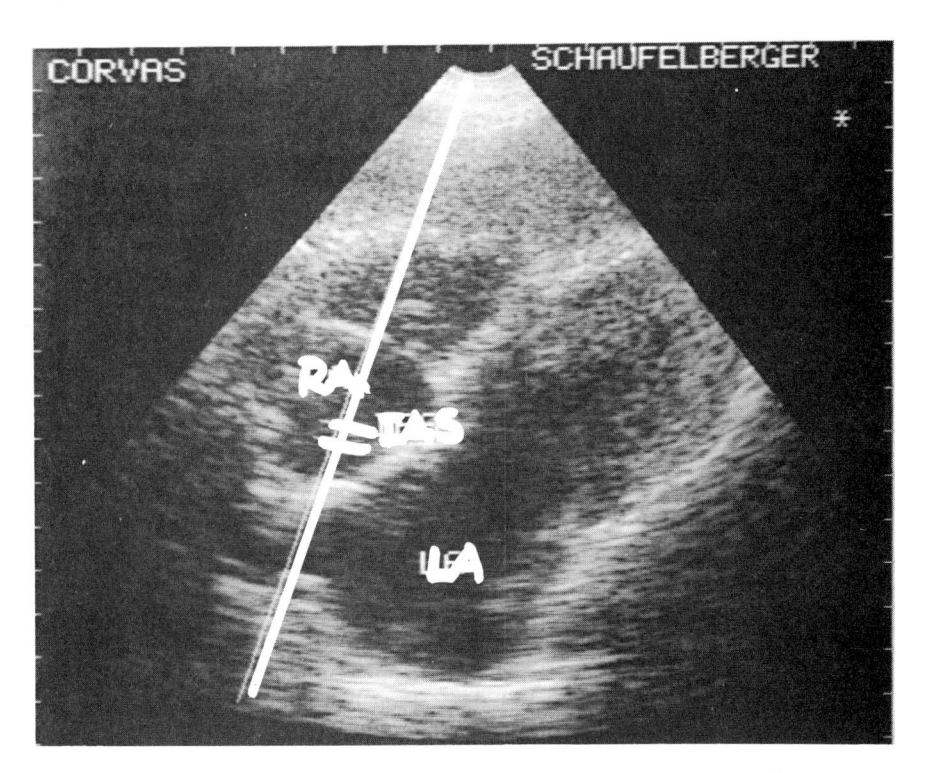

Figure 10-40 The subcostal approach demonstrates how the right atrium is sampled for an ASD.

278 Basic Doppler Echocardiography

Other Uses of Cardiac Doppler

A number of other uses of the cardiac Doppler that are gaining acceptance in research centers include calculating pulmonary artery pressure, determining cardiac outputs, and detecting outflow tract abnormalities. Reliable and reproduceable estimates of pulmonary artery pressures can be performed by analyzing tricuspid regurgitation displays. Cardiac outputs can be estimated by measurements of aortic valve flow and aortic root dimensions. Left ventricular outflow abnormalities and, in particular, obstructive hypertrophic cardiomyopathy can be quantitated by analyzing spectral displays from the left ventricular outflow tract.

Color-flow Doppler imaging has recently been developed with present two-dimensional format of intracardiac flow patterns. Spacial relationships of these flow patterns can be useful in determining regurgitant jets, atrial and ventricular shunting patterns, and analysis of wall motion abnormalities.

Basic Doppler Terminology

Aliasing: (Usually associated with Pulsed Doppler). If the velocity exceeds the maximum limit, the signals appear to reverse direction. The peak of the velocity wraps around the graph in the wrong direction. Sampling a signal too slowly makes the high-frequency components of that signal impersonate lower frequencies.

Artifact: A signal that appears in the normal signal mix from tissues but that does not have an anatomical correlate in the tissues. Artifacts can come from reverberations, multipath reflections, external noise, and maladjusted equipment.

Calibration Markers: Usually located on the side of the spectral display, the calibration markers represent velocity in kHz or m/sec, depending on the unit used. The value of each cal marker depends on the range and depth of the velocity.

Hertz: A unit of frequency equal to one cycle per second.

Pulsed Repetition Rate: Depends upon the transmission of a burst of energy and the reception of returning echoes. The number of times per second that transmit-receive cycles occur is the pulse repetition frequency (PRF).

Velocity: Blood flow velocity is directly proportional to the Doppler Shift and is expressed by the following formula:

$$V = \frac{C \pm \Delta f}{2 f^0 \cos 0}$$

V = Blood flow velocity in m/sec
C = Speed of tissue that is approximately 1540 m/sec
± Δf = Doppler shift frequency in Hertz
f^0 = Transmitted frequency of the scanhead in Hertz
Cos 0 = Cosine function of the angle between the ultrasound beam and the blood flow vector

Zero-Shifting: The zero-shift display moves the baseline to the bottom or the top of the display. This can help when limited Doppler shifts are obtained and aliasing occurs. By zero-shifting, the maximum frequency display limits are doubled in either direction.

Chapter 11

Cardiac Catheterization

Linda Humston

Cardiac catheterization is the technique in which small tubes called *catheters* are passed through an artery and/or vein to measure oxygen levels and pressures in the heart. As catheters are moved through the heart and major vessels, pressures are measured from the catheter tip and a permanent pressure tracing is recorded. Blood samples are drawn through the catheter to measure oxygen saturation. Angiograms can then be performed by injecting dye through the catheter and filming its flow through the heart and major vessels. This allows the cardiologist to view the patient's cardiac anatomy.

Data collected at catheterization can be used to calculate cardiac output, shunts (abnormal blood flow), valve areas, resistance, stroke volume, and ejection fraction. Based on angiograms and hemodynamic calculations, the patient may be referred for open heart surgery or treated medically.

The concept of passing a catheter through the venous system into the right heart was developed in 1929 by Werner Forssmann of Eberswald, Germany. He was looking for a means of injecting drugs for cardiac resuscitation and other grave medical situations. When forbidden to study a patient, Dr. Forssmann skillfully tricked a nurse into assisting while he performed the first right heart catheterization on himself!

Following Dr. Forssmann's experiment, research continued at a slow pace until the war years following 1940. Treatment of shock became a major concern and researchers began seeking a way to perform hemodynamic studies using a catheter. In the early 1940's, papers were published on pressures in the right heart and pulmonary artery, determination of cardiac output in man, normal standards for cardiac output, and the effect of intravascular infusions and bleeding. In 1945, the first congenital cardiac anomaly, an atrial septal defect, was identified at catheterization. The first left heart catheterization was not performed until 1950.

Since that time, the field of invasive cardiology has virtually exploded. Catheters are used now for monitoring, diagnosis and, in some cases, actual treatment of cardiovascular diseases.

Catheterization: A Diagnostic Tool

Since its development, cardiac catheterization has been accepted as the "gold standard" for diagnosing cardiovascular problems. Although new non-invasive tests are continually being developed, there is still no single test that can provide as much information as catheterization. Cardiac catheterization remains the only way to measure intracardiac pressures. Surgeons will rarely consider performing open heart surgery without the availability of catheterization data.

Catheterization: A Therapeutic Tool

Cardiac catheterization is no longer used merely as a diagnostic tool. Through the development of new catheters and techniques, some cardiac problems that previously required open heart surgery can now be treated successfully in the catheterization laboratory. Listed below are procedures currently being performed or developed using catheters.

Swan-Ganz Catheterization. A monitoring catheter is placed in the right or left pulmonary artery to monitor pulmonary wedge pressure. Using the same catheter, cardiac output can be measured by thermodilution technique and the data can be used to control medication and fluid levels in the critically ill patient.

Rashkind Balloon Atrial Septostomy. A septostomy catheter is used to create an opening between the two atria in neonates with transposition of the great arteries. Before this technique was developed, most neonates with transposition died shortly after birth.

Cardiac Biopsy. A catheter with biopsy forceps is passed into the right or left ventricle and tissue samples are taken. This is performed frequently in heart transplant patients to detect early signs of rejection.

Coronary Artery Angioplasty. The angioplasty catheter can be advanced across an area of partial obstruction. Its balloon is then inflated to a pressure high enough to break the plaque causing obstruction and force it into the vessel wall. This procedure is proving highly successful.

Angioplasty for Pulmonary Artery Stenosis and Coarctation. An angioplasty catheter can be advanced across the narrowed area and inflated to a pressure high enough to break the band of tissue obstructing blood flow. This procedure has proven successful in reducing the pressure gradient in some patients, although complications have been reported. At present this remains an experimental technique.

Valvuloplasty. This procedure is now used to open stenotic valves on both sides of the heart; however, there is a marked difference in the success rate. Valvuloplasty for pulmonic stenosis has proven very successful with few complications reported. Valvuloplasty for aortic stenosis is currently being tried, with some early success, but remains an experimental procedure.

Atrial Septal Defect. Researchers are currently developing techniques and catheters to place patches through a catheter on atrial septal defects.

It is anticipated that the need for open heart surgery will decrease in the future as new therapeutic catheterization procedures are developed.

Catheterization: An Invasive Technique

Because the catheter actually enters the body, cardiac catheterization is an invasive procedure. This also means that there are significant risk factors not usually associated with noninvasive cardiac testing. Listed below are complications that can occur, either during or after cardiac catheterization.

Infection. This can be as mild as a skin infection at the catheter entry site or as serious as sepsis or endocarditis. The catheter enters the bloodstream directly; therefore, catheterization laboratory personnel must be careful to use sterile technique at all times.

Vessel Damage. During catheterization, it is possible to puncture a vessel with the catheter or guidewire. It is also possible to puncture the free wall of the atrium, resulting in hemopericardium and cardiac tamponade. Following catheterization, vessels used can become permanently occluded.

Hemorrhage. This can occur if a catheter penetrates the wall of the heart or a major vessel. Serious hemorrhage has also been reported with the use of streptokinase and during balloon atrial septostomy if the atrial wall is torn.

Infarction. Myocardial infarction can occur if the catheter breaks off a piece of plaque, causing it to occlude coronary blood flow. It is also possible to induce ischemia and infarction by occluding coronary blood flow with the catheter. Pulmonary infarction has been reported after a tiny blood clot is flushed through a catheter in the pulmonary artery.

Stroke. Stroke can occur if a tiny blood clot is flushed through a catheter and goes to the brain. This is most common following left heart catheterization.

Persistant Arrhythmia. As the catheter is moved through the heart, arrhythmia is induced. Usually this will subside if the catheter is moved away from the irritable focus; however, occasionally, arrhythmia persists and must be treated appropriately.

Dye Reactions. Usually reaction to dye consists of skin rash or hives; however, serious complications such as airway obstruction, shock, or cardiac arrest have been reported. To date, tests are not available that would positively identify those patients who will react to contrast injection.

Death. Death can occur as a result of the complications listed above or from the patient's original disease process.

The complications listed above are all very serious in nature but it must be emphasized that the actual occurrence of these complications is rare. Catheterization is generally considered a very safe procedure.

Anatomy and Physiology

Before beginning a discussion of the details of cardiac catheterization, it is necessary to understand cardiac anatomy. Chapter 1 covered structural anatomy of the heart and how it functions. In this chapter, emphasis is placed on circulatory systems, intracardiac pressures, oxygen saturations, and how the anatomy can be viewed on angiograms.

First, the two types of circulatory systems must be defined. They are referred to as *systemic* circulation and *pulmonic* circulation, and correspond to the left and right sides of the heart, respectively.

Systemic Circulation

Systemic circulation begins in the left ventricle (LV), which pumps blood into the aorta (Ao) and through the major arteries of the body. The deoxygenated blood is then returned to the right atrium via the superior vena cava (SVC) and inferior vena cava (IVC). This route of circulation is shown in Figure 11-1.

Pulmonic Circulation

Pulmonic circulation begins in the right ventricle (RV), which pumps blood into the pulmonary arteries (PA). The pulmonary arteries carry blood through the lungs where it is oxygenated, into the pulmonary veins (PV), and back to the left atrium (LA). See Figure 11-2.

Once the circulatory patterns are defined, the physiology and hemodynamics of the heart must be considered. Physiology is the study of the actual function of an organ, and hemodynamics is a study of the forces

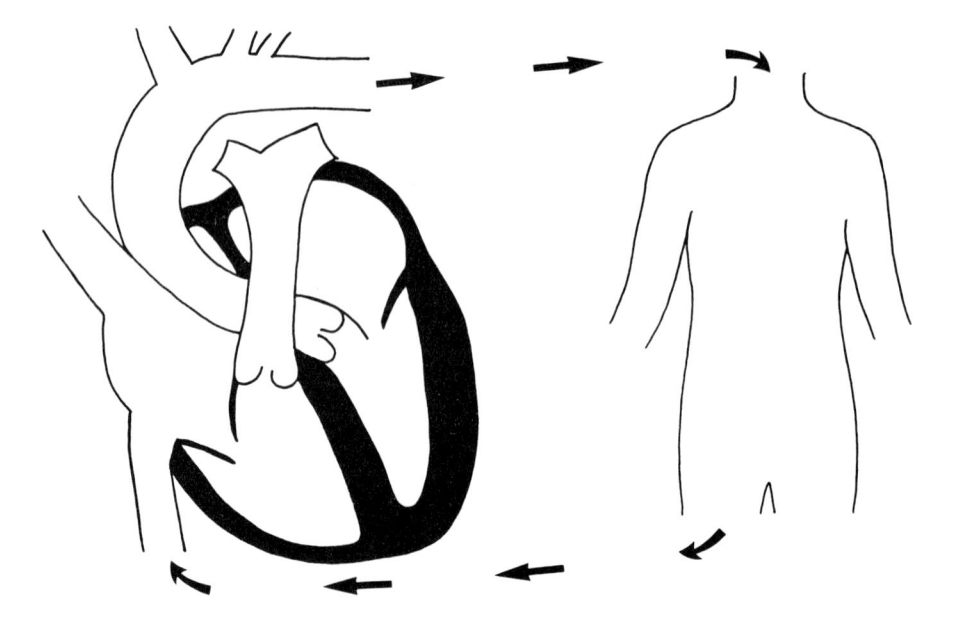

Figure 11-1 Systemic circulation.

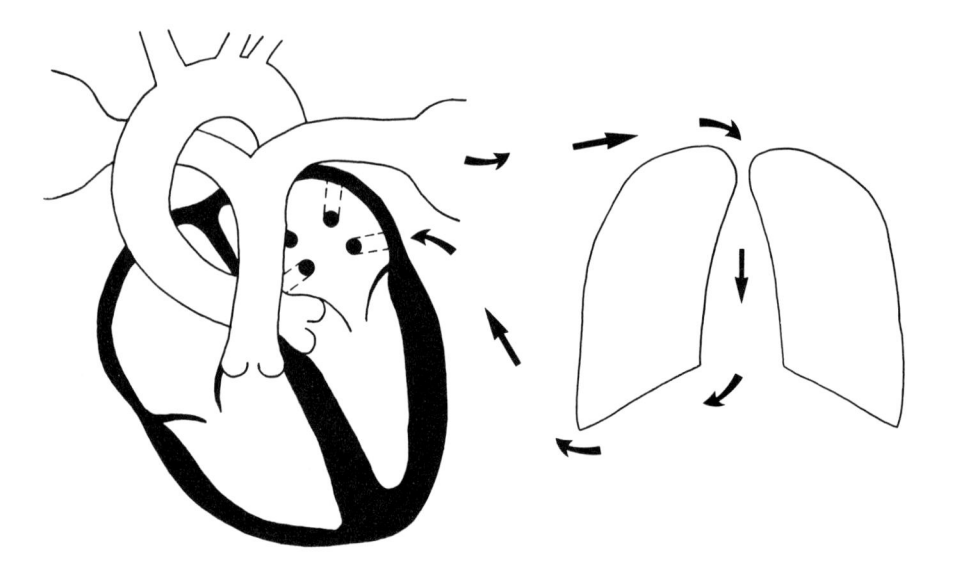

Figure 11-2 Pulmonary circulation.

involved in circulating blood through the body. Both are interrelated and will not be discussed separately in this chapter.

Intracardiac Pressures

One of the most important pieces of information collected at catheterization is the measurement of *intracardiac pressure*. Pressure measurement is the only part of cardiac catheterization that cannot be performed noninvasively. As a technologist in the catheterization laboratory it is necessary to know what the normal pressure values are for the heart and major vessels and be able to recognize each pressure by its wave form. Table 11-1 lists the normal pressures in the heart. Notice that pressures on the right side of the heart are significantly lower than those on the left. Right ventricular systolic pressure should always be equal to the pulmonary artery systolic pressure. Likewise, left ventricular systolic pressure should always equal the systolic pressure in the aorta. The a wave in the left atrium should equal the end diastolic pressure in the left ventricle.

Table 11-1   **Normal Pressures in the Heart and Great Vessels**

	Range
Left Atrium	
Mean	<12
Left Ventricle	
Systolic	90–140
End diastolic	<12
Aorta	
Systolic	90–140
Diastolic	60–90
Mean	70–105
Venae Cavae	
Mean	1–10
Right Atrium	
Mean	<8
Right Ventricle	
Systolic	15–28
End diastolic	<8
Pulmonary Artery	
Systolic	15–28
Diastolic	5–16
Mean	10–22
Pulmonary Artery Wedge	
Mean	6–15

286 Cardiac Catheterization

To measure pressure, the catheter is connected either directly to a transducer or to a manifold (a series of three-way stopcocks) that, in turn, connects to the transducer. When the catheter tip is in the desired location, a pressure tracing can be recorded.

To evaluate stenosis, many physicians perform "pullback" pressures. With the recorder running, the catheter is pulled from one area to another and pressures are measured in each location. For example, a right heart pullback would begin in the right or left pulmonary artery with a pressure tracing being recorded as the catheter is pulled through the main pulmonary artery, right ventricle, and right atrium. Written, the pullback would be shown as follows:

$$RPA \rightarrow MPA \rightarrow RV \rightarrow RA =$$

This one tracing can be used to evaluate peripheral pulmonic stenosis, valvular and subvalvular pulmonic stenosis, and intraventricular anomaly such as anomalous right ventricular muscle bundles and tricuspid stenosis. Other examples of common pullback pressures are those measured from the left ventricle to ascending aorta to descending aorta, to evaluate valvular and subvalvular aortic stenosis and coarctation of the aorta; and from the left atrium to the right atrium to evaluate atrial septal defect versus patent *foramen ovale*.

Later in this chapter, pressure wave forms will be discussed, in particular, their appearance and how each one is measured.

Oxygen Saturations

Oxygen saturation is the amount of oxygen absorbed in the blood. In the normal heart, deoxygenated blood returns to the right heart where it is pumped out to the lungs for oxygenation; therefore, oxygen saturations will

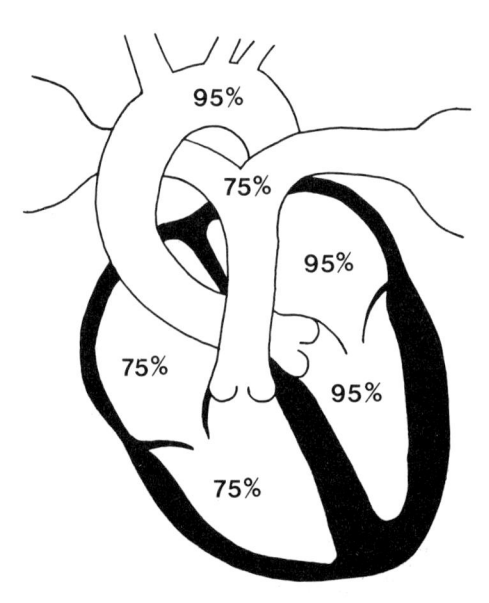

Figure 11-3 Normal oxygen saturation in the heart.

remain essentially the same throughout the right side of the heart. From the lungs, oxygenated blood returns to the left heart via the pulmonary veins and is circulated to the body. Oxygen saturations remain essentially the same throughout the left side of the heart (Figure 11-3).

Oxygen data become most valuable whenever intracardiac shunts are present. For example, if a ventricular septal defect is present, blood will flow from the left ventricle (high pressure) to the right ventricle (low pressure). This is called *left-to-right shunting*. When oxygenated blood from the left ventricle mixes with deoxygenated blood from the right ventricle, the saturation in the right ventricle will be higher than that of the right atrium. The increase in saturation from one chamber to another is referred to as an *"oxygen step-up."* Oxygen step-ups are directly proportionate to the degree of shunting present. In other words, the larger the oxygen step-up, the larger the shunt.

Technical Aspects of Catheterization

Catheter Placement

Before cardiac catheterization can be accomplished, a vessel must be isolated and a catheter placed in the vessel. Two techniques are commonly used to isolate a vessel for catheterization. The least invasive way to introduce a catheter is by the percutaneous Seldinger technique. The steps are illustrated in Figure 11-4.

1. A percutaneous needle is inserted through the vessel and drawn back until blood appears from the hub of the needle.

2. A guidewire is threaded through the needle into the vessel.

3. Using care not to draw out the guidewire, the needle is removed completely.

4. A catheter or sheath is placed over the guidewire into the vessel.

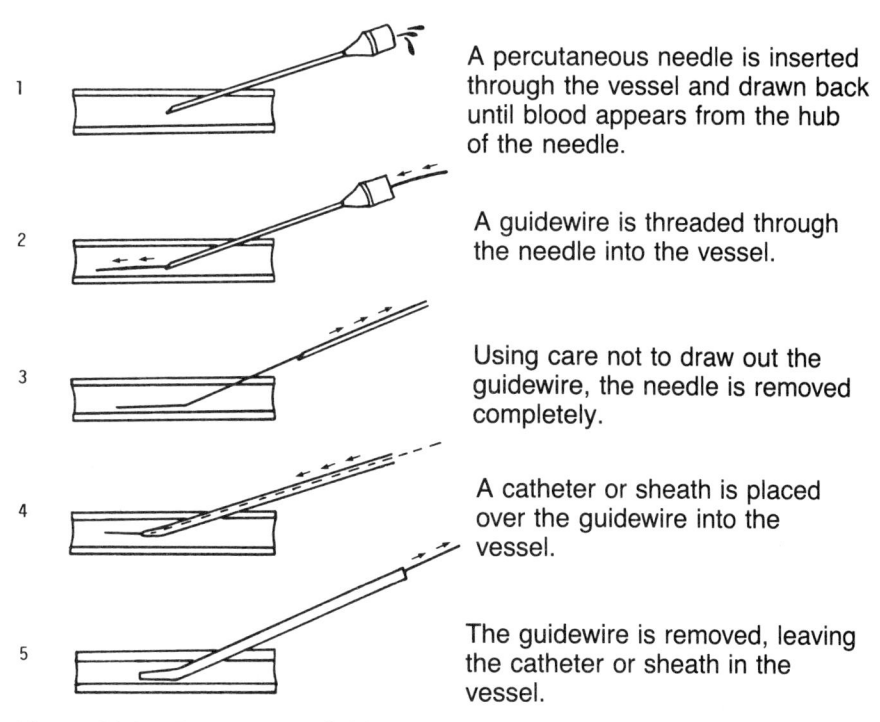

5. The guidewire is removed, leaving the catheter or sheath in the vessel.

Figure 11-4 Percutaneous Seldinger technique.

The Sone's technique involves performing a cutdown on the antecubital fossa to isolate the brachial artery or vein using the following steps:

1. The artery is located by palpation.
2. Local anesthesia is injected.
3. The vessel is isolated, using an incision and blunt dissection.
4. Two ligatures are placed to stabilize the vessel.
5. Incision is made into the vessel and the catheter is introduced.

Of the two methods described above, the most popular is the percutaneous Seldinger technique. Because it uses no incision, there is no scar, there are no sutures to remove, and the chance of infection is significantly lowered. After a cutdown is performed, the vessel must either be repaired, which is a delicate procedure, or tied off completely. The skin then has to be sutured. When the Seldinger technique is used, pressure is held over the catheter entry site until bleeding stops and a pressure dressing is placed over the site. The patient can then be returned to his room or sent to the recovery room depending on hospital protocol.

Catheters and Their Uses

Cardiovascular catheters come in many sizes and shapes. The cardiologist must choose which catheters to use according to the patient's size and the type of catheterization to be performed.

Catheters used on the right heart are distinctly different than those used on the left heart. One reason for this is the difference in the way the ventricles are entered. When performing right heart catheterization, the catheter enters the right atrium via the SVC or IVC and is then advanced across the tricuspid valve into the right ventricle. Right heart catheters are always advanced in the direction of normal blood flow. Some right heart catheters have a balloon that can be inflated to help "float" the catheter into the right ventricle, across the pulmonic valve, and into the pulmonary artery. These catheters are referred to as *flow directed*. When a left heart catheterization is performed, the catheter enters the left ventricle in retrograde fashion from the aorta. To cross the aortic valve against blood flow at high pressure, a pigtail catheter is used. The pigtail curve allows the catheter to catch in the aortic valve and to be advanced into the left ventricle (Figure 11-5).

In adults, the most common reason for catheterization is to assess the presence and severity of coronary artery disease. Special catheters have been designed to make selective coronary artery catheterization easier. Coronary artery catheters have a curve that allows them to be manipulated from the aorta into the selected coronary artery without difficulty. Before the development of preformed coronary artery catheters, contrast was injected into the aortic root and the coronary arteries visualized simultaneously. This technique was not optimal because the detail was not as good as selective coronary artery visualization, where each artery can be seen individually.

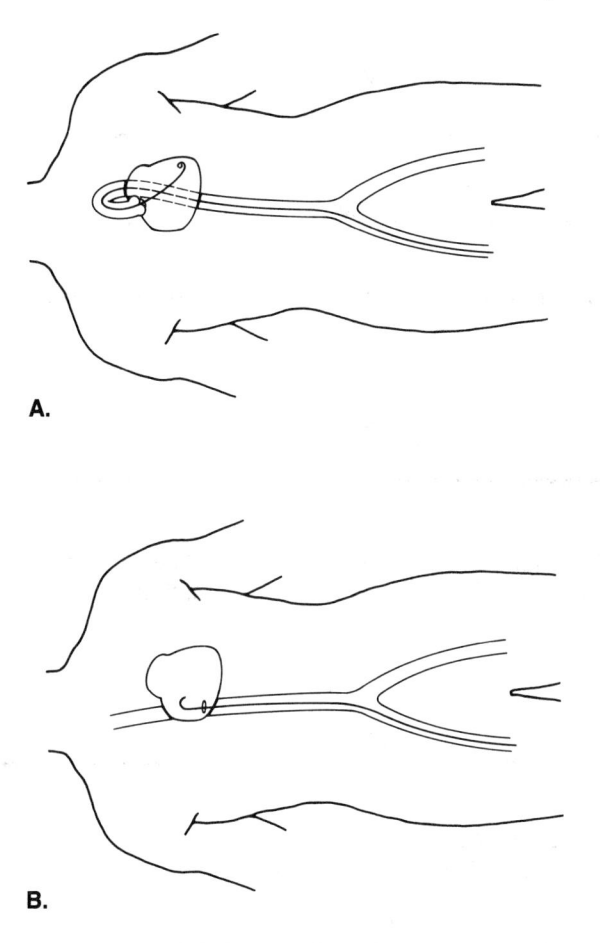

Figure 11-5 (A) Retrograde catheter approach through the aorta and into the left ventricle. (B) Direct catheter approach into the right atrium via the inferior vena cava (IVC).

Many catheters used on the left side of the heart and coronary arteries are thin-walled, requiring use of a guidewire to advance the catheter. The guidewire is advanced through the catheter and provides additional stiffness so that the catheter can be moved safely. Failure to use a guidewire when recommended can result in kinking and actual knotting of the catheter within a vessel. Various catheters and their uses are illustrated in Figure 11-6.

When selecting catheters, contrast injection rate becomes an important consideration. Optimal angiograms are obtained when large amounts of contrast are injected rapidly into the vessel or area of the heart to be visualized. The cardiologist must choose a catheter that will allow him to use the amount of contrast necessary to visualize the desired anatomy. Table 11-2 shows how much injection rates can differ without changing catheter size.

290 Cardiac Catheterization

Sone's coronary artery catheters

Judkins coronary artery catheters

Pigtail catheter used for left heart angiography

Rashkind balloon atrial septostomy catheter

Goodale-Luben catheter used for right heart catheterization

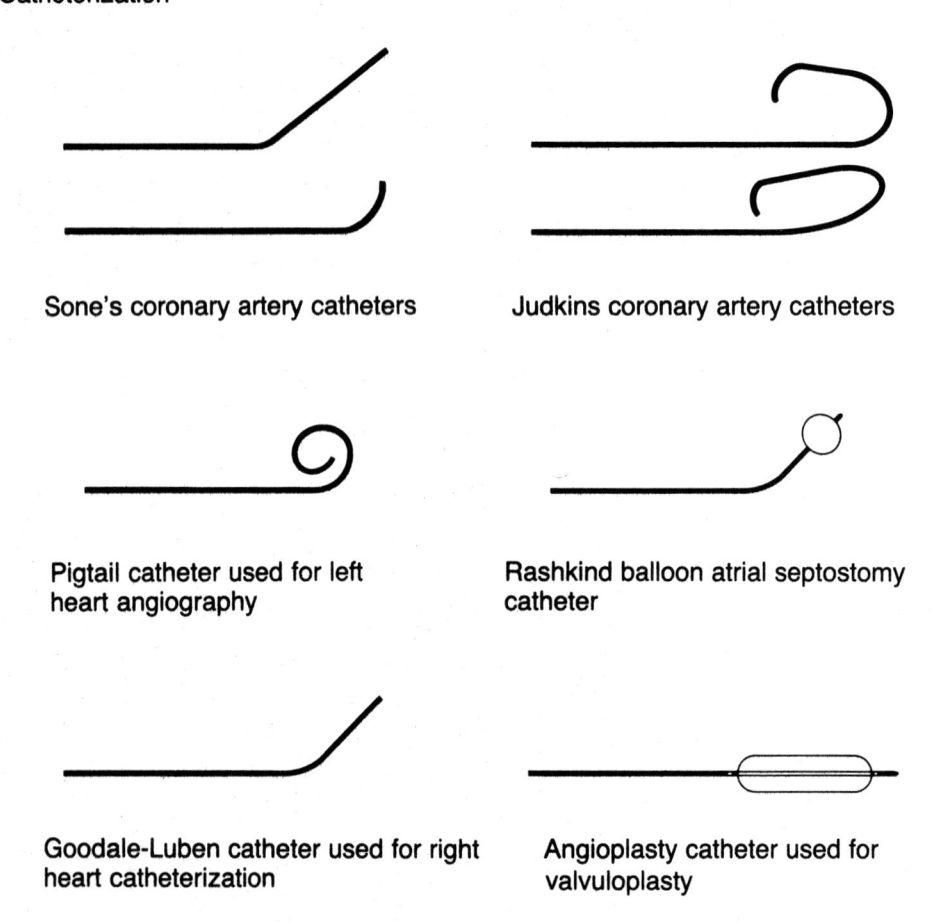

Angioplasty catheter used for valvuloplasty

Figure 11-6 Various catheters and their uses.

    Guidewires have a variety of uses in the catheterization laboratory. When introducing a catheter into the vessel, a guidewire is positioned first and the catheter is then passed over the wire. To advance a catheter into a difficult position, a guidewire can be inserted through the catheter and positioned. The catheter can then be advanced over the wire and the wire removed.

    Guidewires come in many sizes and shapes. Wire sizes are measured in inches, such as .035 or .018, and correspond to the lumen size of the catheter. Most catheter manufacturers include the recommended guidewire size on the catheter label. A guidewire smaller than recommended can be used; however, blood may leak back through the catheter. A guidewire larger than recommended simply will not pass through the catheter. Figure 11-7 illustrates various guidewire shapes.

    Construction of the guidewire is unusual. Rather than one piece of metal that is molded into a certain shape, the guidewire is made of very tightly

Table 11-2   **Injection Rates for Five French Catheters**

Catheter	Rate (ml/sec)
Berman Angiography	9
Cook Pigtail	8–12
Cook High Flow Rate	16–25
Edwards Angiography	8
Goodale–Luben	9–13
UMI Pigtail	12–15

Standard straight guidewire

Straight guidewire with flexible tip

Guidewire with 3 mm curved flexible tip

Guidewire with 6 mm curved flexible tip

Guidewire with 15 mm curved flexible tip

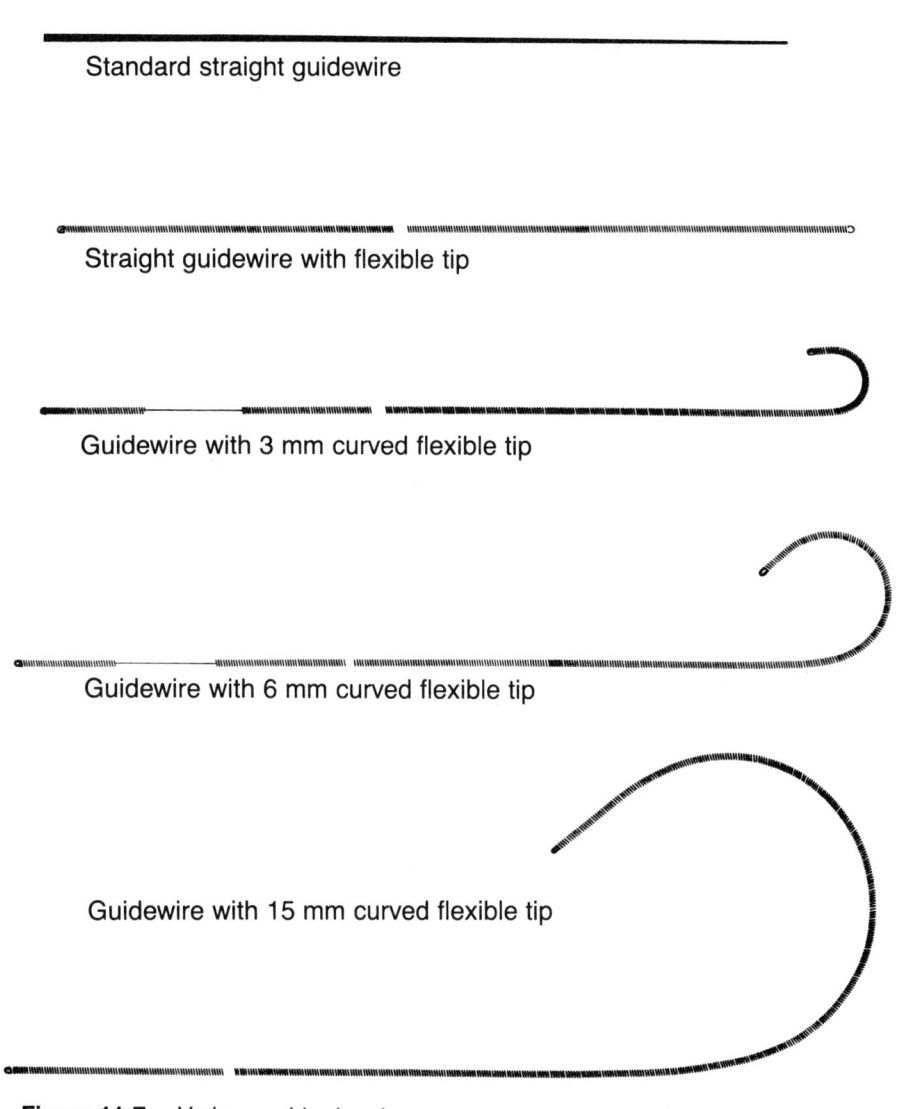

Figure 11-7   Various guidewire shapes.

coiled fine wire. This allows the wire to be flexible and easily manipulated. A stiff wire can puncture a vessel whereas a flexible wire will bend or kink before this happens.

Catheterization Laboratory Instrumentation

Cardiac catheterization requires more than just catheters. Catheters are advanced using fluoroscopic visualization. This allows the physician to view the catheter as it is advanced and to change course when necessary to position the catheter in the desired location. Since fluoroscopy actually involves exposing the patient to radiation, routine radiation safety procedures must be followed. Some of the most important are listed in Table 11-3. The fluoroscope is turned on only when necessary. The physician controls the fluoroscope during catheterization through the use of a foot pedal.

Cineangiography involves the injection of contrast media into the desired area of the heart and then filming its flow. This, too, involves the use of radiation and is, therefore, subject to the safety procedures listed in Table 11-3. Cineangiograms are recorded on 35 mm film at a rate of 30–60 frames per second.

In the early days of catheterization, films could be taken only in limited projections, frequently requiring that the patient be moved or repositioned. Today, both single and biplane cineangiograms are available using C-arms that move around the patient as needed. When biplane cineangiograms are recorded, a single contrast injection can be filmed simultaneously from two different angles (Figure 11-8).

Injection of contrast in the catheterization laboratory is performed using an automated pressure injector (Figure 11-9). The injector can be programmed to provide the desired amount of contrast in a specified period of time. Pressure safety limits must be set to avoid catheter damage. If this is not done, it is possible to rupture a catheter by injecting dye too quickly. For most catheters, the acceptable pressure limit is 600 pounds per square inch. Recommended injection rates and pressure safety limits are packaged with each catheter.

Measurement of hemodynamic data is one of the main reasons for performing cardiac catheterization. It is also necessary to monitor ECG patterns and intracardiac pressures throughout the procedure. To do this, a

Table 11-3 **Radiation Safety Procedures**

1. Always wear a film badge. These are checked monthly and a cumulative record kept of radiation exposure for each person in the cath lab.
2. Always wear a lead apron when X-ray is in use.
3. When possible, stand away from the X-ray table.
4. To protect the patient from receiving excess radiation, keep the tube columnated at all times.

Technical Aspects of Catheterization **293**

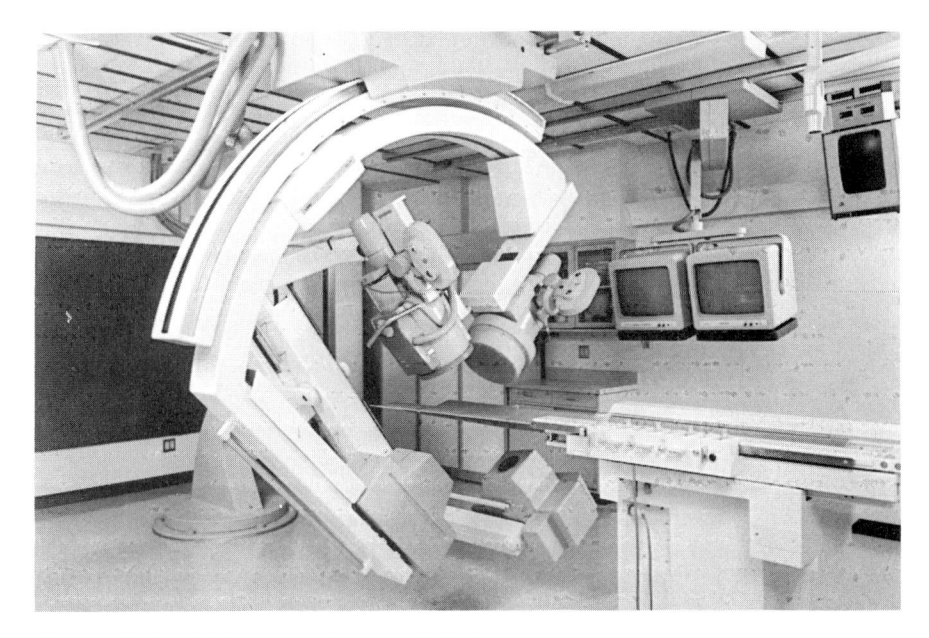

Figure 11-8 Philips poly diagnost C biplane cine unit.

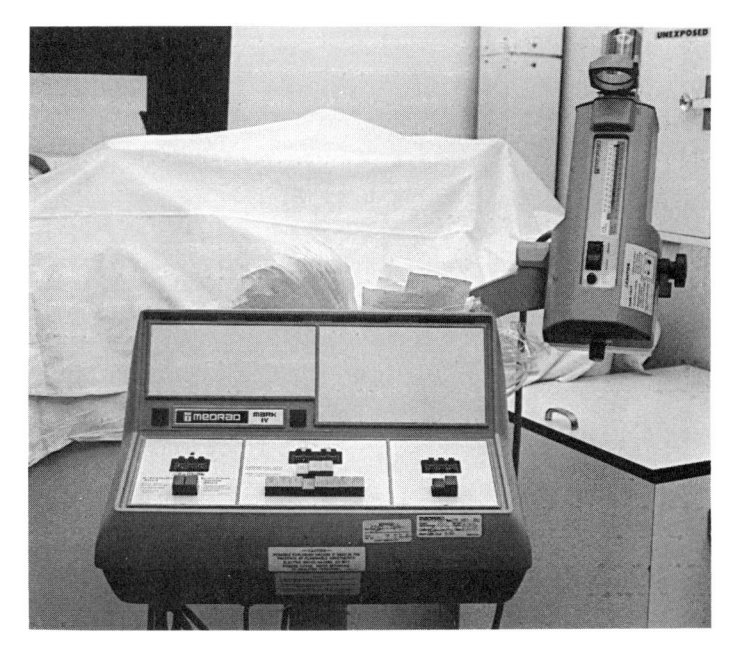

Figure 11-9 Pressure injector.

physiologic recorder is used. The physiologic recorder (Figure 11-10) is a multichannel unit that can perform many different functions. Channels can be ordered individually and interchanged as needed in the recorder. Channels are available to monitor ECG patterns and heart rate, pressures, respirations, EEG, HIS bundle electrograms, and real-time echocardiograms.

The patient is connected to the ECG monitor through the use of a standard cable that plugs into the ECG channel. Some laboratories monitor two ECG leads simultaneously for easier arrhythmia identification.

Pressures are measured using a strain gauge with a transducer on one end. The transducer is covered with a sterile dome and connected to the catheter. The other end connects to the pressure channel. When both right and left heart catheterization is being performed, pressures can be monitored simultaneously from both sides of the heart.

While the catheter is being manipulated, the physician must watch the fluoroscope; therefore, it becomes the responsibility of the technologist to monitor the patient's heart rhythm and blood pressure. If changes occur, the physician must be notified immediately. It is also necessary for the technologist to recognize pressure wave forms and notify the physician if a pressure gradient exists. This gives the physician an opportunity to repeat the pressure measurement for verification of the gradient. Pressure tracings are recorded on paper so that measurements can be made after the catheterization. A variety of actual recording techniques is used. Some machines use liquid chemical developer while others use heat-sensitive dry silver paper.

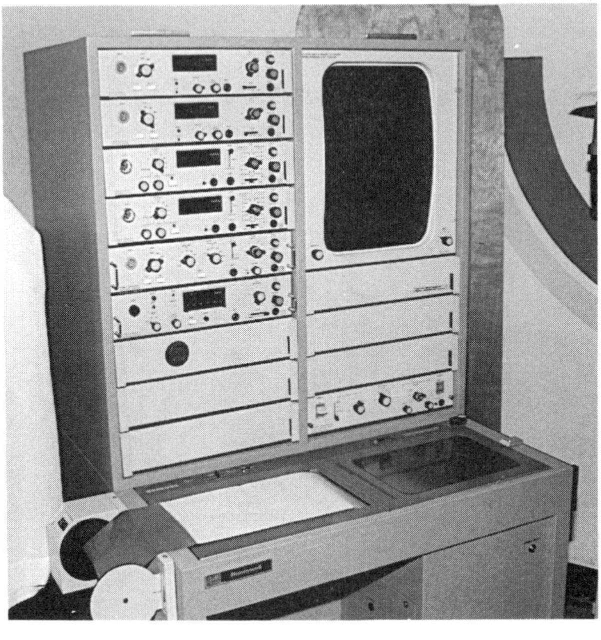

Figure 11-10 Physiologic pressure recorder.

Graph lines are not printed on the paper because the graph is adjustable within the recorder and photographed simultaneously with the ECG and pressure tracing. Paper speeds vary from 25 mm/second to 200 mm/second and amplitude settings vary from 10 to 400 mmHg. This wide range of adjustments allows flexibility to look at very large or very small wave forms (Figure 11-11).

Other small but important pieces of equipment are also used in the catheterization laboratory, as listed below.

Oximeter: Measures the oxygen saturation of blood samples.

Oxygen Consumption Monitor: Uses a flow-through system to measure oxygen consumption. The patient is placed in a hood and room air is drawn

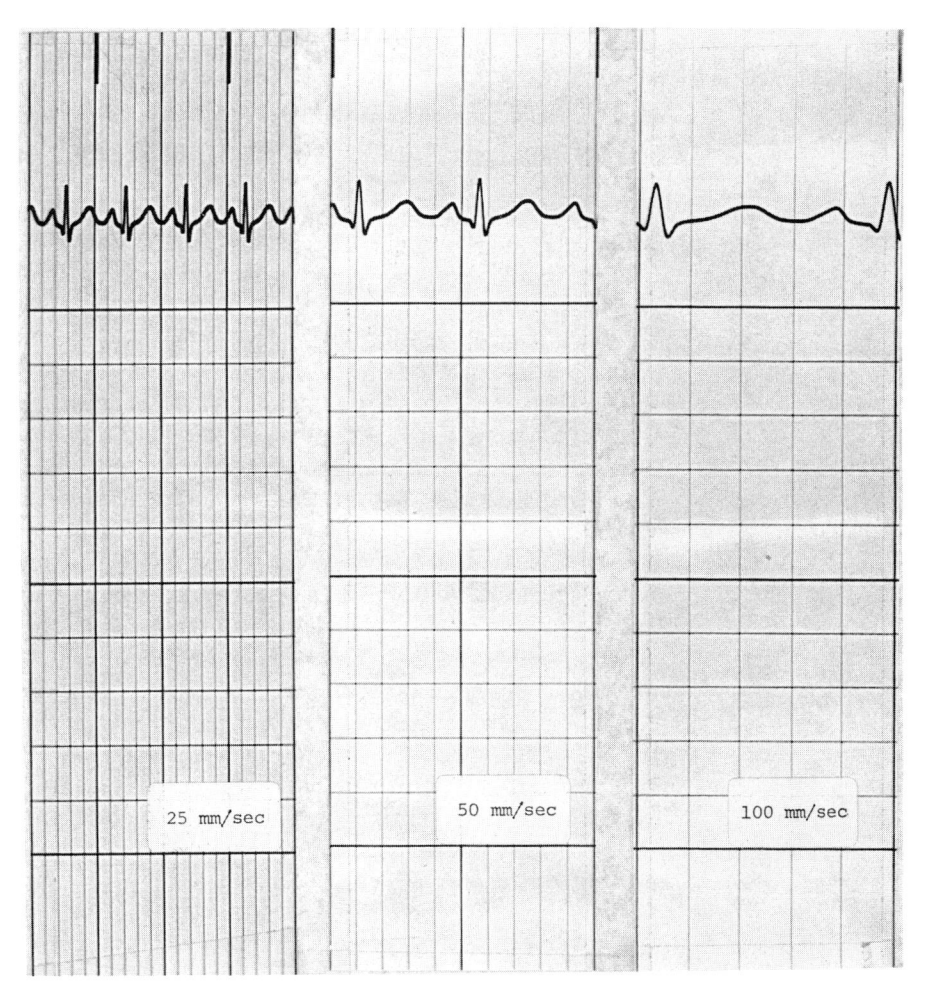

Figure 11-11 Comparison of paper speeds with vertical time lines set at .1 second.

296 Cardiac Catheterization

in at a set speed. The machine calibrates to room air and measures the oxygen difference as the patient exhales.

Defibrillator: This must be available for emergencies. Some defibrillators can be synchronized to the ECG by plugging them into the ECG channel of the physiologic recorder.

Transcutaneous pO_2 Monitor: This unit is able to continuously monitor pO_2 through a probe that is placed on the skin.

Doppler: A Doppler probe can be placed distal to the catheterization site to monitor pulses throughout catheterization or to check for pulses when the procedure is completed.

Pressure Wave Forms

Pressure wave forms are unique in each area of the heart. The catheterization laboratory technologist must be able to recognize where the catheter is by the wave form and pressure reading. For example, both ventricular pressures look somewhat alike; however, one can distinguish which pressure is being recorded because the left ventricular pressure is approximately five times that of the right ventricle (Figure 11-12).

Atrial, venous, and wedge pressures are all measured by a and v waves instead of systolic and diastolic pressures. The a wave occurs as a result of atrial contraction and can be measured by drawing a line straight down from the P wave upstroke on the ECG tracing. After ventricular depolarization, there is a drop in pressure due to atrial volume changes. Venous inflow produces a rise in pressure that peaks with the opening of mitral and tricuspid valves. This peak is the v wave and can be measured by drawing a line straight down from the beginning of the QRS complex. Figure 11-13 illustrates the proper measurement of a and v waves.

Pressure curves from the right and left ventricles have the same configuration; however, the left ventricular systolic pressure is approximately five times that in the right ventricle. On ventricular pressure curves, the systolic and end diastolic pressures are measured as illustrated in Figure 11-14. End diastolic pressure is the point at which the rapid upstroke of the pressure curve begins. If the end diastolic pressure is damped and difficult to measure, a line can be drawn on the rapid upstroke of the pressure curve.

Arterial pressure curves have the same appearance but, like the ventricles, the systolic pressure in the aorta is approximately five times that in the pulmonary artery. Both of these pressures are measured using systolic over diastolic pressures. In the presence of normal circulatory anatomy, the aortic pressure will equal the arm blood pressure measured with a cuff and sphygmomanometer (Figure 11-15).

Pressures recorded in the catheterization laboratory can show significant respiratory variation. Venous pressures drop with inspiration and rise with exhalation. As a rule of thumb, the highest pressures should be measured. The one exception to this rule is when the patient is being ventilated mechanically. The lowest pressure must then be measured.

Technical Aspects of Catheterization 297

RIGHT ATRIUM (20)

LEFT ATRIUM (40)

RIGHT VENTRICLE (40)

LEFT VENTRICLE (200)

PULMONARY ARTERY (40)

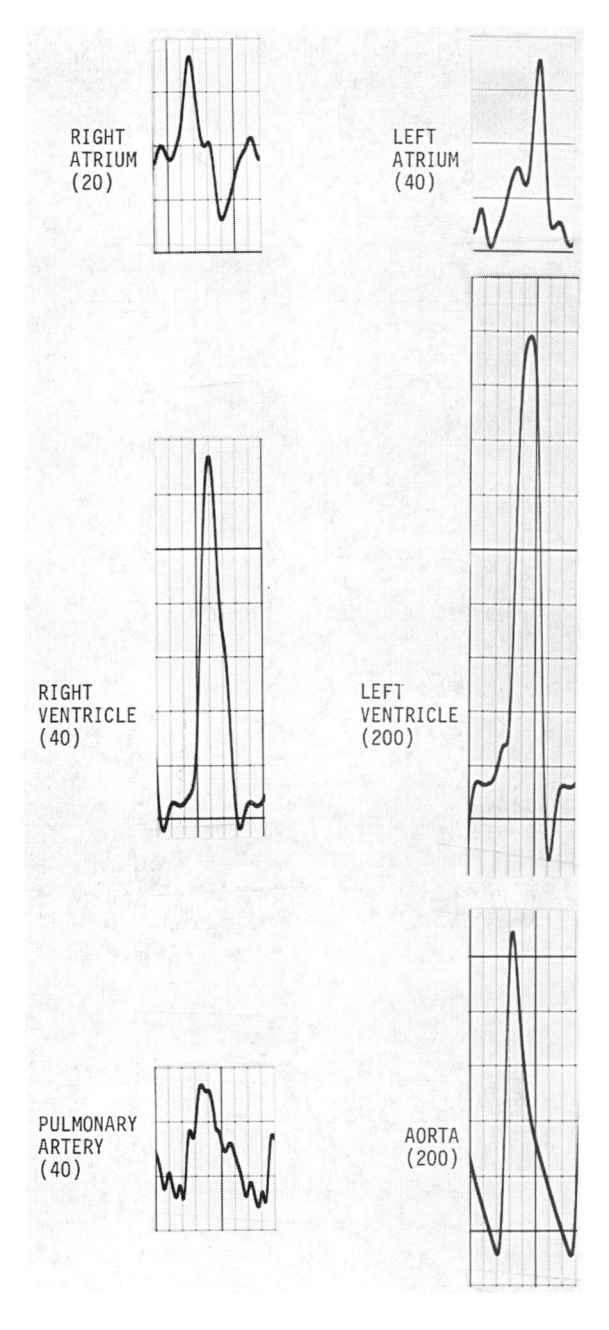

AORTA (200)

Figure 11-12 Pressure wave forms and amplitude settings usually used to record them.

298 Cardiac Catheterization

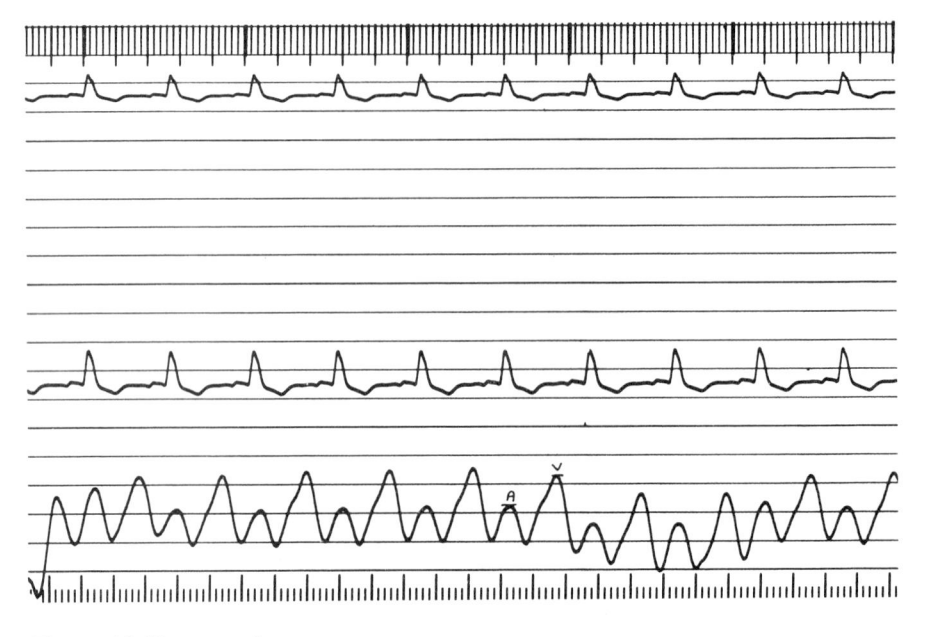

Figure 11-13 *a* and *v* waves.

Catheterization Calculations

Right and left cardiac catheterization provides sufficient data to calculate cardiac output (both pulmonic and systemic), pulmonary and systemic resistances, direction and amount of abnormal shunting, and pulmonary to systemic flow and resistance ratios. Several abbreviations are used as follows:

Qp: Q always stands for flow and the small "p" for pulmonary so Qp is pulmonary flow or pulmonic output. This tells how much blood is flowing to the lungs and is shown in liters per minute (liter/min).

PI: Pulmonic index. This is pulmonary blood flow (Qp) that has been divided by the body surface area (BSA). Results are shown in liters per minute per square meter (liter/min/M^2).

Qs: Q stands for flow and the "s" for systemic. Qs is systemic flow or systemic output. This tells how much blood is flowing to the body in liter/min.

CI: Cardiac index. This is systemic flow divided by the body surface area and shown in liter/min/M^2.

Qp/Qs: This stands for pulmonary to systemic flow ratio and tells how much blood is flowing to the lungs compared to how much blood

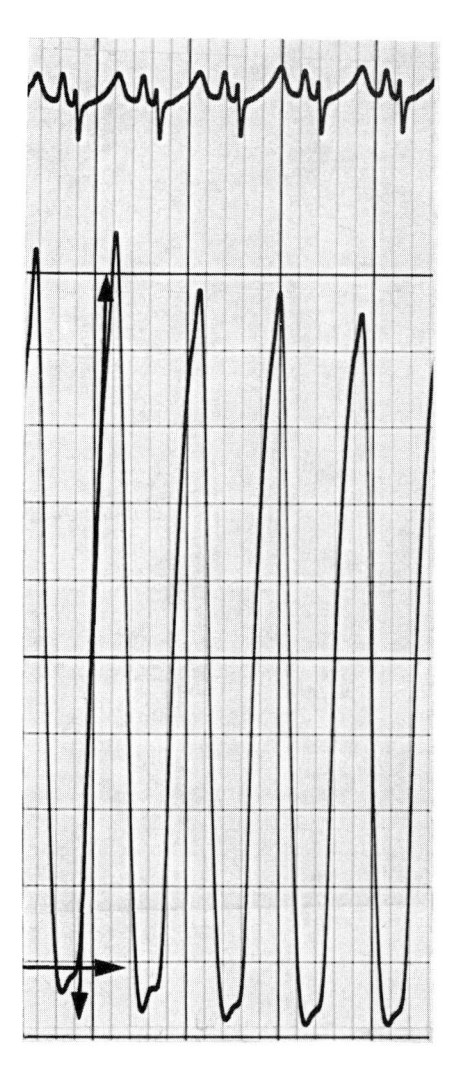

Figure 11-14 Measurement of ventricular end diastolic pressure.

is flowing to the body. In the normal heart, pulmonary and systemic flow are equal, therefore, the ratio is 1:1.

Qep: This stands for effective pulmonary flow and reflects the amount of blood oxygenated in the lungs and actually circulated to the body.

Rp: R always stands for resistance and "p" for pulmonary so Rp is pulmonary resistance. Resistance is expressed in resistance units (RU) or in dynes.

Rs: R stands for resistance and "s" for systemic so this is systemic resistance and is expressed in resistance units or dynes.

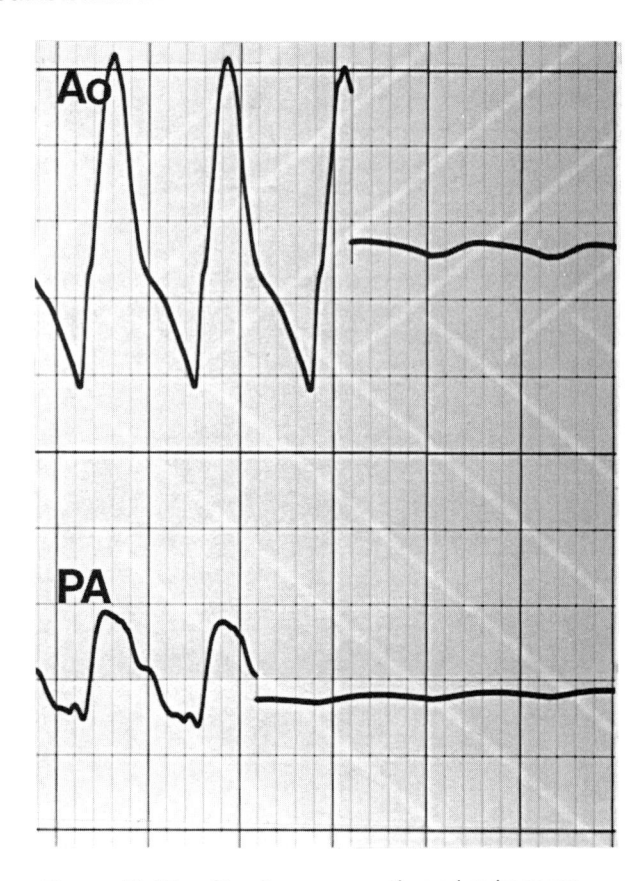

Figure 11-15 Simultaneous aortic and pulmonary artery pressures.

Measurement of Cardiac Output

Three methods are used to determine cardiac output or blood flow. They are the Fick method, the thermodilution method, and the dye dilution method. The following data must be available to calculate blood flow by the Fick method:

O_2 Consumption (vO_2): Oxygen consumption can be measured in the catheterization laboratory using an oxygen consumption monitor, by Douglas bag collection, or can be estimated from a chart based on the patient's sex, age, and heart rate.

O_2 Capacity: This is calculated using the patient's hemoglobin measurement multiplied by 1.36 (ml O_2 STPD/gram hemoglobin) × 10. STPD is standard temperature and pressure dry.

O₂ Saturation: Oxygen saturation is measured in blood samples obtained from the major vessels and chambers of the heart at catheterization. This information is used to determine arteriovenous O₂ content difference.

By definition, the Fick principle states that the quantity of oxygen per minute delivered to the pulmonary capillaries via the pulmonary artery plus the quantity of oxygen per minute that enters the pulmonary capillaries from the alveoli must equal the quantity of oxygen per minute that is carried away by the pulmonary veins. The algebraic equation is as follows:

$$\text{Cardiac Output} = \frac{O_2 \text{ Consumption}}{\text{Arteriovenous } O_2 \text{ Difference (Vol. \%)}}$$

Information needed to complete the above equation is obtained at catheterization. Specifically, oxygen consumption is measured using a monitoring device, or it can be assumed from a chart based on age, sex, and heart rate. Oxygen capacity is calculated using the hemoglobin measurement multiplied by 1.36. Arteriovenous O₂ content difference is determined using oxygen saturation data from both ends of the circulatory system involved. For example, systemic blood flow is calculated using oxygen saturations from the aorta and superior vena cava. Pulmonic blood flow is calculated using pulmonary vein and pulmonary artery saturations. When no abnormal shunting is present, both pulmonary and systemic flow are equal. However, in the presence of a shunt, pulmonary and systemic flow must be calculated separately using the appropriate oxygen saturations. It is also possible to calculate effective pulmonary blood flow using the following equation:

$$Qep = \frac{O_2 \text{ Consumption}}{(\text{PV sat} - \text{SV sat}) \times O_2 \text{ Capacity}}$$

Effective pulmonary flow is the amount of blood that is oxygenated in the lungs and actually circulated to the body. This calculation is necessary to determine the amount and direction of any abnormal shunting that may be present.

Another calculation frequently performed is cardiac index. Cardiac index (CI) equals the cardiac output divided by the patient's body surface area (BSA).

$$CI = \frac{\text{Cardiac Output}}{\text{BSA}}$$

Body surface area is shown in square meters (M^2).

The second method used to determine cardiac output is called *thermodilution*. Thermodilution cardiac outputs are performed by passing a flow-directed thermodilution catheter through the right heart and positioning it in the pulmonary artery. This catheter has four lumens, one for the proximal injection port, one for the distal injection port, one for balloon inflation, and the fourth lumen contains a wire that transmits temperature changes from a thermistor in the catheter to the cardiac output computer.

The first step in determining cardiac output by thermodilution is to tell the computer what size catheter is being used and how much injectate will be given at each determination. Outputs are then performed by injecting solution at a known temperature through the proximal port of the catheter. The output computer senses the change in blood temperature and measures the time it takes for the blood to return to its baseline temperature. Complex algebraic equations are then used to calculate cardiac output. A variety of injectate solutions can be used, but the most common are normal saline and D_5W. Some new output computers have an in-line thermistor that measures the injectate temperature as it enters the catheter, allowing for more accurate calculation of cardiac output and increased flexibility in actual injectate temperatures to be used. There must be at least 10°F temperature difference between the blood temperature and the injectate temperature for a correct output determination to be made. There are three advantages to performing thermodilution cardiac outputs when possible.

1. It is faster than doing saturations in each chamber of the heart and performing Fick calculations.
2. It can be performed at the patient's bedside and can be used to monitor critically ill patients for several days at a time.
3. The patient loses less blood during the procedure.

Resistance is defined as the ratio of the mean pressure drop across a hydraulic system, or segment thereof, to the flow through it. To calculate resistance, it is necessary, then, to know the mean pressure measurements on both ends of the system and the amount of flow. For pulmonic resistance, mean pressures must be measured in the pulmonary artery and pulmonary vein. In the absence of measured pulmonary venous pressure, left atrial mean pressure can be used. If neither of these pressures is available, pulmonary capillary wedge pressure can be used because it is an indirect measurement of the pulmonary vein pressure. Calculation of systemic resistance requires both systemic arterial and systemic venous mean pressure. The systemic artery is the aorta and the systemic vein is the vena cava. Right atrial mean pressure can also be used as the systemic vein. Pressures measured at catheterization are shown in millimeters of mercury (mmHg). Mean pressures are shown with a line above the pressure ($\overline{PA}$ or $\overline{Ao}$). Now the information above can be applied to actual patient cases.

Case 1 The patient is a 65-year-old female who presented to the hospital with chest pain.
BSA = 1.4 M²
Hemoglobin = 13.2 gm
O_2 Consumption (nonindexed) = 151.71 cc/minute
O_2 Capacity = 13.2 hgb × 1.36 × 10 = 179.52 cc/Liter

O₂ Saturations: Superior vena cava (SV) = 73%
Pulmonary artery (PA) = 73%
Pulmonary vein (PV) = 97%
Aorta (SA) = 97%
Mean Pressures: Right atrium (SV) = 2 mmHg
Pulmonary artery (PA) = 16 mmHg
Pulmonary vein (PV) = 8 mmHg
Aorta (SA) = 85 mmHg

$$Qp = \frac{O_2 \text{ Consumption}}{(PV \text{ sat} - PA \text{ sat}) \times O_2 \text{ Cap}} = \frac{151.71 \text{ cc/min}}{(.97 - .73 \times 179.52} = 3.52 \text{ Liter/min}$$

$$PI = \frac{3.52 \text{ Liter/min}}{1.4 \text{ M}^2} = 2.51 \text{ Liter/min/M}^2$$

$$Qs = \frac{O_2 \text{ Consumption}}{(SA \text{ sat} - SV \text{ sat}) \times O_2 \text{ Cap}} = \frac{151.71 \text{ cc/min}}{(.97 - .73) \times 179.52} = 3.52 \text{ Liter/min}$$

$$CI = \frac{3.52 \text{ Liter/min}}{1.4 \text{ M}^2} = 2.51 \text{ Liter/min/M}^2$$

$$Qp/Qs = \frac{3.52 \text{ Liter/min}}{3.52 \text{ Liter/min}} = 1 \text{ or } 1:1$$

$$Rp = \frac{PA - PV}{PI} = \frac{16 \text{ mm Hg} - 8 \text{ mm Hg}}{2.51 \text{ Liter/min/M}^2} = 2.27 \text{ RU}$$

$$Rs = \frac{Ao - RA}{CI} = \frac{85 \text{ mm Hg} - 2 \text{ mm Hg}}{2.51 \text{ Liter/min/M}^2} = 23.57 \text{ RU}$$

In this case, both pulmonic and systemic flow are equal; therefore, the pulmonary to systemic flow ratio is normal at 1:1. Both pulmonary and systemic resistances calculate to be normal. Now consider a case in which shunts are present.

Case 2 The patient is a 3-year-old male with a Grade III/VI pansystolic murmur.
BSA = .60 M²
Hemoglobin = 15.4 gm
O₂ Consumption (nonindexed) = 97.38 cc/min
O₂ Capacity = 15.4 hgb × 1.36 × 10 = 209.44
O₂ Saturations: Right Atrium (SV) = 63
Pulmonary Artery (PA) = 84
Pulmonary Vein (PV) = 95
Aorta (SA) = 92
Mean Pressures: Right Atrium (SV) = 3 mmHg
Pulmonary Artery (PA) = 70 mmHg
Pulmonary Vein (PV) = 10 mmHg
Aorta (SA) = 76 mmHg

$$Qp = \frac{O_2 \text{ Consumption}}{(\text{PV sat} - \text{PA sat}) \times O_2 \text{ Cap}} = \frac{97.38 \text{ cc/min}}{(.95 - .84) \times 209.44} = 4.22 \text{ Liter/min}$$

$$PI = \frac{4.22 \text{ Liter/min}}{.6 \text{ M}^2} = 7.03 \text{ Liter/min/M}^2$$

$$Qs = \frac{O_2 \text{ Consumption}}{(\text{SA sat} - \text{SV sat}) \times O_2 \text{ Cap}} = \frac{97.38 \text{ cc/min}}{(.92 - .63) \times 209.44} = 1.60 \text{ Liter/min}$$

$$CI = \frac{1.60 \text{ Liter/min}}{.6 \text{ M}^2} = 2.66 \text{ Liter/min/M}^2$$

$$Qp/Qs = \frac{4.22 \text{ Liter/min/M}^2}{1.60 \text{ Liter/min/M}^2} = 2.64 \text{ or } 2.64:1$$

$$Qep = \frac{O_2 \text{ Consumption}}{(\text{PV sat} - \text{SV sat}) \times O_2 \text{ Cap}} = \frac{97.38}{(.95 - .63) \times 209.44} = 1.45 \text{ Liter/min}$$

L → R Shunt = Qp − Qep = 4.22 Liter/min − 1.45 Liter/min
= 2.77 Liter/min

R → L Shunt = Qs − Qep = 1.60 Liter/min − 1.45 Liter/min
= 0.15 Liter/min

$$Rp = \frac{\text{PA} - \text{PV}}{\text{PI}} = \frac{70 \text{ mm Hg} - 10 \text{ mm Hg}}{7.03 \text{ Liter/min/M}^2} = 8.53 \text{ RU}$$

$$Rs = \frac{\text{SA} - \text{SV}}{\text{CI}} = \frac{76 \text{ mm Hg} - 3 \text{ mm Hg}}{2.66 \text{ Liter/min/M}^2} = 27.44 \text{ RU}$$

Figure 11-16 is a graphic representation of this case. The calculations performed above give valuable information about the patient. To begin, the amounts and patterns of blood flow should be analyzed. Pulmonic flow is not equal to systemic flow. The Qp/Qs of 2.64 indicates that for every 1 liter of blood that is circulated to the body, 2.64 liters are circulated to the lungs. Blood is shunting from left to right within the heart at a rate of 2.77 liters per minute. Notice that the shunt flow is actually greater than the patient's systemic flow. Resistance calculations show pulmonary hypertension with normal systemic resistance. Left untreated, it is likely that this patient would develop congestive heart failure and eventually the pulmonary capillary beds could become irreversibly damaged. Blood is returned to the left atrium at the rate of 4.22 Liter/min. Of this blood, 2.77 Liter/min flows abnormally to the right heart. 0.15 Liter/min flows back to the left heart as a right-to-left shunt. The combination of the Qep of 1.45 Liter/min and the right-to-left shunt of 0.15 Liter/min equals the total calculated systemic flow of 1.60 Liter/min.

The calculations illustrated here are routinely performed after catheterization and give the physician important information with which a treatment plan can be developed.

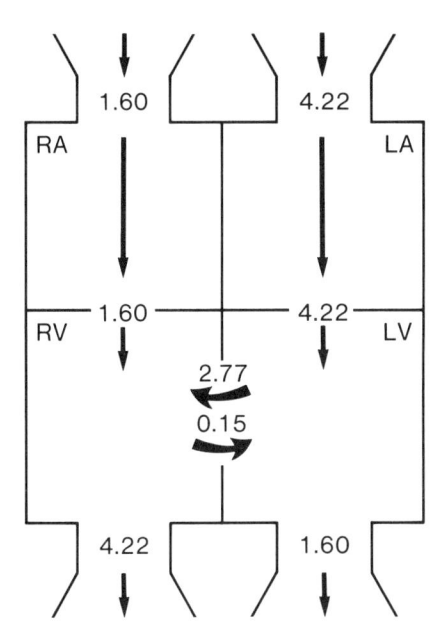

Figure 11-16 *Case 2:* Illustration of blood flow calculations in liters/min/M².

Disease Processes Confirmed

Coronary Artery Disease

The most common reason for performing cardiac catheterization in adults is to confirm the diagnosis of coronary artery disease and to determine its severity. Coronary artery disease (CAD) has many causes and community educational programs are teaching people today how to decrease their chances of developing this disease. The most familiar risk factors are elevated cholesterol, hypertension, obesity, and smoking. Other factors that can lead to CAD are heredity (family history), chronic hypertension that is poorly controlled, lifestyle in general, and variation in coronary anatomy.

The coronary arteries carry oxygenated blood to the heart muscle. Occlusion of a coronary artery causes blood flow to be decreased or totally blocked to the area of heart muscle it feeds. Without oxygenated blood flow, this area of muscle will become hypoxic and die. Coronary flow can be blocked by plaque, blood clot, or a combination of the two. Another form of coronary occlusion is being seen today; that is, coronary artery spasm. The arterial walls are very elastic and can develop spasm just as a muscle does. If a spasm is short in nature, the patient may have only a short episode of chest discomfort or no symptoms at all; however, if the spasm persists, infarction can occur. At catheterization, coronary occlusion can be seen on cineangiograms (Figures 11-17 and 11-18).

306 Cardiac Catheterization

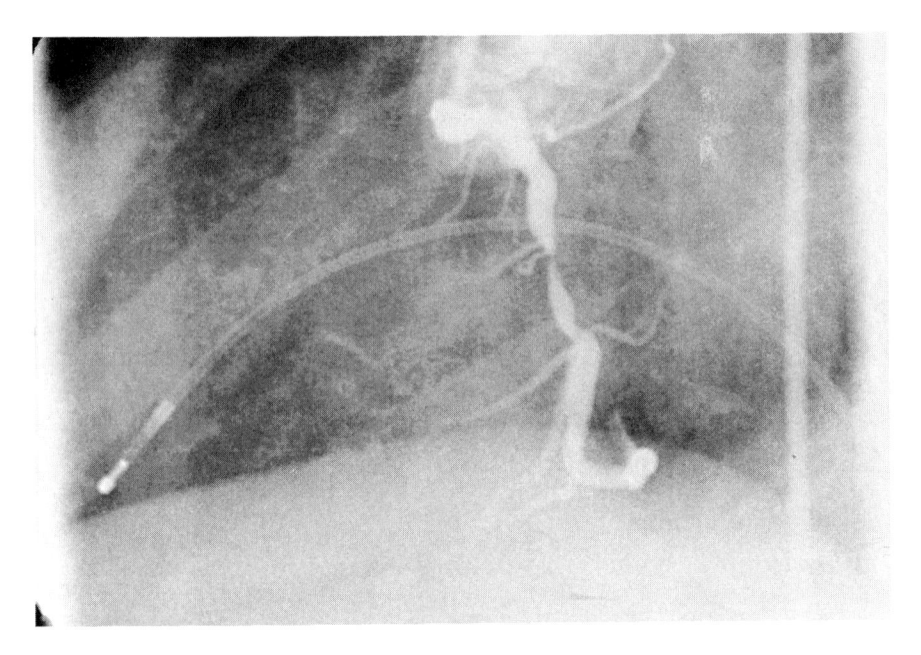

Figure 11-17 Abnormal right coronary artery injection.

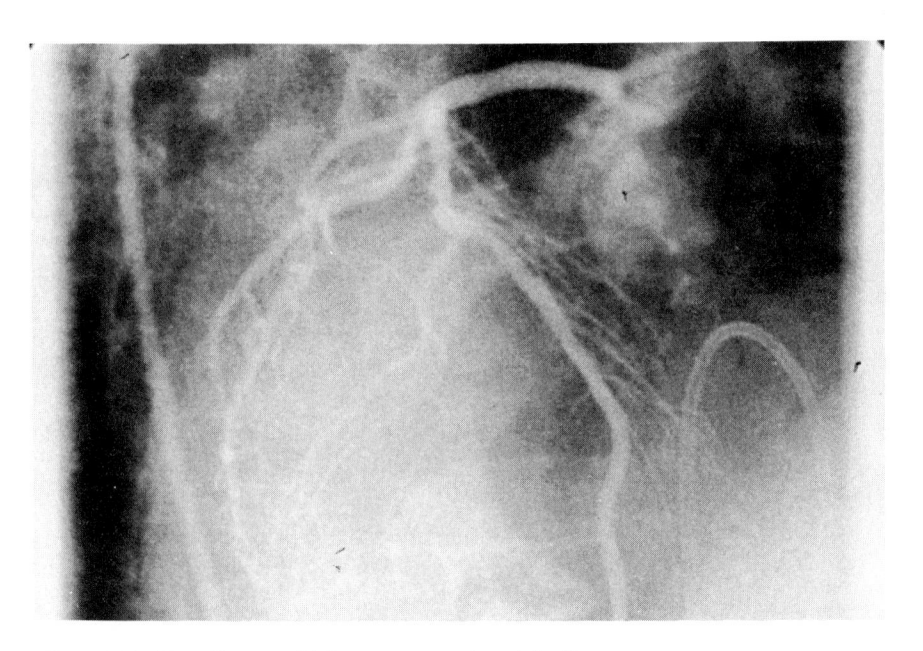

Figure 11-18 Abnormal left coronary artery injection.

Today, treatment for coronary artery disease is quite sophisticated. Medications are available to control various cardiac functions as well as patient symptoms. When invasive treatment becomes necessary, it is often possible to open an occluded vessel by angioplasty, negating the need for bypass surgery. When bypass surgery is necessary, techniques have been perfected and the success rate is excellent. After an infarction or surgery, cardiac rehabilitation programs are available that teach diet, exercise, and how to decrease the risk factors that could lead to further cardiac problems.

When working with infants and children, coronary artery circulation is rarely considered to be a source of difficulty; however, it is possible for an infant to have a myocardial infarction secondary to decreased coronary blood flow. This condition is known as *anomalous left coronary artery* and occurs in only 1 out of 300,000 births. Rather than arising from the aorta, the left coronary artery arises from the pulmonary artery. Flow into the anomalous left coronary artery is poor because the pulmonary artery pressure is lower than that of the aorta. Infarct, then, occurs secondary to insufficient coronary blood flow. In some cases, large collateral vessels from the right coronary artery fill the left coronary artery in retrograde fashion. Because the right coronary artery pressure is systemic (equal to aortic pressure) and the left coronary artery pressure is lower (equal to pulmonic pressure), blood naturally flows from the right coronary artery, through the collateral vessels, and into the left coronary artery. Over a period of time, infarctions occur and ischemic cardiomyopathy develops from lack of sufficient blood flow to the ventricles (Figure 11-19).

Valvular Stenosis

Stenosis can occur in any of the four heart valves and can be congenital or acquired. For many years, mitral stenosis has been recognized in patients who recovered from rheumatic fever. Another cause of valvular stenosis is calcification of the valve leaflets or cusps. The hemodynamic effects of valvular stenosis span a wide range from very mild, requiring no treatment, to critical, requiring immediate intervention.

It is not uncommon for patients with valvular stenosis to develop valvular insufficiency. The reason for this is simple. As stenosis develops, valve leaflets are fused and shortened. Insufficiency occurs if the valve leaflets are shortened sufficiently to keep the valve from closing completely. As the chamber before the valve enlarges, further distortion of the valve can occur. For example, a postrheumatic fever patient is found to have mitral stenosis with no insufficiency. Six months later, a check-up by echo reveals that the left atrium is enlarged and mitral regurgitation is noted. Careful echo evaluation of the valve reveals that the stenotic leaflets have been displaced posteriorly as the left atrium enlarged, causing the mitral insufficiency.

A common complication of mitral stenosis is left atrial thrombus. This occurs because the atrium cannot empty completely with each heart beat. As old blood remains in the atrium, it clots and further blocks the flow of fresh blood.

Normal Coronary Circulation

1. Right coronary artery
2. Right marginal artery
3. Conus artery
4. Posterior interventricular artery
5. Left circumflex artery
6. Left anterior descending
7. Left marginal artery

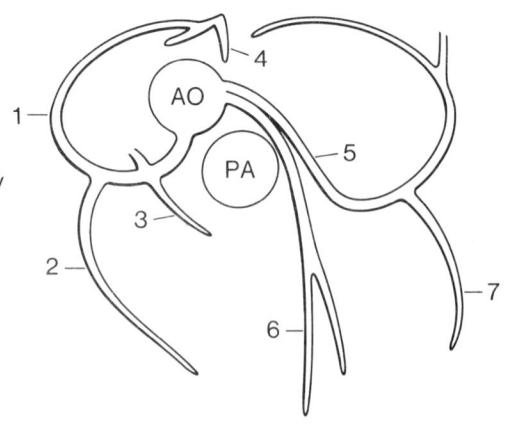

Circulation With Anomalous Left Coronary Artery (LCA)

1. Right coronary artery
2. Right marginal artery
3. Conus artery
4. Posterior interventricular artery
5. Left circumflex artery
6. Left anterior descending
7. Left marginal artery

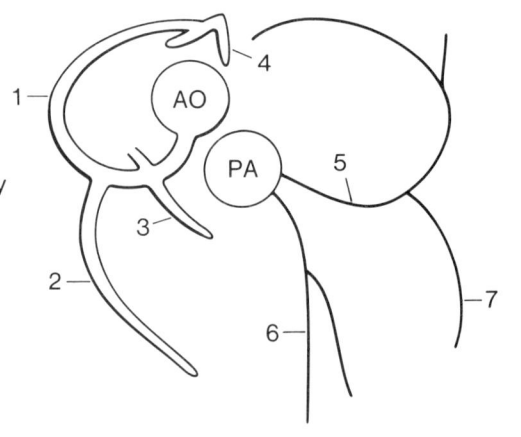

Figure 11-19 When the left coronary artery (LCA) arises from the pulmonary artery (PA), blood from the PA that is at a lower pressure (25–28 mm Hg) fills the LCA poorly. The LCA will appear thin and threadlike while the right coronary artery (RCA) will be dilated and tortuous.

Until very recently, the diagnosis of valvular stenosis and measurement of the pressure gradient was almost always made at catheterization. Today, however, echo Doppler techniques are permitting a prediction of valve gradients noninvasively. In the catheterization laboratory, stenosis is diagnosed by measuring the valve pressure gradient. Remember, a valve pressure gradient is the pressure difference on both sides of the valve. For example, in the normal heart, right ventricular systolic pressure equals the pulmonary artery systolic pressure. If valvular pulmonic stenosis is present, the right ventricular pressure could be 80/10 and the pulmonary artery pressure 25/12. The valve pressure gradient would equal 55 mmHg, the difference between

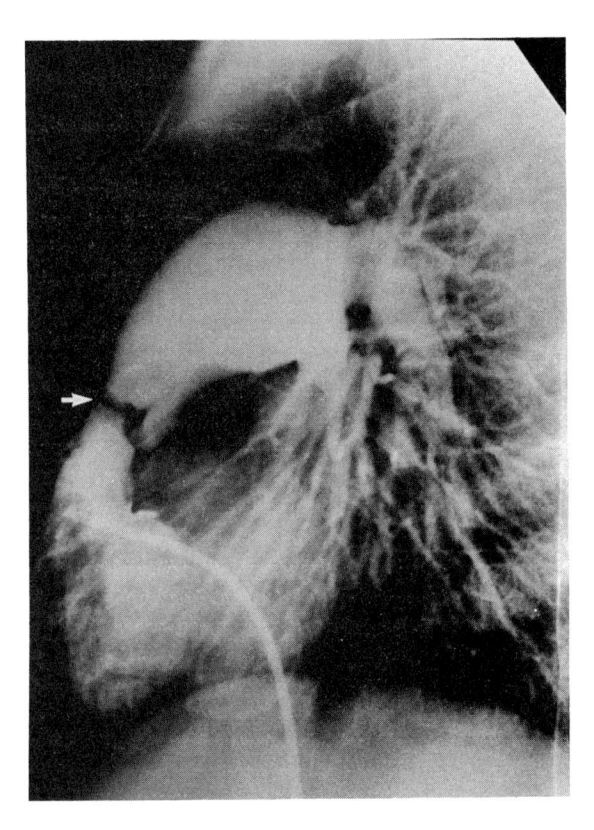

Figure 11-20 Pulmonic stenosis with mild post-stenotic dilatation.

the systolic pressures. Contrast is then injected and flow through the stenotic valve is observed.

Figures 11-20 and 11-21 both show valvular pulmonic stenosis. Notice that the pulmonary artery bulges out above the valve in Figure 11-21. This is caused by a small jet of blood coming through the valve at very high pressure and hitting the vessel wall. You may hear this referred to as the *jet effect* or *poststenotic dilatation*.

Treatment for valvular stenosis can be as simple as taking daily therapeutic medications or as complex as total replacement of the valve. In some patients, surgery can be performed to open the fused valve leaflets.

Congenital Cardiac Anomalies
Congenital cardiac anomalies occur in many different forms and degrees of severity. The purpose of this section is to explain how the common anomalies are diagnosed at catheterization and what their impact is on circulatory function.

Atrial Septal Defect (ASD). An ASD is a defect or hole in the atrial septum that allows blood to flow across the septum. Two major types (there are others) of ASD are identified according to their location in the septum; they

310 Cardiac Catheterization

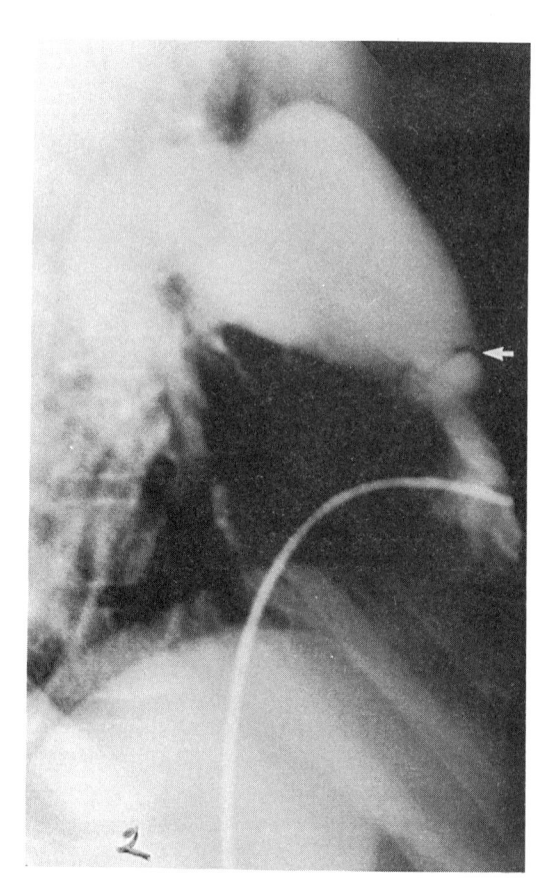

Figure 11-21 Valvular pulmonic stenosis with marked post-stenotic dilatation.

are called *ostium secundum* and *ostium primum*. Ostium secundum ASD's are one of the most frequently seen congenital cardiac anomalies. Patients with secundum ASD may be diagnosed during childhood, because of a heart murmur, or they may go undetected into adulthood. These patients are acyanotic and are rarely symptomatic. Catheterization is elective and sometimes performed in children around age 5 so that surgical correction can be carried out before the child begins school. Some centers do not feel the need to perform preoperative catheterization in patients with simple secundum ASD.

Ostium primum ASD's are usually larger and of greater concern than secundum ASD's. The resulting left-to-right shunt causes pulmonary blood flow to be markedly increased. Left untreated, the right atrium and right ventricle will hypertrophy and pulmonary arteries will enlarge. The left atrium does not enlarge because excessive pulmonary venous return readily flows to the right side of the heart.

Case 3 The patient is a 5 year old female with a secundum ASD confirmed at catheterization.
BSA = .70 M^2

Hemoglobin = 12.4 gm
O$_2$ Capacity = 168.6
O$_2$ Consumption (nonindexed) = 86.8
O$_2$ Saturations and Mean Pressures are shown in Figure 11-22.

$$QP = \frac{86.8}{(.95 - .75) \times 168.6} = 2.57 \text{ Liter/min}$$

$$PI = \frac{2.57 \text{ Liter/min}}{.7 \text{ M}^2} = 3.67 \text{ Liter/min/M}^2$$

$$Qs = \frac{86.8}{(.95 - .67) \times 168.6} = 1.84 \text{ Liter/min}$$

$$CI = \frac{1.84 \text{ Liter/min}}{.7 \text{ M}^2} = 2.63 \text{ Liter/min/M}^2$$

$$Qp/Qs = \frac{2.57 \text{ Liter/min}}{1.84 \text{ Liter/min}} = 1.40 : 1$$

$$Qep = \frac{86.8}{(.95 - .67) \times 168.6} = 1.84 \text{ Liter/min}$$

L → R Shunt = 2.57 Liter/min − 1.84 Liter/min = 0.73 Liter/min

R → L Shunt = 1.84 Liter/min − 1.84 Liter/min = 0

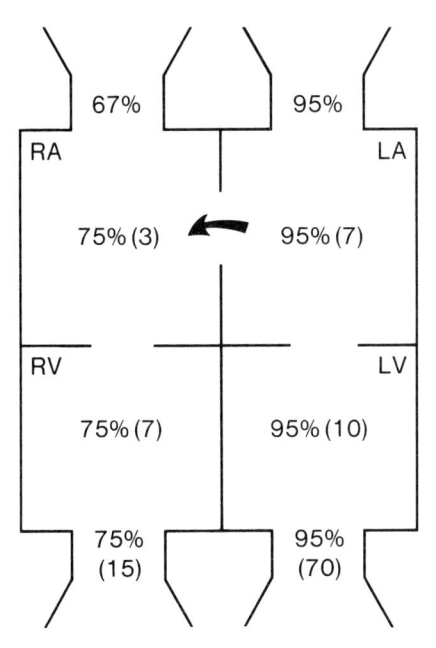

Figure 11-22 Oxygen saturation percentages with mean pressures in parentheses.

$$Rp = \frac{15 \text{ mm Hg} - 7 \text{ mm Hg}}{2.63 \text{ Liter/min/M}^2} = 2.18 \text{ RU}$$

$$Rs = \frac{70 \text{ mm Hg} - 3 \text{ mm Hg}}{2.63 \text{ Liter/min/M}^2} = 25.48 \text{ RU}$$

$$Rp/Rs = \frac{2.18 \text{ RU}}{25.48 \text{ RU}} = .09$$

This patient had a small left-to-right shunt at the atrial level, consistent with an atrial septal defect. No right-to-left shunt was present. Pulmonary resistance was within normal limits. Qp/Qs calculated at 1.40:1. Based on the hemodynamic findings, it was decided that surgery was not necessary for this patient.

Ventricular Septal Defect (VSD). A ventricular septal defect is a hole or defect in the septum between the two ventricles. The most common congenital anomaly is the membranous VSD. This is located in the ventricular septum, just below the aortic valve. VSD's can also be located in the muscular portion of the septum.

In general, ventricular septal defects are of more concern than atrial septal defects because ventricular pressures are higher; therefore, the degree of shunting is greater. Infants with large VSD's fail to grow normally, have difficulty feeding, and frequently develop congestive heart failure secondary to a large left-to-right shunt. These infants require catheterization and surgery to repair the defect. In some cases, a VSD will close spontaneously or become smaller as the child grows.

At catheterization, the VSD can be visualized by injecting contrast into the left ventricle and filming its flow across the ventricular septum.

Physiologic measurements will vary from patient to patient, depending on the size and location of the defect. Generally, the right ventricle and pulmonary artery pressures and oxygen saturations are elevated, as illustrated in the case below.

Case 4 The patient is a one-year-old male with a Grade IV/VI pansystolic murmur. He has been hospitalized twice for congestive heart failure.
BSA = .43 M^2
Hemoglobin = 14.3 gm
O$_2$ Capacity = 194.5
O$_2$ Consumption (nonindexed) = 67.08
O$_2$ Saturations and Mean Pressures are shown in Figure 11-23.

Using the information above, blood flows and resistances were calculated. Results are as follows:

$$Qp = 4.31 \text{ Liter/min}$$
$$Qs = 1.28 \text{ Liter/min}$$
$$PI = 10.03 \text{ Liter/min/M}^2$$

```
              63%              95%
         RA                         LA

              65% (2)          95% (8)


         RV                         LV

              84% (8)  ←  93% (10)


              87%              90%
              (63)             (65)
```

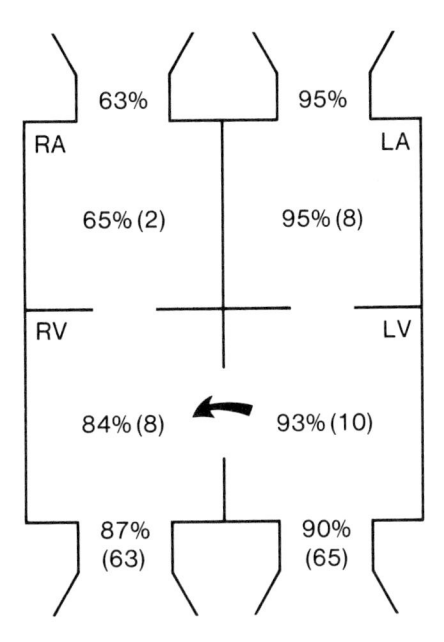

Figure 11-23 Oxygen saturation percentages with mean pressures in parentheses.

$$CI = 2.97 \text{ Liter/min/M}^2$$
$$Qep = 2.51 \text{ Liter/min/M}^2$$
$$Qp/Qs = 3.38$$
$$L \rightarrow R \text{ Shunt} = 7.52 \text{ Liter/min/M}^2$$
$$R \rightarrow L \text{ Shunt} = 0.46 \text{ Liter/min/M}^2$$
$$Rs = 5.48 \text{ RU}$$
$$Rp = 21.21 \text{ RU}$$

Notice the relationship between pulmonary flow and systemic flow. The left-to-right shunt across the VSD is more than twice the total systemic output. With the degree of shunting present, it is easy to see why this youngster has had congestive heart failure.

When studying ventricular septal defects, it is important to note that adults may develop VSD's and when this occurs, the consequences are very serious. When an infant is born with a congenital VSD, the heart is usually well compensated because the hemodynamic abnormalities occurred gradually as the heart was developed *in utero*.

VSD's in the adult population can occur as the result of blunt chest trauma or after an acute myocardial infarction (MI). During the course of an acute MI, areas of the septum may be involved and become hypoxic. The tissue can then become necrotic and blood at high pressure will rupture the already weakened septum. Because the adult heart is accustomed to its normal hemodynamics, the sudden change that occurs can be life threatening. The lungs are suddenly flooded with excess blood flow and congestive heart failure develops rapidly (Figure 11-24).

Cases have been reported where adults with acquired VSD's were taken to surgery for immediate repair of the defect and did well postoperatively.

Coarctation of the Aorta. Coarctation is a congenital narrowing of the aorta that usually occurs in the area of the *ductus arteriosus*. This narrowing may be very mild, causing no symptoms, or very severe, requiring immediate intervention. Occasionally, coarctation is not diagnosed until adolescence or adulthood because patients develop significant collateral circulation to the descending aorta. Patients with good collateral circulation to the distal descending aorta may be totally asymptomatic. Severe or critical coarctation of the aorta does occur in infants, although this finding is rare.

Anomalies of the aortic valve are associated with coarctation of the aorta. Approximately 80% of the patients with coarctation will also be found to have some anomaly of the aortic valve.

Clinically, the coarctation patient can be challenging to diagnose and treat. On routine physical examinations, coarctation can be suspected if there is a difference in the pulses between the arms and legs. Supine arm and leg blood pressures can then be measured and compared. If coarctation is suspected, the patient can be exercised with supine arm and leg blood pressures measured simultaneously immediately postexercise. If coarctation is present, arm blood pressures will be higher than the leg pressures after exercise. The electrocardiogram may show left ventricular hypertrophy or may be totally normal.

Although symptoms are not always present, some coarctation patients complain of headaches or coldness of the feet. In adults, the symptoms are primarily due to long-standing hypertension. Infants with severe coarctation may appear to be normal until the second week of life when they present with

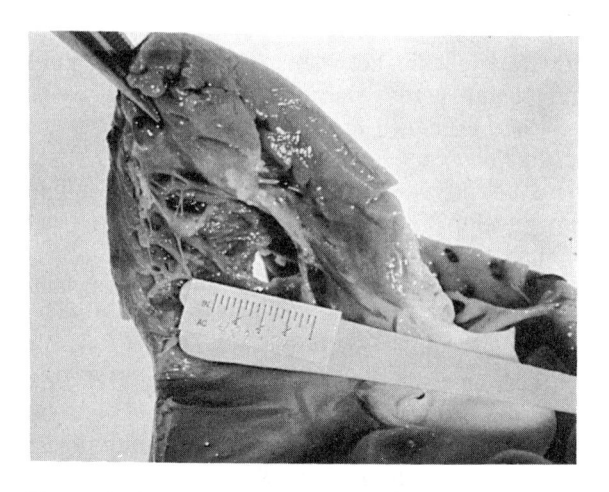

Figure 11-24 Ventricular septal defect.

very severe congestive heart failure. At that point, immediate intervention is necessary to prevent permanent damage to the left ventricle or possibly sudden death.

At catheterization, the diagnosis of coarctation is made by performing a pull-back pressure recording from the ascending aorta to the descending thoracic aorta. A pressure gradient will be measured at the coarctation site. Contrast can then be injected into the left ventricle and flow through the aortic valve and the aorta can be filmed. If the left ventricle is not entered, supravalvular aortic injection can be made, injecting contrast just above the aortic valve.

Figures 11-25 and 11-26 demonstrate coarctation of the aorta, using left ventricular injection and supravalvular aortic injection, respectively. In both cases, the coarctation site is distal to the *ductus arteriosus*. Notice the tortuosity of the vessels coming off the aorta. Blood is forced through these vessels at pressures higher than normal, causing upper body hypertension. In both of these cases, the coarctation is discreet or limited to a small portion of the aorta. Surgical repair for discrete coarctation can be carried out using subclavian flap angioplasty or by resecting the narrowed area and reconnecting the aorta using end-to-end anastomosis. If the coarcted segment is long, a tubular graft may be inserted to replace the narrowed aortic segment.

Patent *Ductus Arteriosus* (PDA). The *ductus arteriosus* is a connection between the aorta and left pulmonary artery that, *in utero*, allows right

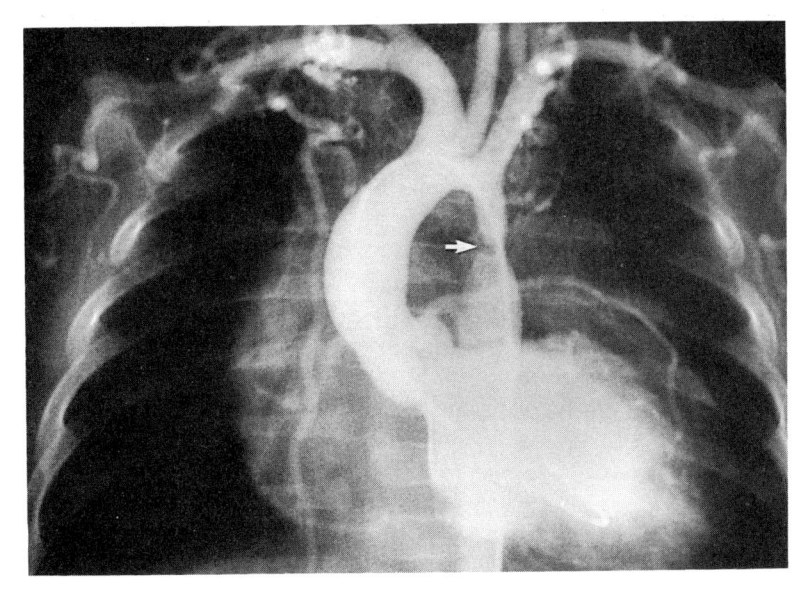

Figure 11-25 Coarctation of the aorta filmed after left ventricular injection.

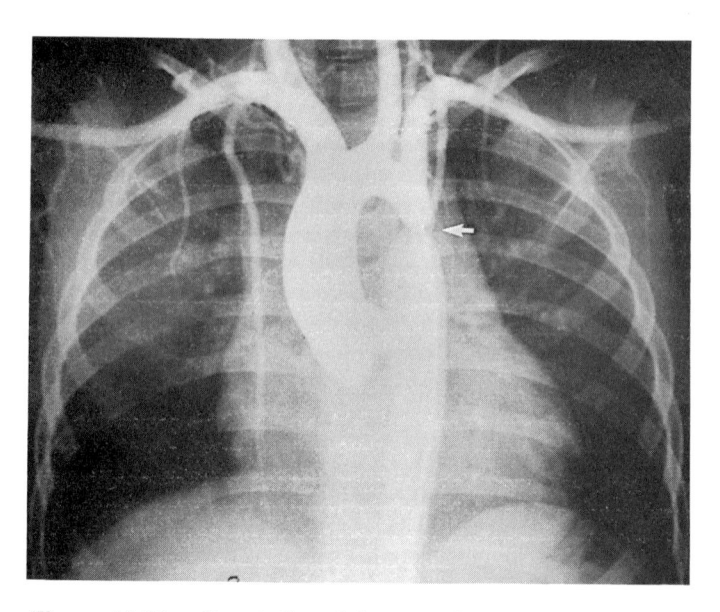

Figure 11-26 Coarctation of the aorta following supravalvular aortic injection.

ventricular blood to bypass the nonfunctioning lungs. When respiration begins at birth, usefulness of the *ductus arteriosus* ends and usually the *ductus* will close within the first few days of life. For some unknown reason, the *ductus arteriosus* remains patent in some patients. As an isolated anomaly, the PDA is one of the most common congenital cardiac anomalies. Usually patients with PDA are asymptomatic although infants with very large PDA's can develop congestive heart failure. This is due to the large amount of blood being shunted from the aorta at high pressure to the pulmonary artery and lungs, which are at a lower pressure.

At catheterization, hemodynamic findings are generally normal except for increased PA saturation, increased PA pressure (if the *ductus* is large) and increased aortic pulse pressure. Pulse pressure is the difference between the systolic and diastolic pressures. For example, if aortic pressure is 110/60, the pulse pressure is 50 mmHg. In the PDA patient, the diastolic pressure in the aorta is lower than normal, causing the pulse pressure to be greater.

The arrow in Figure 11-27 shows the patent *ductus arteriosus*. Contrast was injected into the left ventricle and filmed as it flowed into the aorta and through the patent ductus arteriosus. In many institutions, it is agreed that catheterization is not necessary to confirm the diagnosis of PDA. Repair consists of surgical ligation of the ductus.

Tetralogy of Fallot (TOF). This is by far the most common form of cyanotic congenital heart disease that, untreated, is compatible with a somewhat

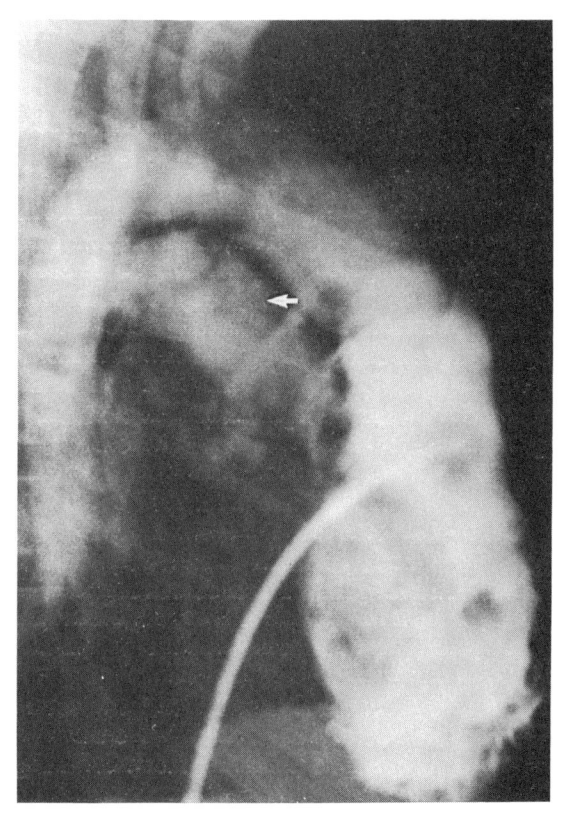

Figure 11-27 Patent *ductus arteriosus*.

normal life span. Described by Fallot, the tetralogy consists of four cardiac defects. They are pulmonary stenosis or atresia, ventricular septal defect, overriding of the aorta, and right ventricular hypertrophy.

The ventricular septal defect is generally large, allowing blood to shunt freely from the right ventricle to the left ventricle. The aortic valve is displaced over the VSD, so that the aorta appears to arise from both ventricles. This allows blood to flow from both ventricles into the aorta. The presence of cyanosis in the TOF patient is dependent upon how much blood is flowing from the right ventricle into the aorta. If the pulmonic valve is atretic or nearly so, the total right ventricular output will shunt right to left across the VSD as well as into the aorta, making these patients very cyanotic. Right and left ventricular pressures are equal in such patients.

Case 5   A 1-year-old male, known to have tetralogy, is being catheterized because of increased cyanosis and sweating when he feeds.
BSA = .30 M^2
Hemoglobin = 17.8 gm
O_2 Capacity = 242.1
O_2 Consumption (nonindexed) = 60.3

318 Cardiac Catheterization

$$O_2 \text{ SATURATIONS:} \quad SVC = 63\%$$
$$PV = 95\%$$
$$Ao = 85\%$$
$$RV = 63\%$$
$$\text{MEAN PRESSURES: } RA = 2$$
$$LA = 6$$
$$AO = 70$$

Calculations are illustrated in Figure 11-28.

In this patient, the degree of shunting is not great. The Qp/Qs ratio was calculated to be .68. In the absence of pulmonary artery saturation, the right ventricular saturation was used to calculate pulmonary flow. Pulmonary resistance could not be calculated because no mean pressure was measured in the pulmonary artery.

Treatment for tetralogy in early infancy consists of a surgical shunt between the pulmonary artery and aorta to improve pulmonary blood flow. Later in life, the patient must then undergo complete surgical repair of his defects.

Transposition of the Great Arteries. For an infant born with D-transposition of the great arteries, cardiac catheterization becomes a life-saving procedure. In D-transposition, the aorta comes off the right ventricle and the pulmonary artery comes off the left ventricle. Essentially, the patient has two totally separate circulatory systems. Figure 11-29 illustrates the blood flow patterns of D-TGA.

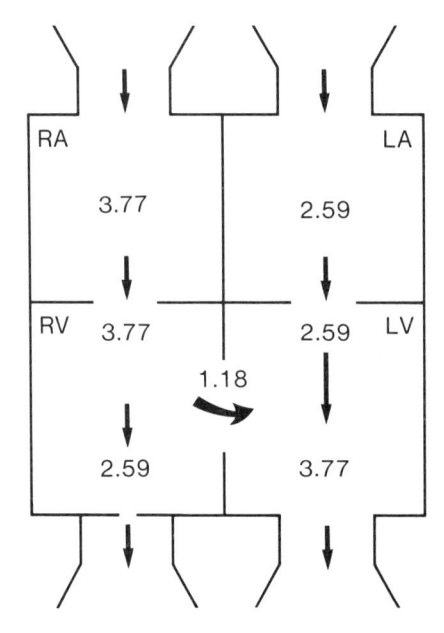

Figure 11-28 Tetralogy of Fallot catheterization calculations shown in liters/m/M^2.

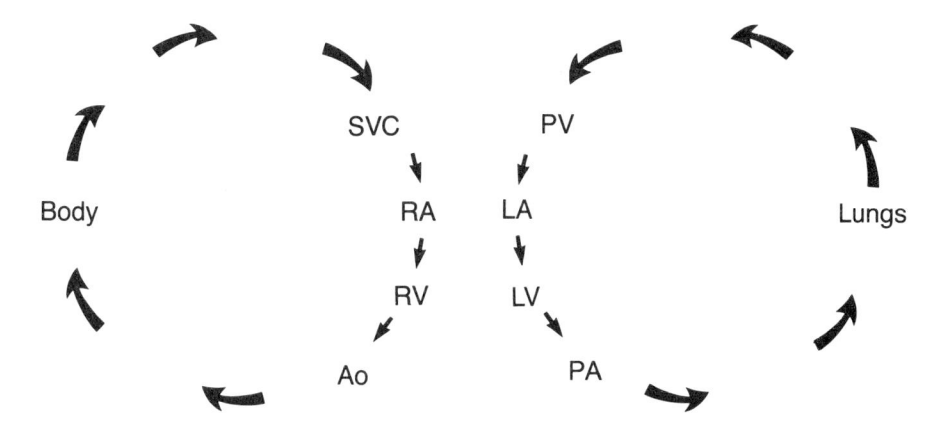

Figure 11-29 Circulatory patterns in D-transposition of the great arteries.

Infants with D-TGA usually present within the first few hours of life with severe cyanosis. The cyanosis worsens quickly because oxygenated blood from the lungs is not reaching the body. Before therapeutic catheterization procedures were developed, infants with D-TGA died very early in life. Today, balloon atrial septostomy can be performed to preserve life.

As with any medical diagnosis, it is important to note that not all patients with D-transposition fit the description above. Some infants are born with associated atrial septal defects or ventricular septal defects that allow blood to mix within the heart. These defects relieve some of the early severe cyanosis and allow the infant to stabilize prior to catheterization. After initial intervention, the infant can usually wait for 6 to 12 months before surgical repair is carried out. The additional months of growth make the patient a better surgical candidate. Some centers are now attempting an arterial switch operation that must be performed in the first month of life in children with simple D-TGA.

Another form of transposition is L-TGA or also referred to as *congenitally corrected transposition*. Patients with L-TGA may not be diagnosed until adolescence because their blood flow is not really abnormal. The circulatory pattern for L-TGA is illustrated in Figure 11-30.

Although the circulatory pattern appears almost normal, complications can arise from L-TGA, the most common being arrhythmia and complete heart block requiring pacemaker insertion.

Therapeutic Catheterization Procedures

Catheterization today provides more than diagnostic information. Many patients who would have required open heart surgery are now being helped in the catheterization laboratory.

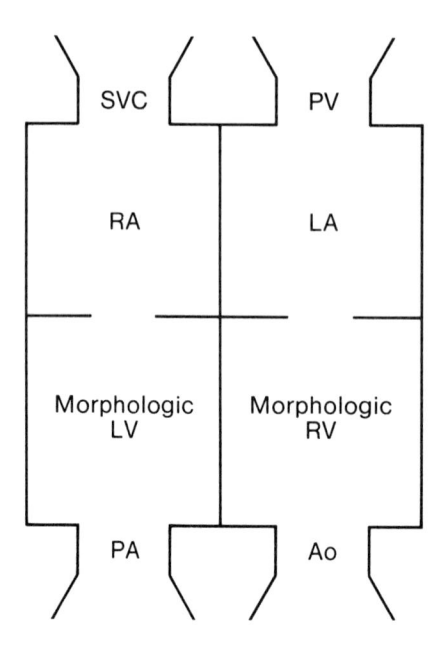

Figure 11-30 Circulatory pattern in L-transposition of the great arteries.

Streptokinase

Streptokinase was introduced several years ago as a medication to dissolve blood clots. Since myocardial infarction can be caused by a blood clot at the site of a coronary artery lesion, this drug was readily accepted as a method of quickly reopening blocked coronary vessels.

Initially streptokinase was administered through a catheter directly into the coronary arteries; however, this limited the drug's usefulness. By the time a patient could be prepared and taken to the catheterization laboratory, infarction had already occurred. It has now been discovered that streptokinase can be administered intravenously in the emergency room, allowing the medication to begin dissolving a blood clot sooner, and minimizing or preventing damage to the myocardium. Today streptokinase can be used to dissolve a blood clot, then angioplasty can be performed to open the coronary artery lesion.

Angioplasty

Without a doubt, one of the most exciting new therapeutic catheterization procedures is the angioplasty. Originally developed to open occluded coronary vessels, angioplasty is now being used to open stenotic valves as well as aortic coarctations.

In the coronary artery, angioplasty can open specific sites of occlusion caused by plaque. To do this, a guidewire is passed through the narrowed vessel and positioned. A balloon dilatation catheter is passed over the guidewire and positioned so the catheter markers are on each side of the occlusion. The balloon is then inflated to a pressure high enough to break the plaque and force it into the vessel wall. The vessel wall then heals over the plaque. Figure 11-31 illustrates the coronary artery before and after angioplasty.

When performing angioplasty on a stenotic valve, the procedure is sometimes called *valvuloplasty;* it is basically the same as coronary angioplasty. The primary difference is in balloon size. Coronary arteries are small and, therefore, require a small balloon. On the other hand, valvuloplasty and aortic angioplasty are performed using very large balloons, up to 25 mm in diameter. During valvuloplasty, extra care must be taken to select the appropriate balloon site. If the balloon is too large, the valve annulus can be damaged. Currently pulmonary valvuloplasty is proving to be very successful.

Figures 11-32 and 11-33 illustrate successful balloon angioplasty for coarctation of the aorta. The patient is a 18-month-old girl in whom subclavian flap repair had been performed at 6 months of age. On follow-up exam, she was again noted to have evidence of coarctation (decreased pulses in the legs and upper body hypertension). Successful balloon dilatation was accomplished as seen in Figure 11-33.

Swan-Ganz Catheterization

Hemodynamic monitoring began a little over 20 years ago with the introduction of central venous pressure (CVP) measurement. This measurement enabled the clinician to estimate crudely preload (the amount of blood presented to the heart). The major break came in 1970 when Doctors Swan and Ganz developed a flow-directed pulmonary artery catheter. This permitted measurement of pulmonary capillary wedge pressure, which is equal to left atrial and left ventricular end diastolic pressures and provides an accurate assessment of left ventricular preload. By using a flow-directed thermodilution catheter positioned in the pulmonary artery and a cardiac output computer, the full range of hemodynamic calculations can be per-

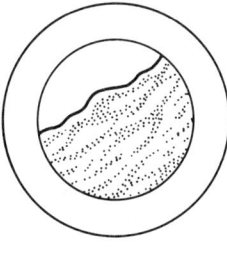

Coronary occlusion before angioplasty

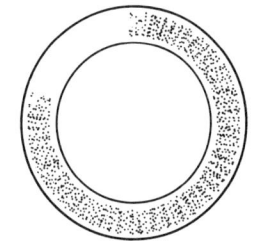

Coronary artery after angioplasty

Figure 11-31 Coronary artery pre- and post-successful balloon angioplasty.

322 Cardiac Catheterization

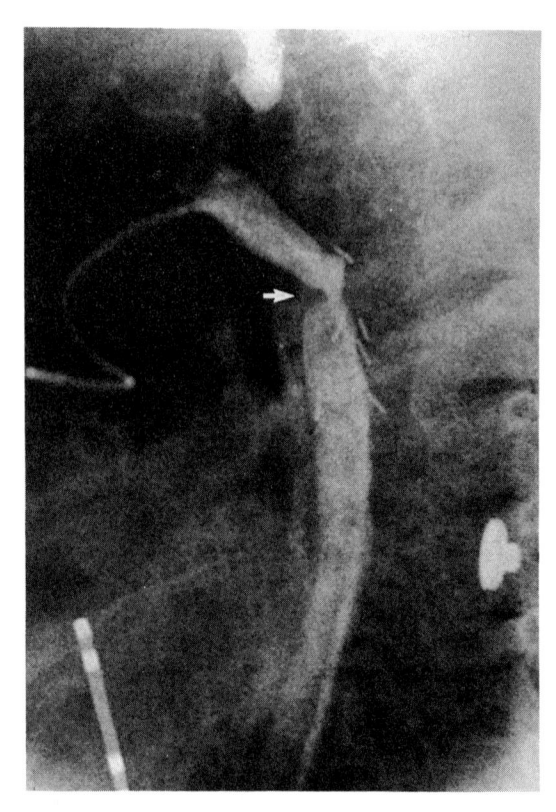

Figure 11-32 Coarctation before balloon angioplasty.

formed at a patient's bedside. Thermodilution cardiac outputs are performed by injecting fluid at a known temperature through the proximal catheter port. The cardiac output computer then uses complex algebraic equations to calculate cardiac output. The catheter balloon can be inflated for short periods of time to measure pulmonary capillary wedge pressure.

The most common risk factor with Swan-Ganz catheterization is infection. With a catheter in the heart for several days at a time, sterile technique must be followed at all times. Of course, there are many advantages, including the ability to perform the entire procedure at the patient's bedside.

Rashkind Balloon Atrial Septostomy

Performed in infants with D-transposition, the Rashkind procedure creates an opening in the atrial septum that allows blood to mix at the atrial level. Septostomy is performed by advancing the septostomy catheter into the right atrium, across the patent *foramen ovale,* and into the left atrium. The balloon is then filled with contrast and pulled back through the atrial septum to create an atrial septal defect. The balloon used to do this is very large (4 cc capacity) and must be filled completely so that it will be hard enough to

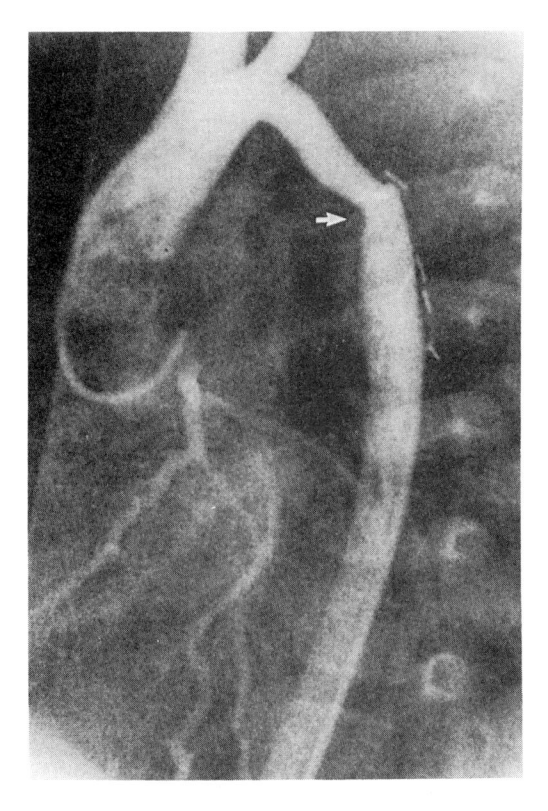

Figure 11-33 Coarctation post-balloon angioplasty.

tear the septum. When successful septostomy is performed, the very cyanotic infant with D-TGA immediately turns pink and begins to stabilize. Corrective surgery can then wait for 6 to 12 months when the infant has grown and is a better surgical candidate.

Summary

The first cardiac catheterization was performed a little over 50 years ago in an effort to treat dying patients. Since that time, many new types of catheterization have been perfected, including therapeutic techniques for treating heart disease. As progress continues in this field and new catheterization procedures are developed, the need for open heart surgery will likely become less frequent.

Bibliography

Grossman W: Cardiac Catheterization and Angiography. Philadelphia, Lea & Febiger, 1980
Hurst WJ: The Heart. New York, McGraw-Hill, 1982
Keith JD, Rowe RD, Vlad P: Heart Disease in Infancy and Childhood. New York, Macmillan, 1967

Moller JH: Essentials of Pediatric Cardiology. Philadelphia, F. A. Davis Co., 1978

Netter F: The Ciba Collection of Medical Illustrations, Volume 5: The Heart. Summit, N.J., Ciba Publications, 1971

Rocchini AP, Kveselis DA, Crowley D et al: Percutaneous balloon valvuloplasty for treatment of congenital pulmonary valvular stenosis in children. J Am Col Cardiol 3:1005, 1984

Slonim NB, Bell BP, Christensen SE: Cardiopulmonary Laboratory Basic Methods and Calculations. Springfield, IL, Charles C. Thomas, 1974

Warren JV: Fifty years of invasive cardiology: Werner Forssmann (1904–1979). Am J Med 69:10, 1980

Yang SS, Bentivoglio LG, Goldberg H: From Cardiac Catheterization to Hemodynamic Parameters. Philadelphia, FA Davis, 1981

Chapter 12

Peripheral Vascular Testing*

Mark A. Oliver

Peripheral vascular testing encompasses the noninvasive evaluation of peripheral arterial, venous, and cerebrovascular disease. Doppler ultrasound, plethysmography, and duplex scanning are techniques utilized in these evaluations.

It must be emphasized that these procedures are not intended to supplant traditional history and physical examinations or more invasive angiographic or venographic procedures in assessing patients with vascular disorders. However, these diagnostic tools have provided more objective information, both physiologically and anatomically, which can help our diagnostic and therapeutic approaches to vascular disease.

This chapter is designed as an introduction for students, technologists, and physicians to the field of noninvasive peripheral vascular testing. It is divided into four basic sections. In the first section noninvasive techniques are described with historical backgrounds, principles, and applications. The remaining sections are divided conveniently into Arterial Evaluation, Cerebrovascular Evaluation, and Venous Evaluation.

Noninvasive Techniques

Doppler Ultrasound

Sound moves through the air in waves or frequencies (cycles per second, cycles/second, CPS). Frequencies may be expressed in Hertz (1 Hertz, Hz, 1 cycle/second). Ultrasound refers to sound having a frequency beyond the capability of human hearing (20,000 Hz or 20K Hz).

*Acknowledgment is made to Joan Dennis for her assistance with this chapter.

The principle of a change in frequency caused by a moving source was first determined by a physicist named Christian Johann Doppler (1842).[1] An everyday example of the Doppler principle is the fact that the sound of a train whistle seems higher when it approaches a person and lower when it moves away.

The ultrasonic flow detector "senses blood flow by the frequency shift of sound reflected from moving blood cells."[2] A piezoelectric crystal in this device emits an ultrasonic beam, usually at a frequency between 5 to 10 MHz (5 to 10 megahertz, 5 to 10 million cycles/second). The transmitted frequency is inversely proportional to the depth of flow. Utilizing the Doppler principle, the frequency shift (transmitted frequency–received frequency) is proportional to the velocity of moving cells; red blood cells moving toward the transducer will produce an increase of received frequency while those cells moving away will produce a decrease in frequency (Figure 12-1). An equation can be established from the above: $\Delta F = \dfrac{2 \cos \theta \times Vft}{C}$ where

F = frequency shift
θ = angle between probe and blood flow axis
V = velocity of moving cells
Ft = transmitted frequency
C = velocity of sound in tissue (1500 meters/second)

This frequency shift may be processed as an audible signal, for wave form analysis, or by a spectrum analyzer.

Satomura developed the first ultrasonic flow detector in 1959[3] and further application of this device in peripheral vascular evaluation was pioneered by Strandness and others in the late 1960's. Further refinements and clinical research have continued to the present time.

Doppler Types

Ultrasonic flow detectors may be continuous or pulsed and unidirectional or bidirectional.

Continuous Wave. These devices contain an emitting crystal that sends a continuous ultrasonic beam sensitive to reflected sound from all moving objects within the range of the beam. The device also has a receiving crystal to accept the back-scattered frequencies (Figure 12-1). These less expensive machines are insensitive to the depth of detectable blood flow.

Pulsed Doppler. Machines with one crystal transmit repetitive bursts of ultrasound and sample the returning signal at selected intervals. Unlike continuous wave Dopplers, these instruments can detect the depth of blood flow. Thus they can be of particular value for ultrasonic flow imaging and duplex scanning with spectrum analysis.

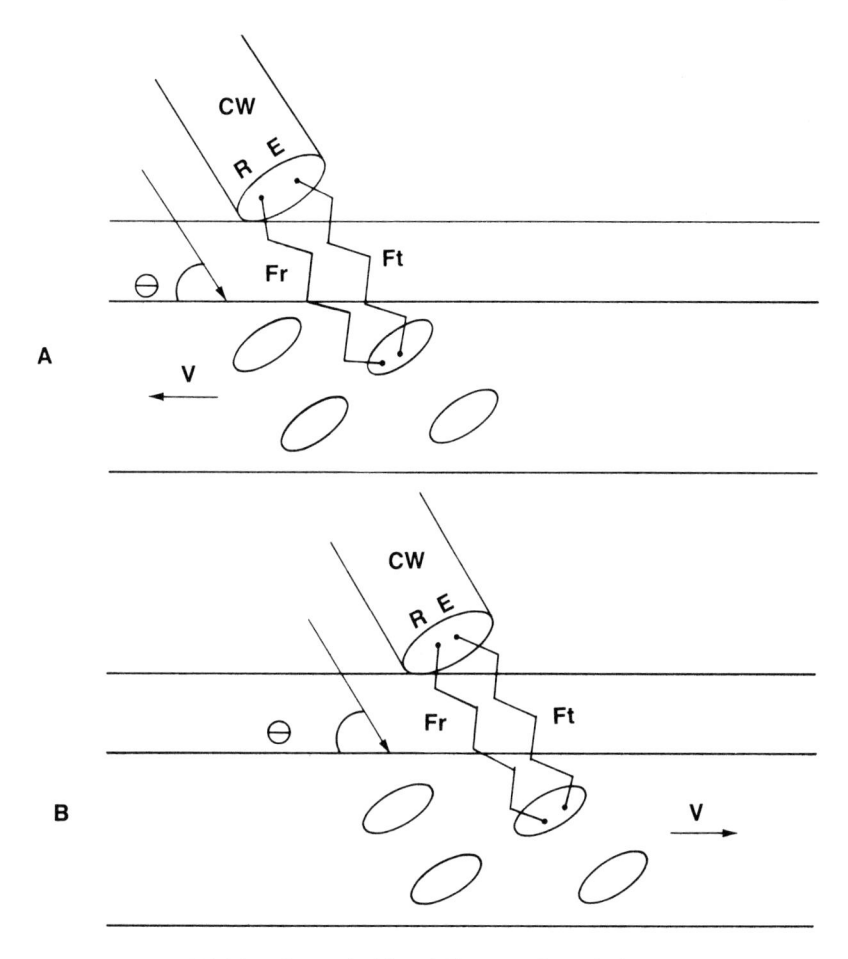

Figure 12-1 (A) Meanings of abbreviations and symbols: CW = Continuous wave Doppler. E = Emitting crystal. R = Receiving crystal. V = velocity. o = Angle between probe and blood vessel axis. Ft = Transmitting frequency. Fr = Receiving frequency. Note increased frequency with cell moving toward probe. *Doppler Principle* $\Delta F = (Ft-Fr)$ is proportional to the velocity of the moving cells. (B) Frequency decreases as cell moves away from probe.

Nondirectional or Unidirectional. These Dopplers are unable to determine the direction of blood flow with respect to the probe, but are less expensive, small, and portable, and may be used effectively in arterial and venous diseases (Figure 12-2).

Directional or Bidirectional. These Dopplers are able to sense whether flow is toward or away from the probe. These devices are more complex and expensive, but have selected advantages in all phases of peripheral vascular testing (Figure 12-3).

328 Peripheral Vascular Testing

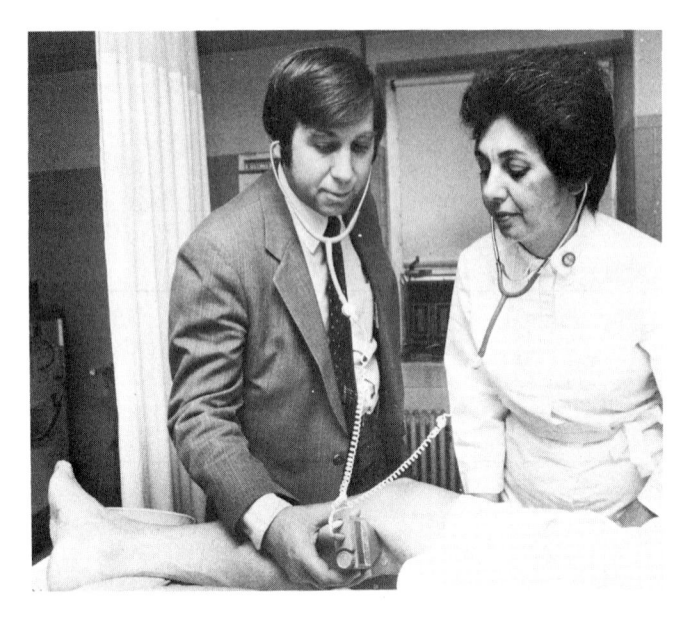

Figure 12-2 Small, portable unidirectional Doppler being utilized in venous disease evaluation.

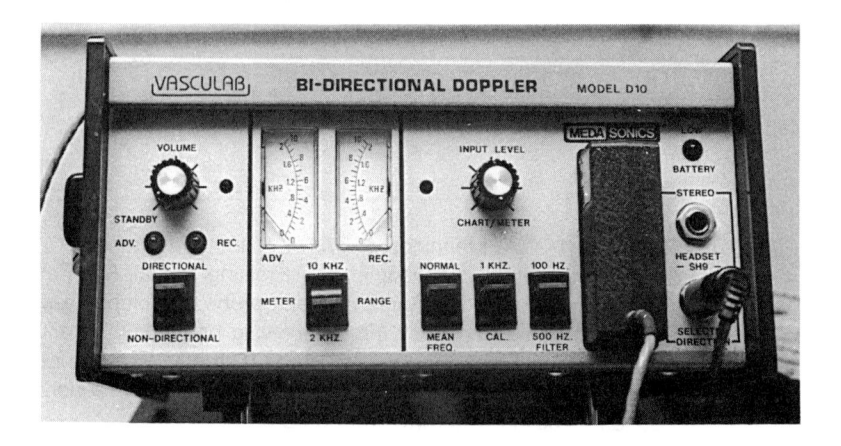

Figure 12-3 Bidirectional Doppler. ADV. = Signal detected toward probe. REC. = Signal detected away from probe.

Signal Detectors

Doppler signals can be processed in four different ways: *audio, analogue recording, spectral analysis,* and *imaging.* Audio is a simple, rapid technique but requires a technician to interpret correctly the arterial and venous signals. Analogue recording is accomplished with a zero crossing detector (conversion of a signal frequency to a corresponding voltage on a strip chart recorder). With spectral analysis, the frequency spectrum of a Doppler signal can be graphically displayed in real-time (Figure 12-4). Ultrasonic imaging is a technique that can image the vessel lumen by accumulating Doppler flow-detected signals on a memory storage oscilloscope.[4] This technique can exist either in the continuous mode with color (such as Echoflow) or with gated pulsed Doppler mode (such as Hokanson's Ultrasonic Arteriograph) (Figure 12-5). Both of these are static systems; currently systems are being developed that will have real-time color Doppler capabilities within a transducer where red may reflect toward the probe (such as arterial flow) and blue may reflect away from the probe (*e.g.*, venous flow).

Doppler ultrasound is a technique that can provide information about blood flow, pressures, and images. Although many of the uses of Doppler ultrasound may be subjective and experience-dependent, it remains a reliable noninvasive tool for screening peripheral vascular disease.

Plethysmography

Plethysmography is a measurement of change in volume in a limb or organ. As early as the 1600's, Johann Swammerdam designed a device that recorded changes in volume associated with animal cardiac contractions.

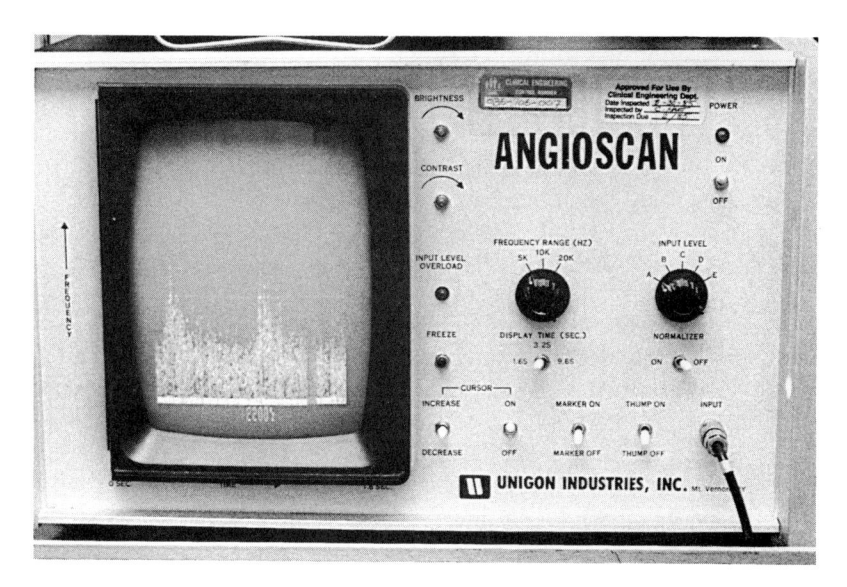

Figure 12-4 Spectrum analyzer graphically displaying blood flow.

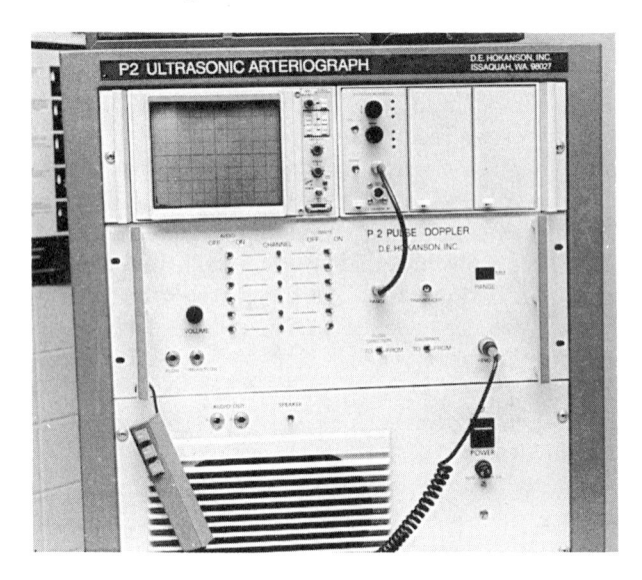

Figure 12-5 Hokanson's P2 ultrasonic arteriograph.

Recording blood flow of an extremity was accomplished by the principle of venous occlusive plethysmography that was introduced by Brodie and Russell in the early 1900's.[5] With venous flow obstructed, a change in volume could represent an increase of flow (arterial). The technique of plethysmography can thus be utilized to evaluate peripheral arterial pulsations, blood flow, blood pressure, and venous filling and emptying.

Plethysmography Types

Air. Air-filled cuffs are placed around an appropriate limb segment and connected to transducers that allow the determination of changes in limb volume. PVR (Pulse Volume Recorder—Lifesciences, Inc.) is an example of this type of machine that can be used in venous and arterial disease (Figure 12-6). An air-filled oculoplethysmograph by Gee can be utilized in cerebrovascular disease.

Strain Gauge. The strain gauge is a Silastic tube that can be placed around a limb or digit and is connected to a circuit that measures electrical resistance. Changes in electrical resistance can be associated with changes in the length of the gauge. The change in gauge length is a reflection of limb volume change. This principle of strain gauge plethysmography can be utilized to evaluate pulse wave forms, limb or digit blood pressures, and limb or digital blood flow.

Impedance. Changes in impedance (electric resistance) can reflect changes in blood volume in limb segments. By attaching the appropriate electrodes

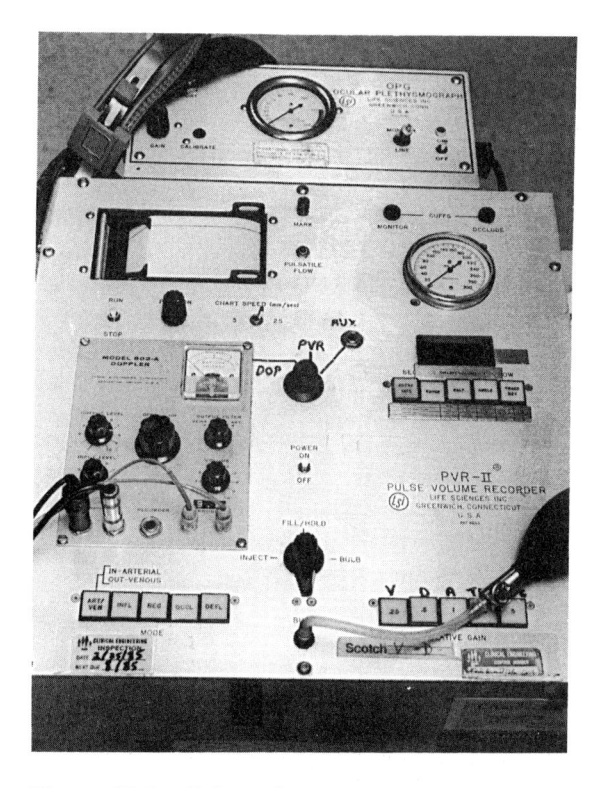

Figure 12-6 Pulse volume recorder (PVR–II).

to the patient's leg or arm, an Impedance Plethysmography (IPG) machine can measure the changes in the resistance of a leg or arm and thus can measure the blood volume changes between these electrodes. Cremer was the first to describe impedance plethysmography in 1907 and Nyboer was credited subsequently for utilizing this procedure to measure changes in limb blood volume.[6,7] This technique is used primarily in the diagnosis of deep venous thrombosis and has been described recently in evaluating venous insufficiency.

Water. In this type of plethysmography a body part is immersed into a water-filled container so that the volume change of the immersed part displaces the same amount of water. This remains the most accurate plethysmograph because of its direct measurement, but is cumbersome and not very portable. The most common present day use of the water plethysmograph for cerebrovascular evaluation is the water-filled oculoplethysmograph of Kartchner–McRae.

Photoelectric. Unlike other forms of plethysmography described thus far, photoelectric plethysmography (PPG) is a pulse recorder. A photo transducer emits infrared light into the skin and a photo cell is able to measure the reflected light from a cutaneous blood vessel, which is recorded as blood flow. In the AC mode, arterial pulse wave forms can be recorded. In the DC mode, PPG can be employed for the evaluation of venous insufficiency (Figure 12-7).

Duplex Scanning

The concept of duplex scanning has provided another dimension for noninvasive peripheral vascular testing. Continuous wave imaging and pulse Doppler imaging have been previously described (see Doppler Ultrasound). Another form of ultrasonic imaging can be produced that is known as *real-time B-mode imaging*. With real-time technology (increasing frames/second) a vessel may be seen pulsating just as it actually is within the body. In B-imaging (Brightness Mode), a reflected ultrasound signal may be displayed as dots (echo strength-dependent) that then may be processed in the gray scale. The gray scale would be affected by different tissue characteristics and a resultant image would then be produced. In order to obtain higher resolution, higher frequency transducers must be used to shorten the wavelength, and depth of penetration must be sacrificed because of increased rate of energy absorption. Despite these shortcomings with higher resolution images, plaques with various characteristics and even more recent clot formations can be visualized (Figure 12-8).

Acoustic properties determine the shades of gray seen on the ultrasonic imaging screen. Because the acoustic property of the newly formed clot is similar to blood, it may not be seen in a vessel and this may erroneously lead to a normal interpretation of a clotted artery. It is also possible that certain parts of a plaque may not be seen totally by ultrasonic imaging alone. New transducers were thus developed that contained both B-mode imaging and

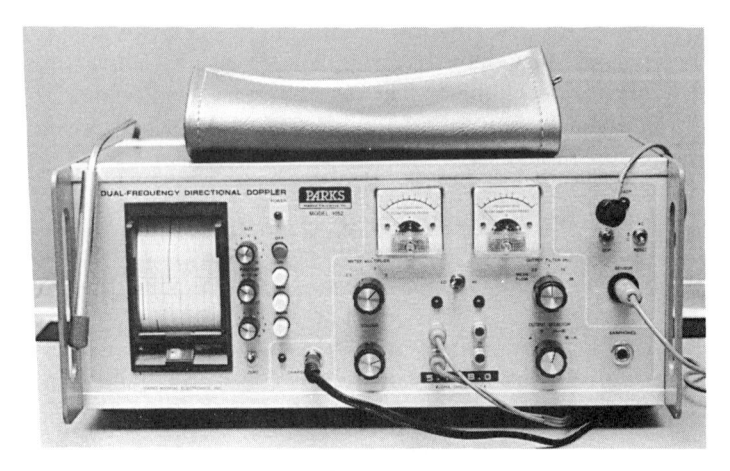

Figure 12-7 PPG small flat transducer seen to left of AC-DC mode switch.

pulsed Doppler (with spectrum analysis) capabilities. As a result, anatomic and physiologic data can be determined and many of the above problems could be resolved. Although the carotid artery evaluation was the first popular use of this technique, further studies have now shown the usefulness of duplex scanning in peripheral arterial and venous evaluations (Figure 12-9).

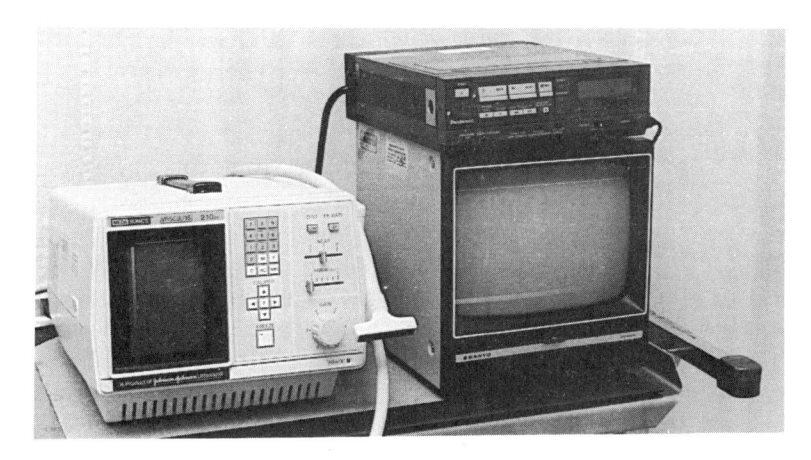

Figure 12-8 Portable real-time high resolution B-mode image with receiver and VCR.

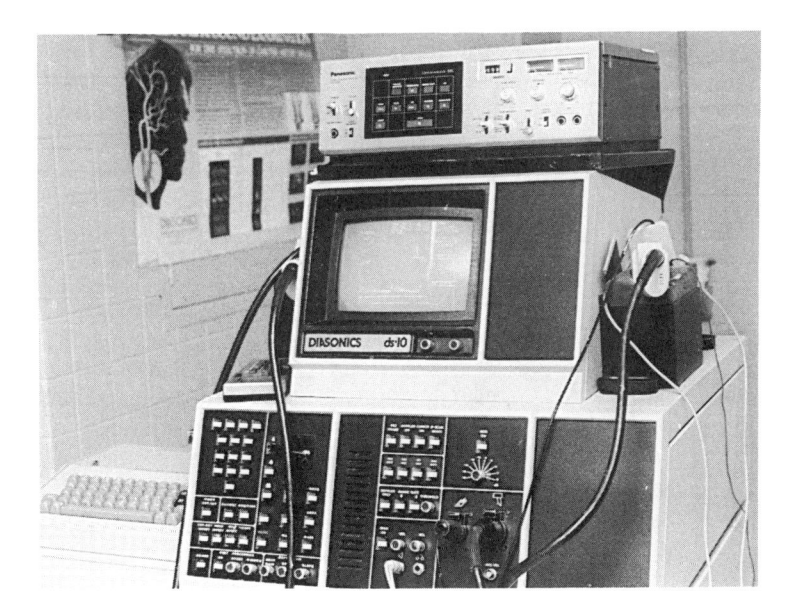

Figure 12-9 Diasonics (DRF 10) duplex scanner.

Arterial Evaluation

A vascular chart report is developed for all patients who enter the laboratory (Figure 12-10).

Documentation

The history taking and documentation are extremely important and in arterial disease vary from the asymptomatic patient to gangrene and potential limb loss. It is interesting to note a direct parallel in this regard between coronary arterial disease and peripheral vascular disease. Whereas in coronary artery disease there may be a spectrum of disease ranging from asymptomatic to angina to myocardial infarction, in peripheral arterial disease there may be a similar spectrum from asymptomatic to claudication to gangrene.

The patient, therefore, will usually present to the laboratory asymptomatic or complaining of some form of pain. With the asymptomatic patient, disease is suspected on physical examination. True claudication refers to the "arterial" condition in which discomfort (generally calf, thigh tightness) occurs on exercise and is relieved by rest. The degree of disability and its effect on life-style are important factors to be determined. Pseudoclaudication may present in a similar fashion, but is not a vascular etiology, such as hip pain, secondary to osteoarthritis. Pain at rest occurs mostly in the foot at night, is made worse by elevation, and is improved by leg dependency. True rest pain reflects previous arterial disease that may be a harbinger of gangrene, ischemic ulceration, or actual limb loss. Finally, the patient may present with the most advanced form of arterial disease—gangrene with eventual limb loss.

Pertinent past history pertains mostly to significant risk factors such as hypertension, diabetes, hyperlipidemia, and smoking. Family history and medication are also recorded.

To discuss clinical conditions at length would be beyond the scope of this text, but some common conditions will be considered briefly at this time.

In an *acute arterial occlusion*, the patient presents with a 6 "P's": *P*ain, *P*aresthesias, *P*aralysis, *P*allor, *P*ulselessness, *P*olar (cold). These may be secondary to local thrombosis (such as underlying atherosclerosis) or proximal emboli (such as in the heart).

Chronic arterial occlusive disease is most often secondary to atherosclerosis (fatty intimal plaques that may narrow the artery) and may range from asymptomatic to gangrene, as described earlier.

Aneurysms refer to an abnormal arterial bulging or enlargement with associated arterial wall thinning that may be secondary to degeneration, trauma, or infection most often found in the lower abdominal aorta and less frequently in lower extremity vessels.

A–V Fistulas are abnormal artery–vein connections that may be congenital or acquired, small or large; they may be hemodynamically significant.

MORRISTOWN MEMORIAL HOSPITAL
SECTION OF CARDIOLOGY
PERIPHERAL VASCULAR LABORATORY
ARTERIAL EVALUATION - EXTREMITIES

LOG #__________

NAME: __________ SEX: _____ DATE: __________

UNIT #: __________ AGE: _____ PHYSICIAN: __________

LOCATION: __________ CLINICAL DIAGNOSIS: __________

VASCULAR HISTORY: [ ] HYPERTENSION [ ] DIABETES [ ] HYPERLIPIDEMIA

[ ] OBESE [ ] ANGINA [ ] M.I. [ ] CVA [ ] TIA

SMOKER: [ ] NON-SMOKER [ ] PREVIOUS [ ] CURRENT

S/P __________

LESIONS __________

RESTING SYMPTOMS __________

EXERTIONAL SYMPTOMS __________

		CAROTID	BRACHIAL	ABD. AORTA	FEMORAL	POP	DP	PT
PULSES	LEFT							
	RIGHT							
BRUITS	LEFT							
	RIGHT							
DOPPLER SIGNAL	LEFT							
	RIGHT							

SUMMARY – OBSERVED HEMODYNAMIC DATA

BP R ARM ____ / ____ L ARM ____ / ____

R Psys L R PVR CATEGORY L

LOCATION				
THIGH				
CALF				
ANKLE				
TM				
DIGIT ( )				

EXERCISE: MAXIMUM WALKING TIME: _____ MIN. RATE _____ MPH DISTANCE _____

FEET GRADE _____ % SYMPTOMS: _____

$\bar{p}$ EX ANKLE						

COMMENTS:

EXAMINED BY: __________

D-SF 5839 10-84

Figure 12-10 Sample of lower extremity arterial evaluation form.

(Continued)

336 Peripheral Vascular Testing

BRACHIAL BLOOD PRESSURE   R ARM _____/_____   L ARM _____/_____

RESTING SEGMENTAL PULSE VOLUME AND SYSTOLIC PRESSURE DATA

RIGHT THIGH P
  sys _____ mmHg

LEFT THIGH P
  sys _____ mmHg

RIGHT CALF P
  sys _____ mmHg

LEFT CALF P
  sys _____ mmHg

RIGHT ANKLE P
  sys _____ mmHg

LEFT ANKLE P
  sys _____ mmHg

Figure 12-10 (Continued)

The remaining conditions may be classified into nonatherosclerotic syndromes.

Vasculitis refers to a group of necrotizing arterial inflammatory diseases of suspected immune etiology (such as polyarteritis *nodosa*, temporal arteritis, Takayasu's and Buerger's disease).

Thoracic outlet syndrome refers to a compression syndrome (neurovascular-bundle compression) that may be indirectly diagnosed by arterial flow obliteration in specific upper extremity positions.

Raynaud's syndrome is a cold-sensitivity syndrome involving digits with tricolor response (blue, white, red) to cold that may be idiopathic, pri-

RIGHT TRANSMETATARSAL   LEFT TRANSMETATARSAL

RIGHT DIGITAL (#   )   LEFT DIGITAL (#   )

EXERCISE EVALUATION

MAXIMUM WALKING TIME _____ MIN   RATE _____ MPH   GRADE _____ %
SYMPTOMS WITH EXERCISE _____

Segmental Plethysmograph and Systolic Pressure after exercise or reactive hyperemia

                                                        exercise _____
Brachial Systolic Pressure _____ _____ mmHg
                                                        reactive hyperemia _____

RIGHT ANKLE P   LEFT ANKLE P
   sys _____ mmHg   sys _____ mmHg

Figure 12-10 (Continued)

mary disease, but usually represents a benign or a phenomenon secondary to other underlying systemic illnesses (usually in their more severe form).

Physical Examination

First of all, it is important to understand the upper and lower arterial anatomy and circulation (Figures 12-11 and 12-12).

Inspection, palpation, and auscultation are the major areas of evaluation in physical examination of arterial disease.

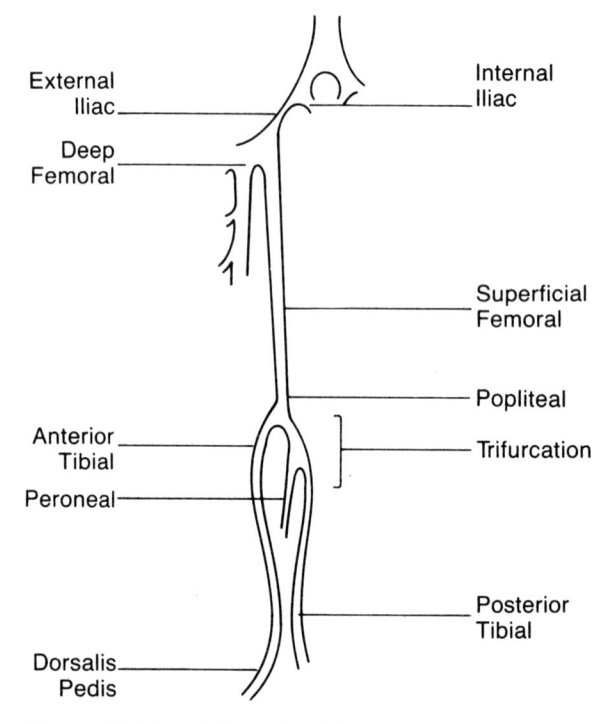

Figure 12-11 Schematic of lower extremity arterial circulation.

On inspection, skin changes (such as shiny, dry, scaly skin), color changes, increased pallor on elevation, increased color on dependency, cyanosis, blue toe and, finally, gangrene may be seen.

On palpation there may be asymmetric temperature differences. Pulses may be palpated as indicated on the evaluation form. The carotid, brachial, radial (added with upper extremity examination), aorta, femoral, popliteal, dorsalis pedis, and posterior tibial areas are palpated with a grading system of 2+ = normal; 1+ = decreased but not absent proximal stenosis; 0 = absent, reflecting occlusion.

On auscultation bruits (a French word meaning *noise*) may be detected in general over the areas of palpation (see the above paragraph), which may reflect stenotic (narrowed) lesions.

Laboratory

After completing the aforementioned history and physical examination, the laboratory studies begin.

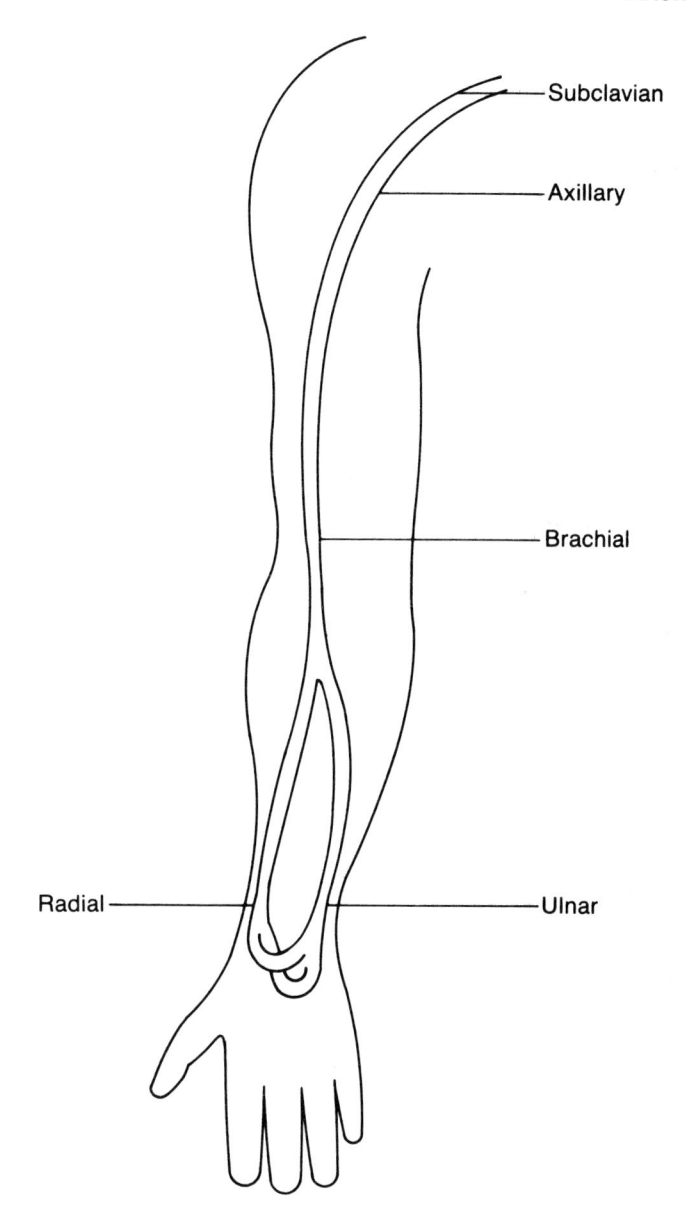

Figure 12-12 Schematic of upper extremity arterial circulation.

Pulse Volume Recorder

Air volume plethysmography, as mentioned earlier, refers to a measurement of volume change that occurs in a limb, for instance, and constitutes the principle utilized in the PVR developed by Raines. Cuffs are applied to bilateral thighs, calves, ankles, and feet and air (65 mm Hg) is forced individually into each cuff with the patient in the supine position. Changes in volume in each limb segment affect the air in the cuff and can be graphically transformed into pulsatile wave forms that have been shown to approximate closely direct intra-arterial recordings.[8]

A normal PVR tracing will have a quick upstroke with a reflected wave on the downstroke. Different degrees of wave forms have been reported by Strandness and Raines and may be applied to PVR results.[9,10] Thus an abnormal tracing will lose the reflected wave and become wider and smoother as the degree of proximal stenosis increases until, in the most severe form, no pulsatile wave form will be recorded (straight line). The calf cuff requires less air than the thigh cuff and thus the calf recording is artifactually greater in amplitude than the thigh. This finding is a very accurate reflection of a patent superficial femoral artery (Figures 12-13 through 12-16). Upper extremity examinations may also be performed using the PVR. Obliteration of wave form in resting, and/or Adson's, 90° and/or military brace position is consistent with thoracic outlet syndrome.

The advantage of the PVR is that it is simple, quick, noninvasive, and nontechnician dependent. It is of special value with calcified arteries that may give falsely elevated pressures and for serial tracings, to follow the natural course of a disease or as follow-up to medial and/or surgical intervention.

Segmental Limb Pressures

Historically Winsor is credited with introducing limb segmental pressure measurement to evaluate peripheral vascular disease.[11]

Segmental limb pressure assessment has proved to be a reliable, noninvasive semiquantitative tool in evaluating the presence and degree of arterial disease.

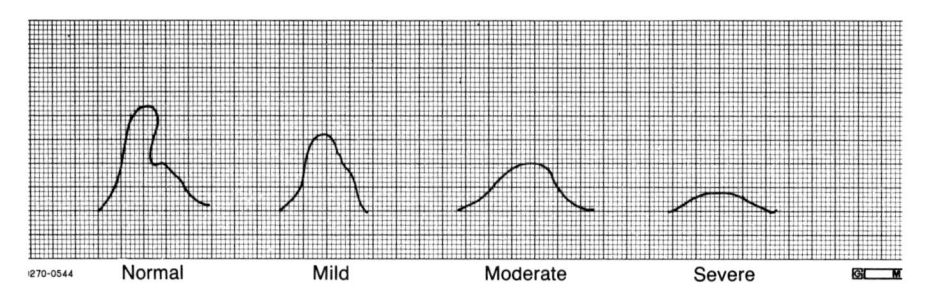

Figure 12-13 Spectrum of PVR wave forms. Raines describes PVR categories. V = straight line (flat).

Arterial Evaluation 341

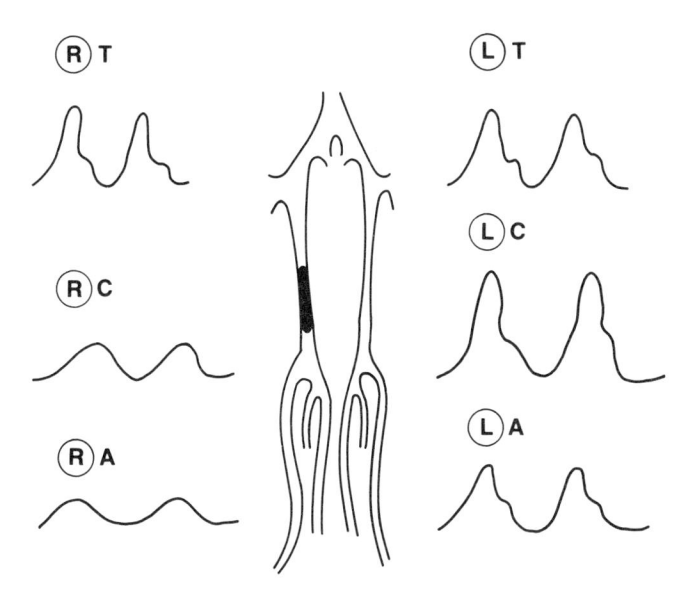

Figure 12-14 Abnormal thigh PVR, reflecting aorto-iliac disease. In patent superficial femoral disease, calf amplitude remains greater than thigh amplitude.

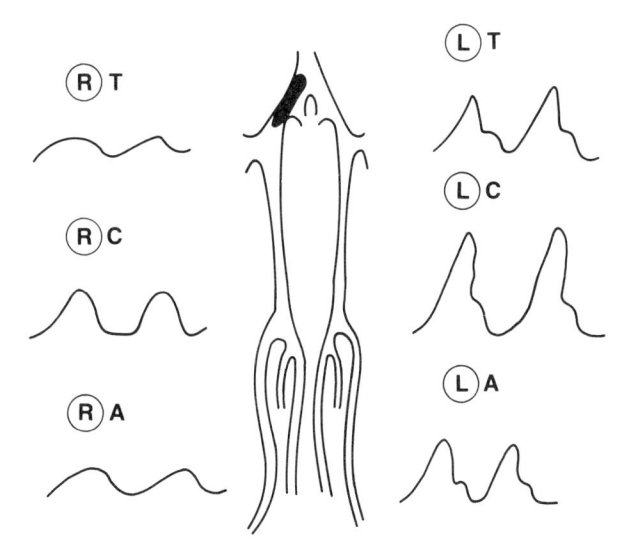

Figure 12-15 On the normal side, the left (L) calf has a sharp upstroke, reflected wave, and is larger in amplitude than the thigh PVR. (T = Thigh, C = Calf; A = Ankle.) On the right calf (R), the wave form has widened with no reflective wave and—in superficial femoral disease—is smaller in amplitude than the thigh PVR.

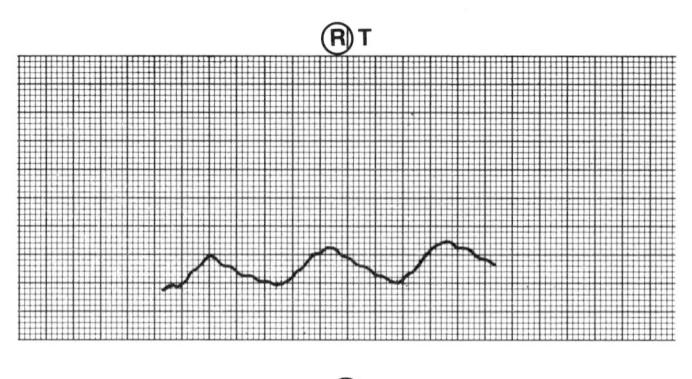

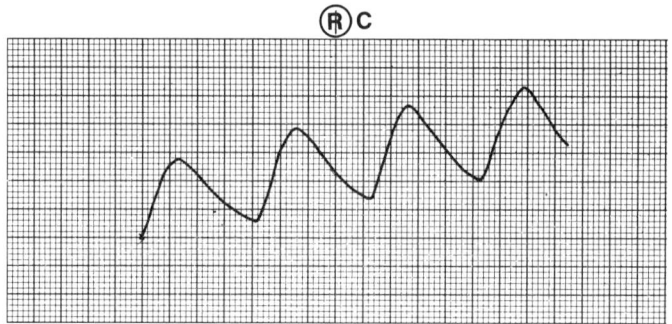

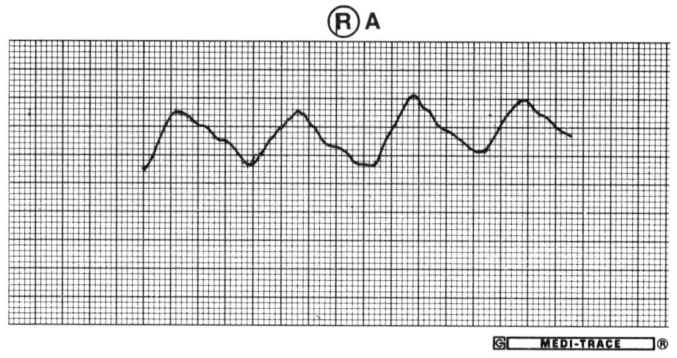

Figure 12-16 (*A*) *Case study:* Patient is a 68-year-old diabetic hypertensive with right thigh and hip pain brought on by exercise. PVR wave forms indicate right aorto-iliac disease with patent superficial femoral artery (SFA). (*B*) Angiograms consistent with right iliac occlusion.

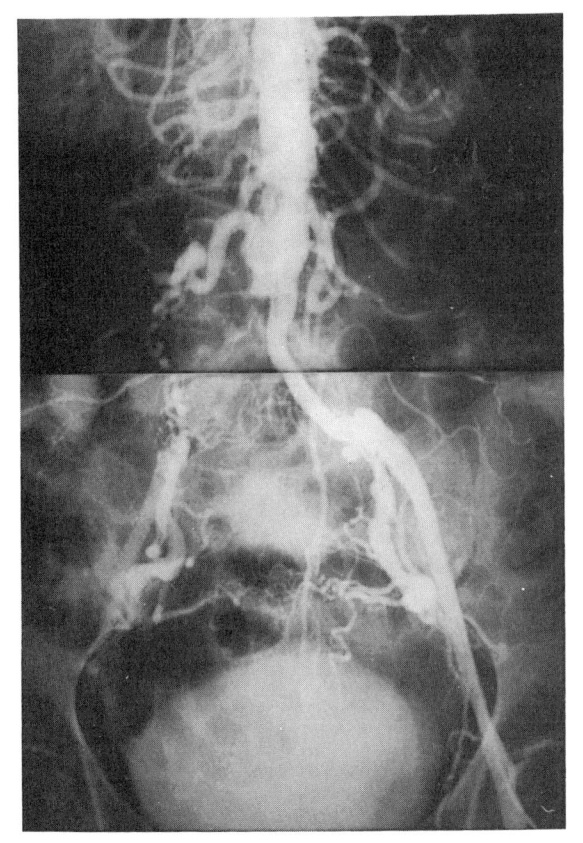

B.

Pneumatic cuffs are placed in either three or four locations when evaluating the lower extremities or two locations for upper extremity disease. Four-cuff technique placements are the most proximal thigh (high thigh); above the knee; on the calf, and on the ankle. Three-cuff technique utilizes just one larger thigh cuff, plus calf and ankle cuffs (Figure 12-17). A simple ultrasound Doppler detector can be used either over the posterior tibial or the dorsalis pedis arteries, and systolic pressures are determined in a similar fashion (Figures 12-18 and 12-19). Brachial systole pressures are also taken on both sides. It should be remembered that the pressure determined in each segment corresponds to cuff occlusion.

It has been shown that an ankle/brachial index (ABI) can be determined that parallels the severity of arterial disease.[12] This index is determined by dividing the ankle systolic pressure by the brachial systolic pressure with a normal value of 1. An A/B index of 0.5 to 0.8 is found in patients with claudication and an A/B index of less than 0.5 is indicative of more severe disease, such as ischemic ulceration. Toe pressures can also be taken (PPG is the most sensitive method) with a normal toe/brachial index (TBI) of 0.6.

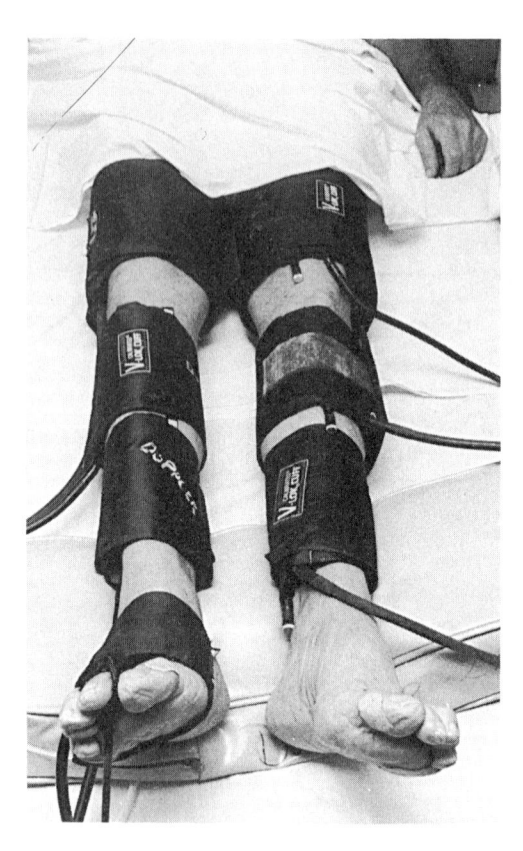

Figure 12-17 Three-cuff technique for segmented limb pressure assessment.

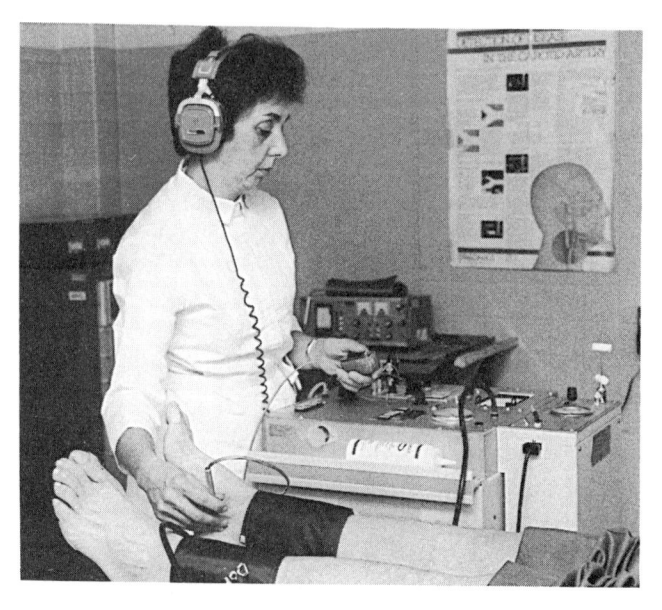

Figure 12-18 Method of measuring systolic ankle pressure, utilizing the posterior tibial artery.

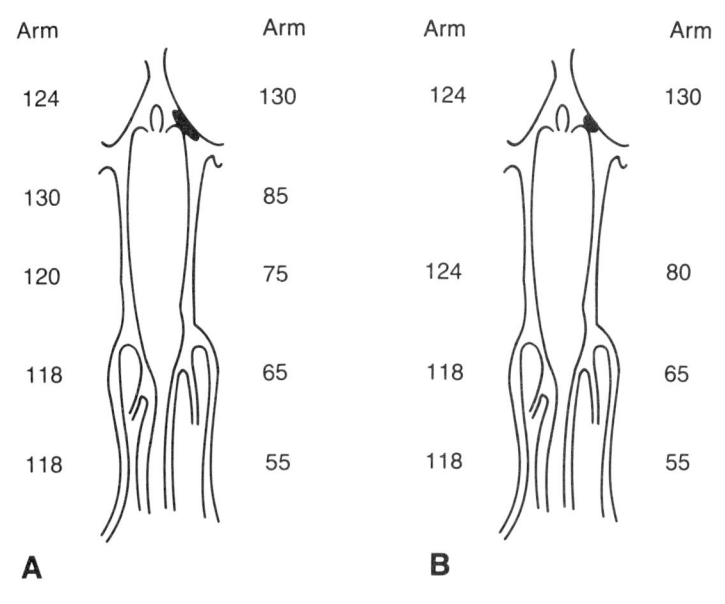

Figure 12-19 (*A*) Four-cuff method. Note difference in arm-thigh pressures. (*B*) Three-cuff method—the same as *A*. Superficial femoral disease may also cause this drop and thus PVR wave form must be combined.

These pressures have been shown to be more accurate in the assessment of healing of ischemic lesions than ankle pressures, with a toe pressure of less than 30 mm Hg generally associated with nonhealing. A penile arterial pressure can also be determined with a normal penile/brachial index (PBI) being 0.7. A PBI less than 0.6 is considered consistent with vasculogenic impotence.[13]

A normal high thigh pressure exceeds the brachial pressure by a factor of 1.2 and, with a regular large thigh cuff (3-cuff method), the ratio is 1:1. A segmental difference of greater than 30 mm Hg generally is consistent with localized arterial disease in the lower extremity. In the upper extremity a brachial BP difference of greater than 15 mm Hg may be associated with more proximal disease, such as subclavian sterosis.

Falsely elevated pressures may be found over calcified vessels, but toe pressures are not generally affected and auscultation of Doppler signals may reveal true disease in the face of these falsely raised pressures.

Despite the aforementioned limitations, this simple noninvasive technique may objectively identify and localize arterial disease and may be used for serial studies.

Doppler Wave Forms

The Doppler velocity detector can be applied directly over specific arterial sites with the use of acoustic gel at an angle of 45° to 60° until the loudest signal is auscultated.

The wave form (Figure 12-20) may be analyzed by simply listening and/or by means of graphic recordings (analog strip recorder vs. spectrum analysis).

A normal peripheral artery signal will be multiphasic and have discrete diastolic sounds on auscultation. The graphic recording will demonstrate a sharp systolic upstroke with an initial reversal diastolic component, depending on peripheral arterial resistance. Significant arterial stenosis or obstruction will be generally monophasic on auscultation and, graphically, there will be a delayed, decreased systolic component and loss of any discrete diastolic component (distal to lesion). At the site of a lesion, the frequency of the signal is increased in proportion to the severity of the lesion and absence of a signal reflects very severe arterial disease.

The signals may be employed in any of the major arteries of the upper or lower extremities. In the lower extremity arterial examination, the most useful signal to record objectively is from the common femoral artery. The loss of diastolic reversal flow may be an indication of inflow disease, while its absence essentially rules out significant aortic or iliac arterial occlusive disease (Figure 12-21).

Doppler wave form analysis by auscultation or graphic recording remains a simple noninvasive tool to indicate whether arterial disease is present, and to qualify its severity and approximate its location.

Treadmill Testing

As has been described earlier, lower extremity arterial disease can be adequately assessed by the laboratory in most situations with techniques such as plethysmography (*e.g.*, PVR) and measuring limb pressures. Stress testing is very beneficial for patients who may present with normal or slightly abnormal ankle pressures and symptoms, patients who may have questionable true claudication, and as a determinant for degree of disability.

Techniques. Brachial and ankle systolic pressures are first measured with the patient in the supine position. The patient then begins to walk on the treadmill, which is set at a 10% grade, 1½ miles per hour (as per Strandness),[14] with or without monitoring, as deemed appropriate. The testing is completed after 5 minutes or when the patient develops claudication. The

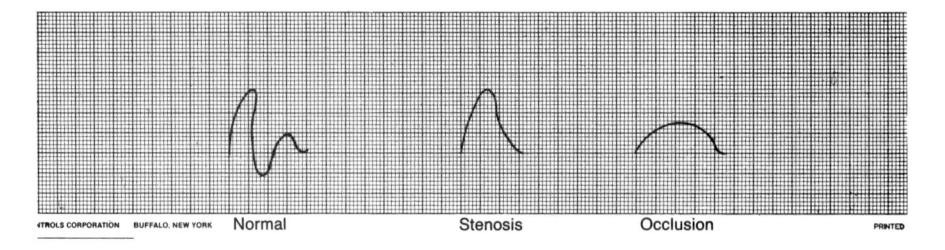

Figure 12-20 Schematic representation of Doppler wave forms.

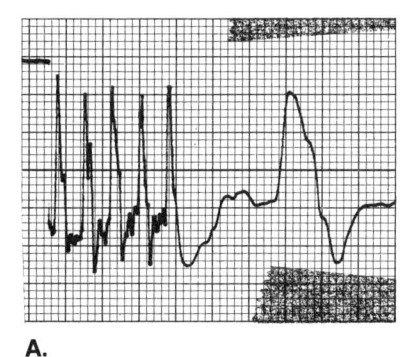

Figure 12-21 (A) Normal Doppler wave form. (B) Abnormal Doppler wave form—right femoral. (From case study: See Figure 12-16.)

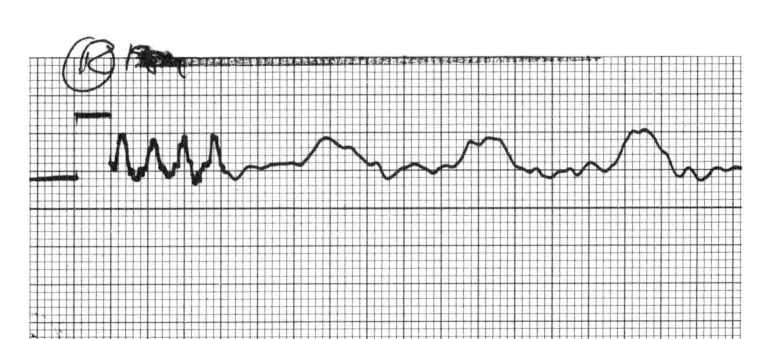

patient is then assisted to the nearby examining table where, once again in the supine position, brachial and ankle systolic pressures are determined. On occasion the test must be discontinued due to other symptomatology such as shortness of breath, chest pain, or dizziness. Other forms of testing may be used, such as ambulating in the hall to induce claudication, as long as the methods are objectively documented for potential comparisons in future testing.

Reactive Hyperemia Testing

With the patient in the supine position, cuffs are applied on the thigh and ankle and ankle systolic pressure is measured. The thigh cuff is inflated to a pressure that is 50 mm Hg greater than the thigh systolic pressure. At the end of 3 minutes, the thigh cuff is deflated and the ankle pressure is measured about every 15 seconds until the pressure returns to the original baseline level.

Interpretation. Normally there should be no change in the ankle pressure after exercise. In patients with true claudication (that is, secondary to peripheral vascular disease) a drop in ankle pressure will occur (Figure 12-22). The amount and length of ankle recovery time (*i.e.*, time necessary for ankle

SUMMARY—OBSERVED HEMODYNAMIC DATA

BP	R ARM_____			L ARM_____		
	R	Psys	L	R	PVR CATEGORY	L
LOCATION						
THIGH						
CALF						
ANKLE						
A/B INDEX						
DIGIT ( )						

EXERCISE: MAXIMUM WALKING TIME: ____ MIN. RATE ____ MPH DISTANCE____
FEET GRADE _____ & SYMPTOMS: _____

$\bar{p}$ EX ANKLE					

Figure 12-22 Ankle pressure drop after limited exercise in hall. (From case study: See Fig. 12-16.)

pressure drop, postexercise, to return to pre-exercise level) is directly related to the severity of disease.

In general reactive hyperemia testing is not done in our laboratory because some patients do have difficulty with pain secondary to thigh occlusion. The ankle pressure should normally fall, but no more than 33% below the initial value, and should return to normal about 1 minute after releasing the thigh cuff. In patients with peripheral vascular disease, there will be a greater drop in pressure and greater ankle pressure recovery time.

The noninvasive laboratory with the above modalities has the ability to determine objectively the presence, location, and severity of disease. Disease states such as neurospinal disease that may mimic claudication can be clarified. Rest pain, which may be secondary to neuropathies (*e.g.*, diabetes mellitus) can be distinguished from true arterial rest pain by means of pressures and wave forms. Primary and secondary Raynaud's may be differentiated and, finally, objective evidence of vascular disability can be elicited.

The presence of a pulsatile wave form is a good indication of digital or foot lesion healing.

Serial studies may be done to determine the effectiveness of medical or surgical therapy. Pressures and repeated stress tests may help in an understanding of the natural course of disease.

Duplex Scanning

As described earlier, this technique combines real-time B-mode scanning (demonstrating anatomy) with pulsed Doppler and spectral analysis (demonstrating physiology). This new noninvasive tool has added another dimension

Cerebrovascular Evaluation

to arterial evaluation and has already been useful in identifying aneurysms (aortic, peripheral arterial) and localizing arterial thrombi. Further applications, such as evaluating aorto-iliac and abdominal vascular disease, are being investigated (Figure 12-23 and Table 12-1).

Cerebrovascular Evaluation

Documentation

Just as in arterial disease, history taking is first in line in a cerebrovascular evaluation and this is documented on the vascular chart (Figure 12-24).

Another parallel can be drawn between coronary, peripheral vascular arterial, and now cerebrovascular presentation. The degree of disease may be from asymptomatic to claudication to gangrene (arterial), asymptomatic to angina to myocardial infarction (coronary), and now the patient may present from asymptomatic to transient ischemic attack (TIA) to stroke.

Atherosclerosis at the carotid bifurcation is the most common pathologic

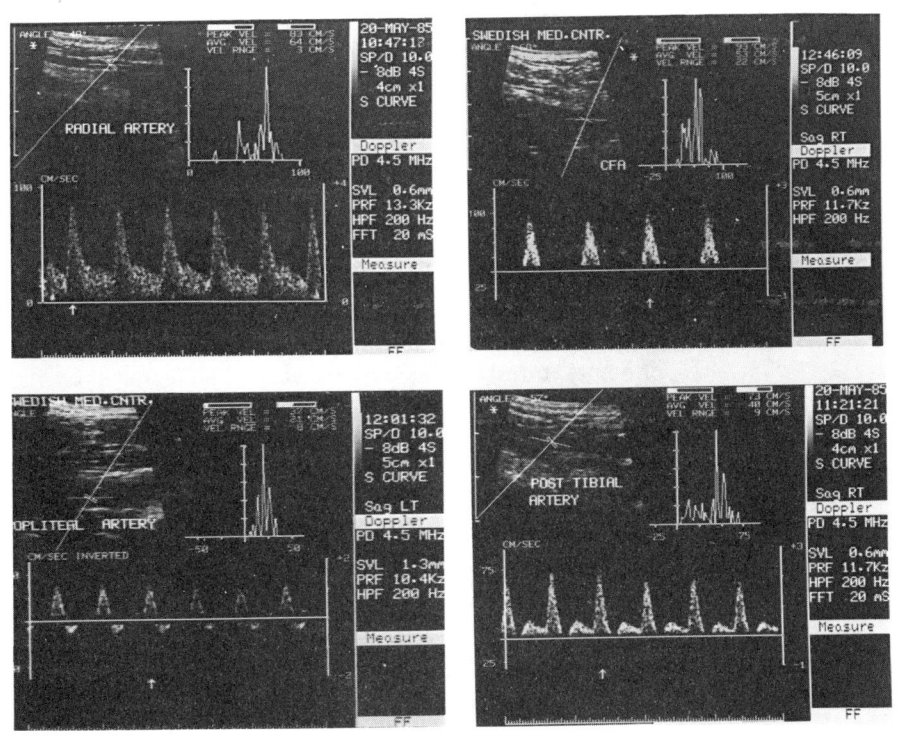

Figure 12-23 Peripheral vascular duplex scanning Doppler cursor shown in vessels with resultant spectral analysis signal that can be analyzed. (Courtesy of Diasonics.)

Table 12-1

Arterial	Normal	Abnormal
PVR	Sharp upstroke Reflected wave	Widened wave form (lesion dependent) Loss of reflected wave
Limb pressure	Segmental difference <30 mm Hg A/B Index about 1 Toe/Brachial index 0.6 or > Toe pressure > 30 mm Hg = heal PBI (penile brachial index ≥ 0.7	Segmental difference > 30 mm Hg A/B index < 0.9 (Parallels severity of disease) Toe/brachial index 0.6 < 30 mm Hg nonhealing < 0.6
Doppler wave form	Sharp upstroke multi-phasic Reversal diastolic component	Loss of sharp upstroke monophasic Loss of diastolic reversal
Treadmill testing	No change in ankle pressure postexercise	Drop in ankle pressure postexercise
Duplex scanning	No plaques, normal configuration Normal flow	Plaques and/or abnormal configuration Flow signal may be abnormal

finding in cerebrovascular disease. The pathophysiology can be divided into ulcerated plaque resulting in emboli versus flow reduction, such as occlusion.

The asymptomatic patient is usually referred to the laboratory because of bruits, questionable decreased or absent pulse, or high risk. The patient with a transient ischemic attack has a neurologic deficit that lasts less than 24 hours. A patient with a reversible ischemic neurologic deficit (RIND) may recover the deficits within a few days to a week following a stroke. A completed stroke thus remains a condition with a fixed neurologic deficit.

The clinical manifestations (TIA or stroke) can be conveniently classified by their anatomic territories (Figure 12-25). The carotid (anterior, hemispheric) manifestations include ipsilateral visual deficit (*amaurosis fugax*— "shade pulled over eye," fleeting blindness), contralateral motor or sensory deficits and, if the dominant hemisphere is involved, speech may also be affected. Vertebrobasilar (posterior, occipital, cerebellum) manifestations may include vertigo, drop attacks, ataxia, unilateral or bilateral motor, sensory, visual, or cranial nerve deficits. Other patients enter a laboratory with atypial symptoms such as dizziness, headache, syncope, or memory loss, which may or may not reflect carotid disease.

Cerebrovascular Evaluation

MORRISTOWN MEMORIAL HOSPITAL
SECTION OF CARDIOLOGY
PERIPHERAL VASCULAR LABORATORY
CEREBROVASCULAR EVALUATION

LOG # _____

NAME _____ SEX: M F   DATE _____

UNIT # _____ AGE: _____ PHYSICIAN _____

LOCATION _____ CLINICAL DIAGNOSIS _____

PRESENTING CONDITION:
- Deficit: ☐ motor ☐ sensory ☐ speech ☐ vision
- Frequency: ☐ once ☐ recurrent duration: _____

ASYMPTOMATIC BRUIT: ☐ Right ☐ Left Known duration: _____

ATYPICAL SYMPTOMS: ☐ dizziness ☐ headache ☐ syncope ☐ memeory loss
☐ other: _____
Duration: _____ Frequency: _____

PAST HISTORY: ☐ hypertension ☐ smoking ☐ Pk. yrs. _____ ☐ heart
☐ hyperlipidemia ☐ diabetes ☐ stroke
☐ medication: _____

SUMMARY OBSERVED DATA:
Blood Pressure: Right Arm _____ Left Arm _____

	RIGHT		LEFT		
TEST:	Normal	Abnormal	Normal	Abnormal	Comment
OPG					
CPA					
DOPPLER DIRECTIONAL					

CONTINUOUS WAVE SPECTRUM ANALYSIS:

ULTRASOUND RESULTS:

IMPRESSION:

EXAMINED BY: _____

D-SF 5838 10/84

Figure 12-24 Cerebrovascular evaluation chart. (Continued)

352 Peripheral Vascular Testing

OCCULAR PLETHYSMOGRAPHY (OPG)

R

L

Blood Pressure:	Right Arm		Left Arm		
			Right		Left
OPG PRESSURES — mmHg					
DOPPLER SIGNALS		O	REDUCED	FORWARD	REVERSED
FRONTAL	Left				
	Right				
WITH TEMPORAL COMPRESSION	Left				
	Right				

Figure 12-24 (Continued)

Figure 12-24 (Continued)

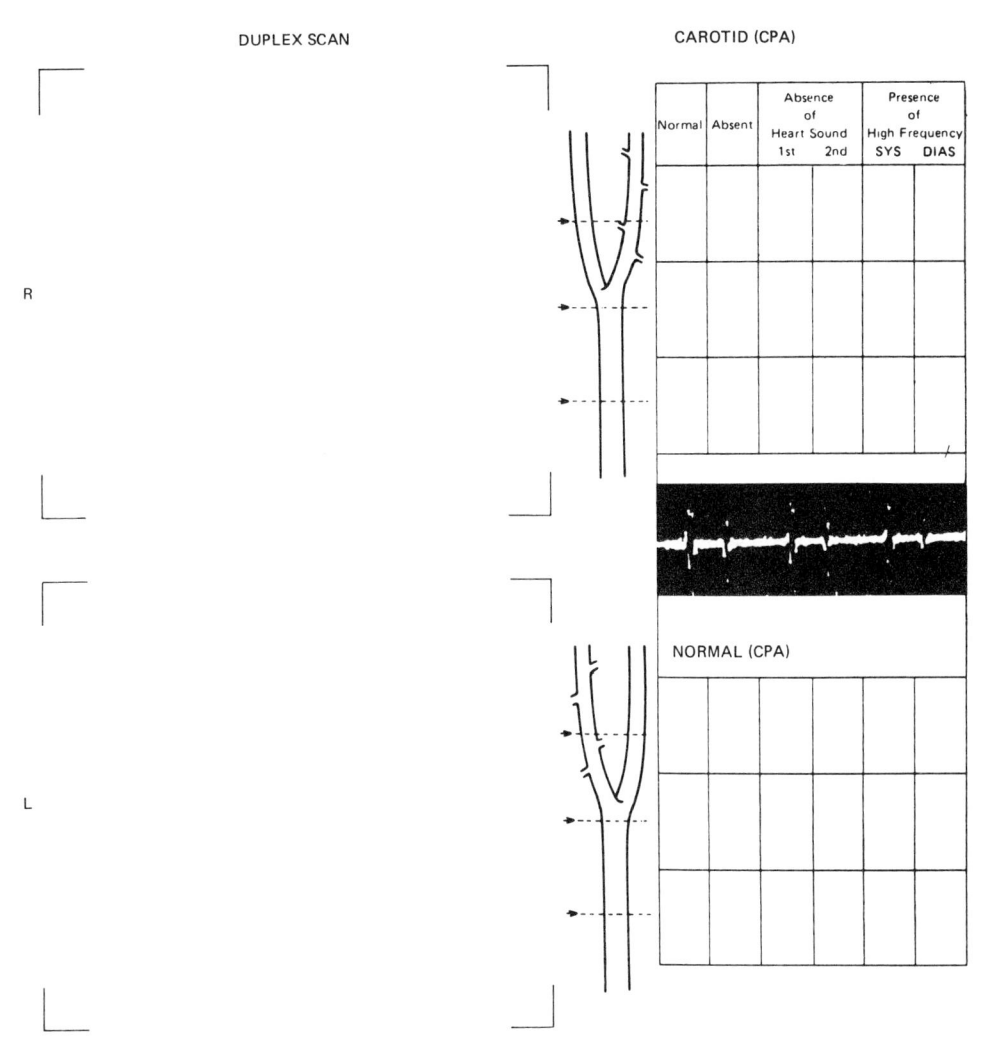

Physical Examination

It is important to take the blood pressures in both arms, especially when a patient presents with dizziness. A difference of each brachial systolic pressure greater than 15 to 20 mm Hg may indicate subclavian stenosis that could steal ipsilateral vertebral blood flow, producing a relative vertebral insufficiency resulting in dizziness (subclavial steal syndrome).

Both carotids are palpated individually in the common carotid area and other arteries (superficial, temporal, radial, subclavian) may also be palpated. Bruits over the subclavian and carotid areas may be auscultated by stethoscope or carotid phonoangiography (CPA; see later in text).

354 Peripheral Vascular Testing

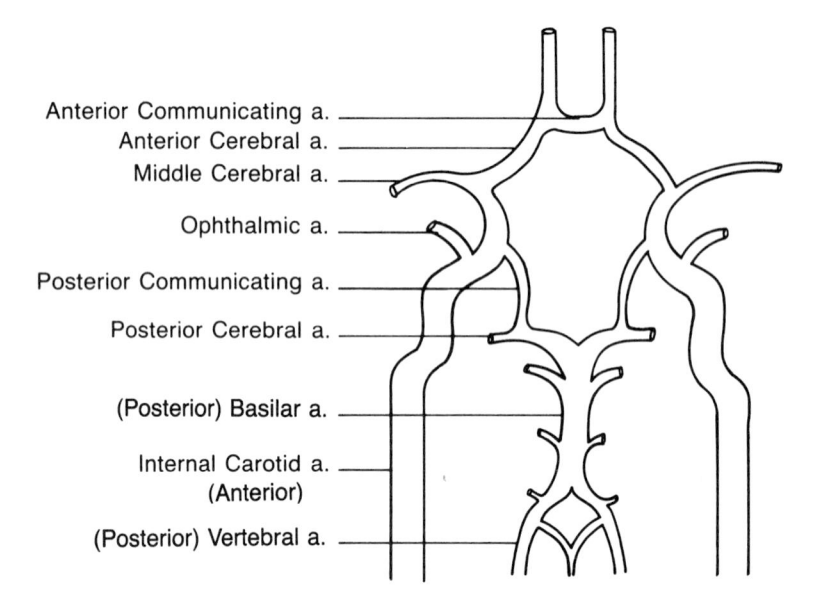

Figure 12-25 Normal extracranial, intracranial anatomy.

A speech or visual deficit may be self-evident, as would localized loss of strength. A retinal examination may also be performed (usually by a medical doctor), to look for Hollenhorst plaques (retina emboli); further neurologic examination may be done as deemed necessary.

Laboratory

The noninvasive testing can be divided into indirect and direct testing. The indirect testing depends on hemodynamically significant abnormalities in the orbital and periorbital circulation, whereas direct testing is not solely dependent on hemodynamics and deals with the extracranial circulation (common carotid, internal, external carotids).

Indirect Testing

Periorbital Doppler. In order to understand the periorbital examination, it is necessary first to understand some anatomy and physiology. The common carotid artery divides into the internal and external carotid arteries. The first intracranial branch of the internal carotid artery is the ophthalmic artery, which itself gives off the frontal artery. The external carotid divides into eight branches and provides orbital collateral flow (Figure 12-26).

Technique. The patient is placed in the supine position with eyes closed. A bidirectional pencil probe is directed over either the supraorbital or frontal artery and the direction of flow is determined. Compression maneuvers may

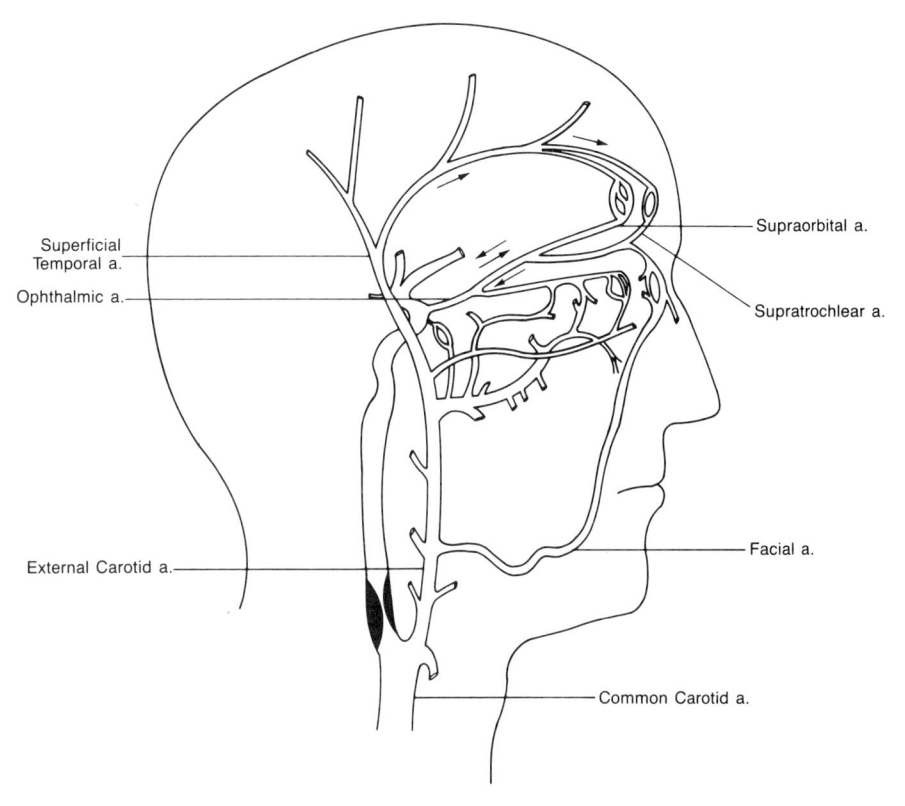

Figure 12-26 Reversal flow by external carotid collateral in severe internal carotid disease.

be performed utilizing external carotid branches (superficial temporal, infraorbital, facial) and, in some centers, common carotid compression may be performed.

Interpretation. Flow in the frontal artery is normally forward. Compression maneuvers of the external carotid will generally not affect the flow. Common carotid compression would result in a decrease in flow. With severe extracranial or intracranial carotid stenosis or occlusion (excluding external carotid) reversed frontal flow may be detected secondary to external carotid collateral flow. The source of the collateral flow may be determined by the external carotid compression maneuvers (Figure 12-26).

Some patients with severe carotid disease will have normal frontal flow as a result of the circle of Willis, which provides intracranial collateral circulation. If this flow comes from the contralateral internal carotid system, contralateral common carotid compression may lead to a decreased periorbital flow on the affected side. However, if flow comes from the vertebrobasilar system, no compression maneuvers will affect the flow.[15]

356 Peripheral Vascular Testing

Although the periorbital examination is quite technician-dependent and is an indirect test, it is quite specific when abnormal and thus may provide a great deal of information in a short time before further studies are completed.

Ocular Plethysmography (OPG). Two basic types of OPG are pulse delay (*e.g.*, Kartchner–McRae or Zira) and the evaluation of retinal artery pressure (Gee technique).[16]

In pulse delay types, ocular transducers are placed over the cornea after local anesthetic drops are used on the eye and photoplethysmograph sensors are placed over each ear.

In OPG-Gee, after a local anesthesic has been applied to the eyes, ocular transducers are placed over the sclera and a vacuum is created (Figure 12-27). The level of this vacuum at which the ocular pulse reenters is the retinal artery pressure. With OPG-PVR, the vacuum is slowly increased and the level that decreases the tracing to ≤2 mm is considered the retinal artery pressure.

Interpretation. Ocular pulse delay between each eye is 10 m/sec and between each ear and between the ear and eye, it is less than 30 m/sec in the normal patient. With severe internal carotid disease, ocular pulse delay is greater than 10 m/sec, and with severe external carotid disease ear, pulse delay is greater than 30 m/sec on the appropriate sides. With severe bilateral

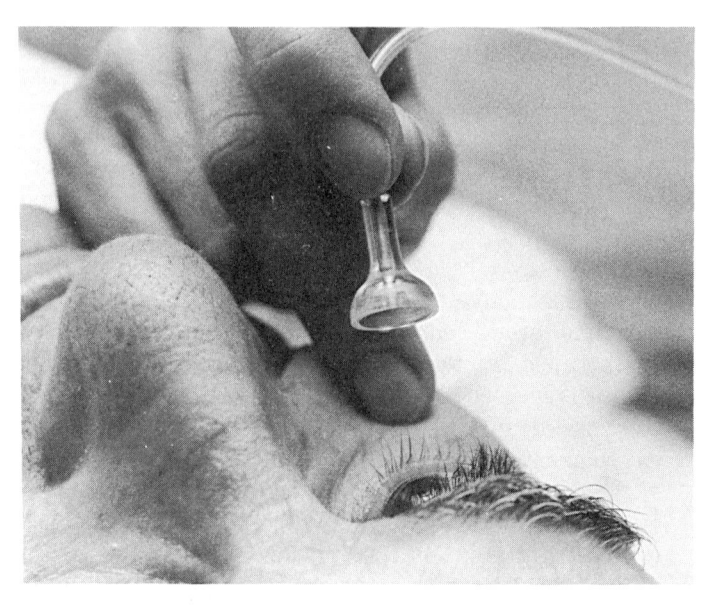

Figure 12-27 Eyecup (OPC-PVR-Gee technique) about to be placed over sclera.

internal carotid disease, the eye pulses in relation to the ear pulses will be greater than 30 m/sec.

General criteria can be applied to the OPG-Gee type machines. The ophthalmic artery pressures should be within 5 mm Hg and pulse size should be within 2 mm's. Other, specific criteria can be utilized that vary with the OPG-Gee and OPG-PVR.

As in the periorbital exam, OPG is an indirect test that will not detect nonhemodynamically significant lesions (<75% area, <50% diameter) and will be falsely negative with well collateralized lesions. On occasion the OPG and/or periorbital examination may be abnormal with a normal direct test that may indicate intracranial pathology.

Direct Testing

Carotid Phonoangiography (CPA). This first example of direct testing utilizes an electric microphone that is positioned over the low, mid- and upper neck areas, reflecting common carotid artery, bifurcation, and distal carotid artery areas respectively. The jugular notch and subclavian areas may also be auscultated for transmitted heart murmurs and subclavian stenosis. The carotid phonoangiography permits enhanced auscultation of these sounds and heart sounds; bruits can also be seen graphically and recorded if so desired for hard copy.[17,18]

Interpretation. Normally the first and second heart sounds will be present with no bruits. Bruits that are loudest over the subclavian area may reflect subclavian stenosis and bruits increased over the mid- and upper neck areas generally reflect carotid stenosis rather than transmitted bruits (*e.g.*, cardiac valvular disease). The increased duration of the bruit indicates increased stenosis and if no bruits are present, this may indicate no disease, disease less than 40%, or disease ≥ 90% (diameter).

Carotid Doppler With Spectral Analysis. *Technique.* A bidirectional Doppler pencil probe is preferable to avoid venous signals, although an unidirectional probe may be used. The probe is placed at approximately a 45-degree angle and, with use of acoustic gel, signals are obtained over the common carotid artery and then the probe is moved slowly up the neck to the bifurcation and finally distally to the external and internal carotid branches. The signals may be auscultated and also interfaced to a sound spectrum analyzer for further analysis (Figure 12-28).

Interpretation. All signals are pulsatile and each vessel has certain characteristics that can be recognized by listening; blood flow can be further analyzed utilizing the spectrum analyzer. The common carotid signal has a prominent diastolic flow signal that is more accentuated in the internal carotid signal, the latter a reflection of lower resistance. The external carotid, being a higher resistance vessel, is more multiphasic with a distinct

358 Peripheral Vascular Testing

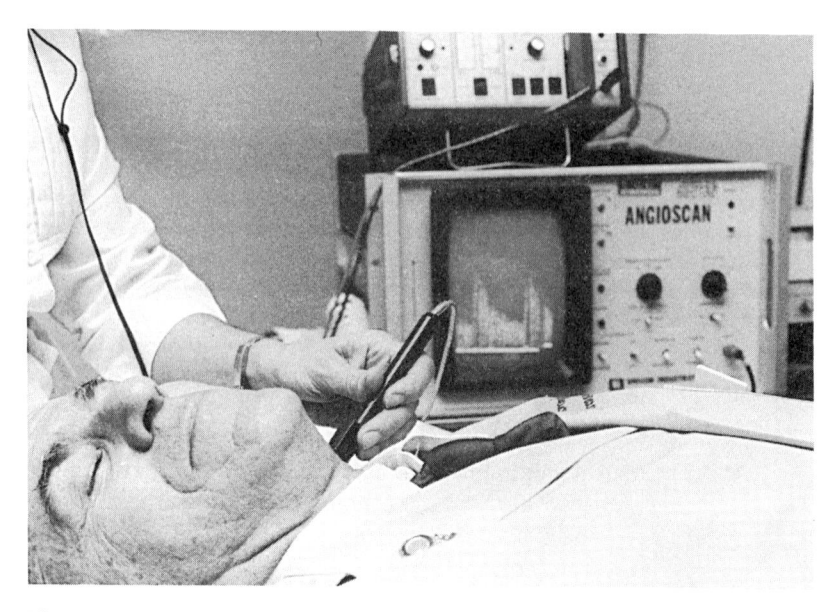

Figure 12-28 Scanning neck with CW Doppler and spectrum analysis.

wave form and lower diastolic flow. The blood flow can be further analyzed graphically by spectrum analysis that displays in gray scale all the resultant frequencies (from moving red cells); with normal laminar flow, a window will be created that will decrease in the face of increased turbulence.

Average and peak frequencies and velocities can also be determined. In fluid dynamics Q (Flow) = V (Velocity) × Area. If flow is constant, as an area decreases the velocity must increase in order to maintain constant flow. Velocity is directly proportional to the Doppler frequency; thus, using the Doppler formula, we can apply this information in the following way. In general if a lesion is greater than 50%, an elevated frequency can be obtained and quantitated. As the lesion approaches greater than 80%, the frequency will increase and, with a very severe lesion, there will be a decrease in the pulsatile signal. Absence of a signal may mean occlusion and a lower diastolic increased-resistant common carotid signal may reflect a high grade lesion further upstream. With lesions less than 50%, the quantitated peak frequency will be normal, but turbulence may be detected with loss of window (spectral broadening) (Figure 12-29).

Ultrasonic Arteriography. *Technique.* The patient is in the supine position with head turned from the examination site. A pulsed Doppler probe attached to a position-sensing arm is placed in the common carotid area with gel having been applied to the neck. After adjusting range gates, a static image is created on the storage oscilloscope based on sampled flow (Figure 12-30).

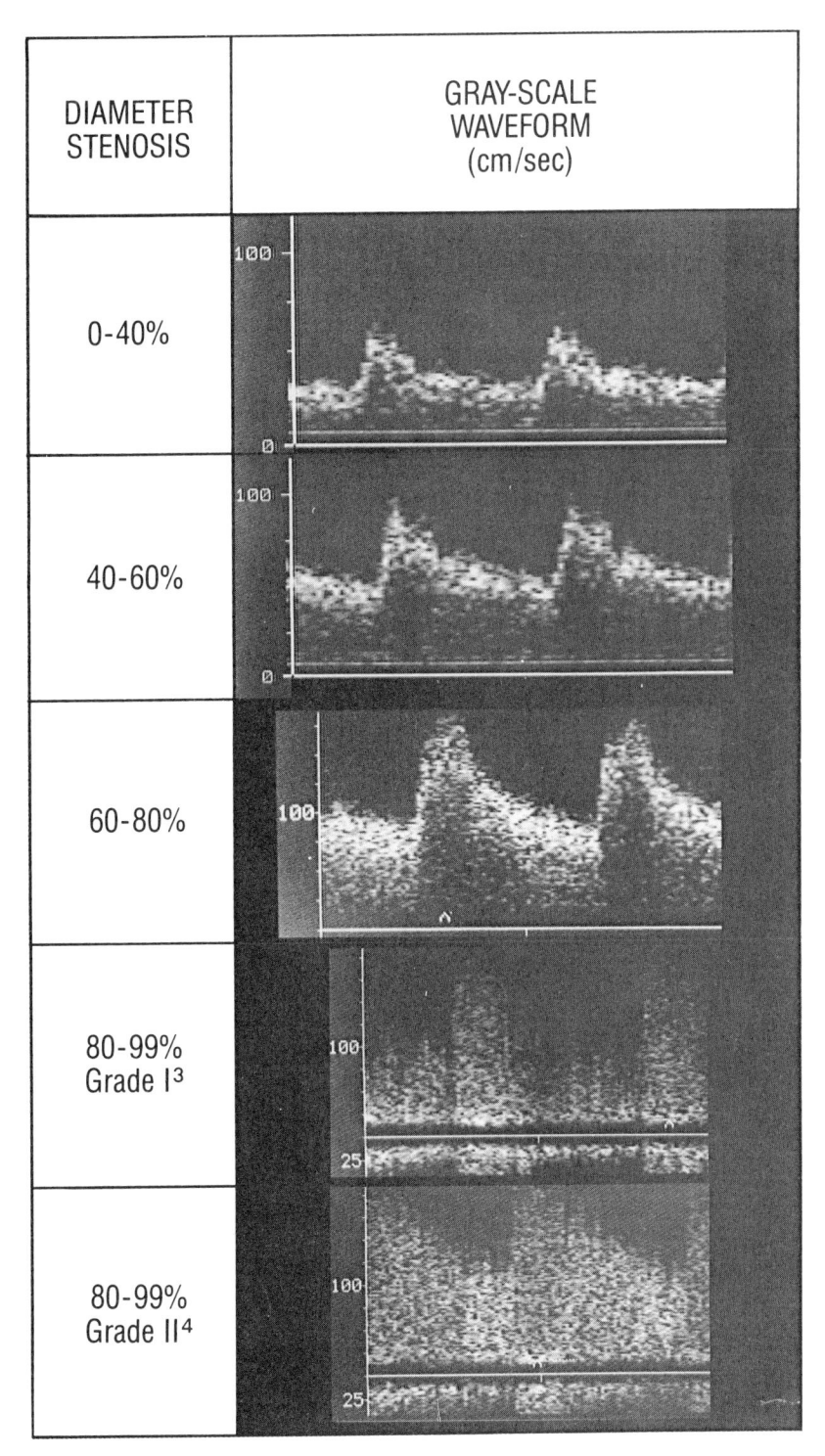

DIAMETER STENOSIS	GRAY-SCALE WAVEFORM (cm/sec)
0-40%	
40-60%	
60-80%	
80-99% Grade I[3]	
80-99% Grade II[4]	

Figure 12-29 Spectrum of spectrum analysis.

360 Peripheral Vascular Testing

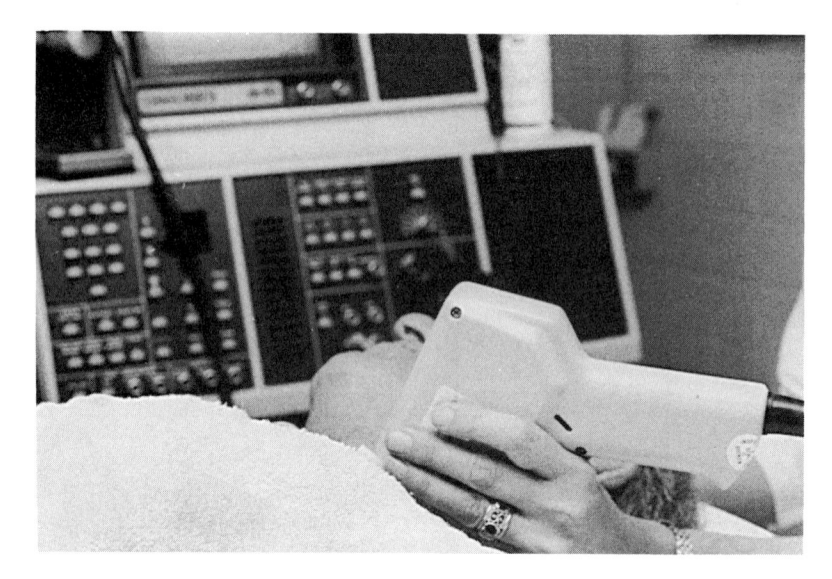

Figure 12-30   Transverse view of neck with Doppler scanner probe.

Interpretation. The normal image appears like an angiograph's oblique view of the common carotid artery and bifurcation. In carotid stenosis there will be a narrowing of this image that can be measured objectively by the concomitant audible spectral analysis. Occlusion can be seen by the lack of a visualized segment of the vessel. Calcification presents a technical problem in this form of evaluation, since ultrasound cannot penetrate calcification. This will be seen as nonvisualized areas of the image, but sound spectral analysis distal to these areas can be evaluated and thus the true patency of the vessel can be assured. It has been shown that the accuracy of ultrasonic arteriography in diagnosing lesions with 50% or greater diameter stenosis is very high.

It is important for the laboratory to determine the accuracy of its results. Although not totally perfect, angiography and venography are generally the gold standards to which the laboratory results are compared.

Five general categories expressed as percentages can be determined for measurements of accuracy.

Sensitivity refers to an ability to determine the existence of disease. This can be calculated by dividing the number of test abnormals that agree with gold standard abnormals by the total number of gold standard abnormals.

Specificity refers to an ability to determine the nonexistence of disease. This can be calculated by dividing the number of test normals that agree with gold standard normals by the total number of gold standard normals.

Positive predictie value refers to the percentage of test abnormals that were gold standard abnormals. This can be calculated by dividing the number of test abnormals that agree with gold standard abnormals by the total number of test abnormals.

Negative predictive value refers to the percentage of test normals that were gold standard normals. This can be calculated by dividing the number of test normals that agree with gold standard normals by the total number of test normals.

Overall accuracy refers to the percentage of all studies correctly assessed by testing. This can be calculated by dividing all the tests and gold standards that agree (normal and abnormal) by all the tests done.[19]

Duplex Scanning. With the development of technology and further understanding of extracranial carotid disease, the duplex scanning concept was formulated and popularized by Strandness and associates in Seattle, Washington.[1,20] Real-time B-mode imaging was able to demonstrate anatomy noninvasively, but due to limitations of ultrasound, fresh clots could mimic normal blood and thus a normal-appearing vessel actually could be as severe as an occlusion. As a result a probe was developed that could combine both anatomy and physiology by superimposing the Doppler signal on the anatomic image and sample flow where desired in the vessel and further analyzing the flow with spectrum analysis.

Technique. With the patient supine and acoustic gel present, a transducer is then placed on the neck along the common carotid artery for transverse section and then moved progressively cephalad (Figure 12-30). Then the sagittal views are obtained and Doppler signals with spectrum analysis are obtained in the common carotid, internal carotid, and external carotid arteries.

Interpretation. Normally no plaques will be seen in these vessels and normal spectrum analysis will be obtained (Figure 12-31).

In mild lesions, mild plaquing that can be categorized as soft, dense or calcified and smooth or irregular, or heterogenous will not affect the spectrum analysis except for some possible spectral broadening. Occasionally ulcerated plaques may be seen. Heterogeneous plaques are believed to have a greater association with symptomatic patients (Figure 12-32). As the stenosis increases to greater than 50%, the frequency and velocity will increase and lesions can be described as above. When no audible Doppler signal is present in an artery with plaquing, a potential diagnosis of occlusion can be made (Figures 12-33 and 12-34).

This technique thus represents the most accurate way of evaluating all degrees of extracranial carotid disease. Further advancements in technology such as real-time color imaging and improved ultrasonic imaging potentially will enhance this testing (Table 12-2).

362   Peripheral Vascular Testing

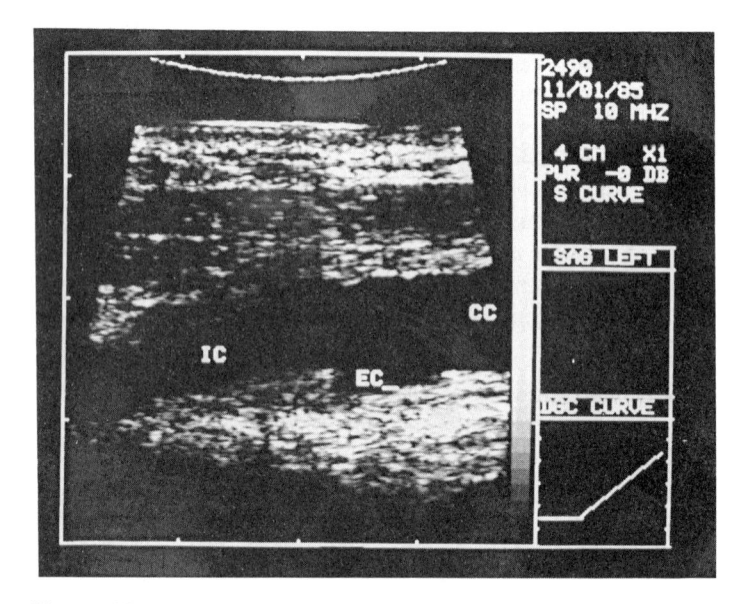

Figure 12-31   Normal internal carotid by duplex scanner.

Plaque Formations

Figure 12-32   Some types of plaqueing.

Figure 12-33   Spectrum of carotid disease.

Venous Evaluation

Documentation and Physical Examination

The venous system can be divided into superficial, perforator, and deep venous systems (Figure 12-35).

The patients that present to the vascular laboratory for venous evaluation will usually present with possible superficial or deep venous disease (acute or chronic) and/or with pulmonary embolus.

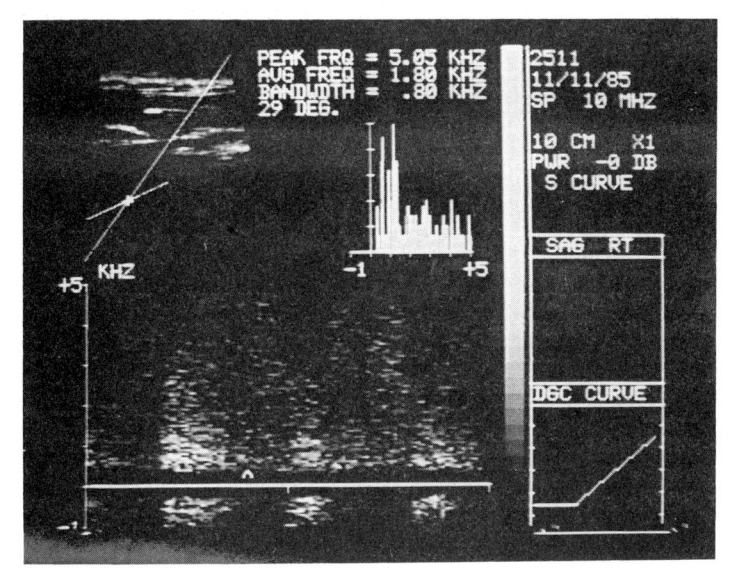

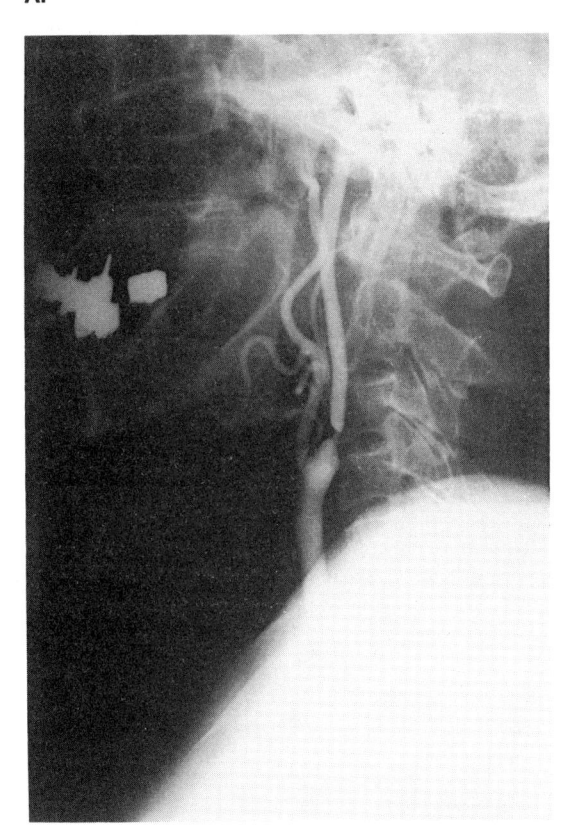

Figure 12-34 (A) Very abnormal spectrum with very high frequency from proximal internal carotid indicating severe stenosis. (B) Angiogram of same patient demonstrating severe lesion.

Table 12-2

Cerebrovascular	Normal	Abnormal
Periorbital	Forward flow	Reverse or forward flow (see text)
OPG-Gee types	OAP's R and L <5 mm Hg	OAP's R and L >5 mm Hg
CPA	ō Bruit	Bruit present or absent
CWSA (5 MHz probe)	<5000 Hz	>5000 Hz Frequency increase with severity of diease Absent = Occlusion
UA	Normal image Normal flow	Abnormal image with Abnormal flow
Duplex scanning	ō plaques Normal spectrum	Plaques Abnormal spectrum

Acute Deep Venous Thrombosis (DVT) is an extremely important condition due to its life-threatening potential and morbidity. Signs and symptoms are usually secondary to obstruction and inflammation and thus include pain, swelling, and tenderness. Chronic disease may present with recurrent swelling, pain (*e.g.*, post-phlebitic syndrome), stasis changes, and ulceration.

Superficial disease may present with primary (superficial venous) or secondary (incompetent perforators with deep venous disease) varicose veins (dilated, tortuous), or superficial prominent veins.

The potential complication of DVT is pulmonary embolism with patient presenting asymptomatic or with chest pain, shortness of breath, hypoxia and, possibly, with hemoptysis.

Most of the risk factors can be related to Virchow's triad—stasis (*e.g.*, immobilization), hypercoagulable state (*e.g.*, pregnancy, malignancy), and trauma (*e.g.*, trauma, postop).

All of the above are included in the present complaint, past history, and examination on the venous evaluation forms (Figure 12-36).

Laboratory

Because of the inaccuracy in physical examination (50%) for the diagnosis of DVT and potential problems with invasive venography, noninvasive tests were developed.

Doppler Ultrasound

Technique. The patient is placed in the supine position with the leg being examined in a slightly externally rotated hip flex position. A 5 MHz portable continuous wave Doppler velocity detector (Medasonics) is utilized in our

(*Text continues on page 369*)

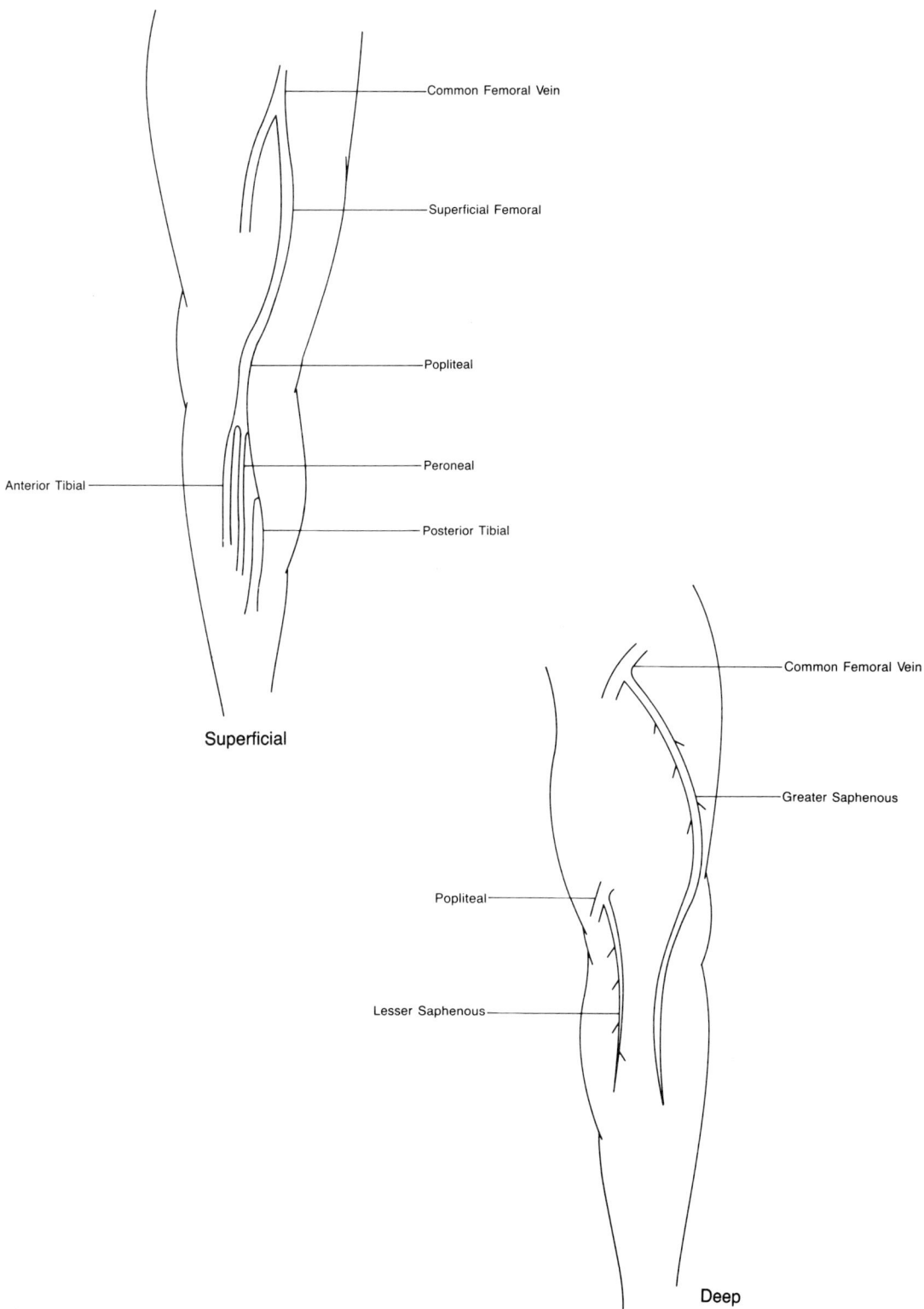

Figure 12-35 Venous system (lower system).

Peripheral Vascular Testing

```
                    MORRISTOWN MEMORIAL HOSPITAL
                         SECTION OF CARDIOLOGY
                      PERIPHERAL VASCULAR LABORATORY
                           VENOUS EVALUATION
LOG # _____

NAME: _____  _____ SEX: _____ DATE: _____

UNIT #: _____ AGE: _____ PHYSICIAN: _____

LOCATION: _____ CLINICAL DIAGNOSIS: _____
```

PRESENT COMPLAINT

Chest pain ☐   fever ☐   dyspnea ☐   hemoptysis ☐
leg symptoms _____
other _____

PAST HISTORY

phlebitis ☐   emboli ☐   previous anticoag ☐   support hose ☐
edema ☐   stasis dermatitis ☐   previous vein surgery ☐
oral contraceptives ☐   trauma ☐   bedrest ☐
malignancy ☐   obesity ☐   heart disease ☐
pregnancy _____ post op _____ other _____

EXAMINATION

	Ulcer	Cyanosis	Prom. Veins	Inflam.	Tenderness	Edema	Varices	Stasis derm.	Homan's
L	☐	☐	☐	☐	☐	☐	☐	☐	☐
R	☐	☐	☐	☐	☐	☐	☐	☐	☐

DATA

	R	L
Maximum Venous Outflow (MVO) mm/sec.		
Segmental Venous Capacitance (SVC) mm		
No respiratory waves		
Abnormal venous doppler signals		
Femoral		
Popliteal		
Post. Tibial		

COMMENTS

EXAMINED BY: _____

D-SF 5840 10/84

Figure 12-36   Venous evaluation form.

Venous Evaluation

PLETHSMOGRAPHY STRIP
right
left

DOPPLER	+ = present		o = absent				↓ = decrease		
Signal	Com. Fem.		Sup. Fem.		Pop.		Post. Tib.		Saph.
	R	L	R	L	R	L	R	L	R	L
Patent										
Spontaneous										
Phasic										
Augmented										
Competent										
Nonpulsatile										

Figure 12-36 (Continued)

368 Peripheral Vascular Testing

VENOUS IMAGING

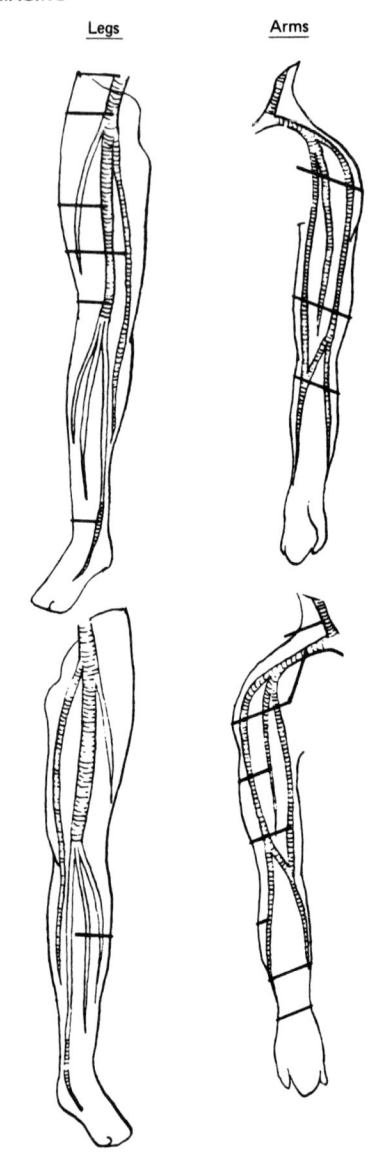

Legs   Arms

Figure 12-36   (Continued)

laboratory for this particular study. Doppler venous sounds are usually evaluated audibly but also may be graphically displayed on an analogue strip chart recorder. The posterior tibial veins are first assessed at the ankle level. A signal may or may not be spontaneous in this listening area and the next step is to compress the foot and listen for venous flow augmentation. Compression of the calf and release maneuvers are then accomplished while listening over the posterior tibial vein area. The popliteal superficial femoral and femoral vein areas are then studied with distal compression and proximal compression and release maneuvers. It is advisable to proceed in an orderly manner, examining an area on one leg and then the same area on the other leg for direct immediate comparisons. The saphenous vein may also be evaluated along its distribution and incompetent perforating veins can be assessed by listening for reflux flow while compressing the calf above a tourniquet applied to the leg.

Finally, veins of the upper extremity, such as the subclavian, axillary, and brachial veins can be examined with similar techniques. The testicular veins may also be evaluated for varicoceles that may play a role in the cause of infertility in selected cases.

Interpretation. The interpretation is based on the subjective evaluation of five basic venous flow characteristics.[21]

Spontaneity: The presence of an audible spontaneous signal. Loss of this signal may indicate occlusive thrombosis over the listening area.

Phasicity: Normal venous flow will vary with respiration (phasicity). A continuous signal (nonphasic) in deep veins is consistent with the diagnosis of DVT (Figure 12-37).

Augmentation: An increase in venous flow produced by compressing distally or releasing proximally to the area being examined (Figure 12-37).

Competence: With normal competent valves, no negative reflux will occur after proximal compression. Incompetent valves will be responsible for negative retrograde flow after proximal compression.

Pulsatility: Unlike arteries, normal veins have a nonpulsatile venous

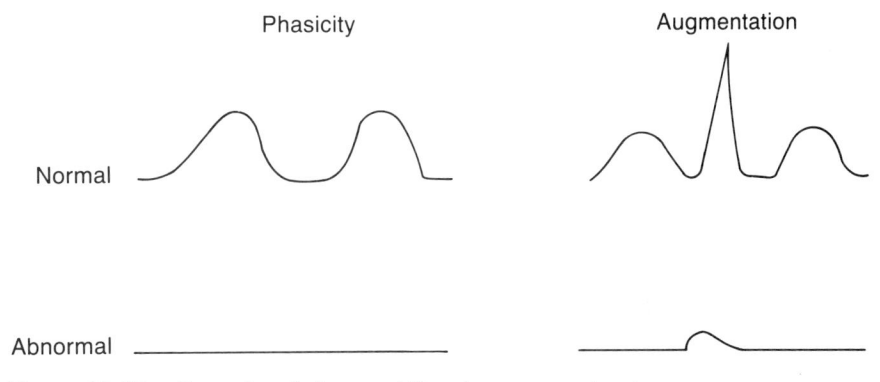

Figure 12-37 Normal and abnormal Doppler venous signals.

signal quality. Pulsatility will be found in conditions where venous hypertension is present (*e.g.*, congestive heart failure).

The Doppler technique is highly sensitive to proximal thrombi and, in expert hands, has a sensitivity of up to 90%. However, it is subjective and technician-dependent, and insensitive to nonocclusive nonhemodynamic thrombi and minor calf thrombi.

Plethysmography (Acute)

Plethysmography is a measure of volume change, as discussed earlier. Two basic types are utilized in deep venous disease—*venous occlusive* and *volume plethysmography.*

In both PVR (Pulse Volume Recorder) and IPG a thigh cuff is occluded to 50–55 mmHg, producing a temporary venous occlusion allowing an increase in volume (SVC-venous capacitance); with deflation of the thigh cuff a venous cutflow (MVO) can be determined. With the PVR, cuffs are applied to both thighs and calves whereas with the IPG, two electrodes are placed on the calf to monitor calf volume change. The leg is externally rotated and knee flexion is repeated three times in order to assure good venous flow and the SVC and MVO are subsequently obtained.

Interpretation. A normogram has been established for the IPG popularized by Wheeler, and Raines has set forth a point system to aid the diagnosis of DVT with the PVR.[22]

In acute DVT with major thrombi, there may be some decrease in the SVC and there will be an abnormal venous outflow, both reflecting venous obstruction (Figures 12-38 and 12-39).

Phleborrheography utilizes volume plethysmography with two different methods to diagnose DVT. Changes in respiration will not be present with

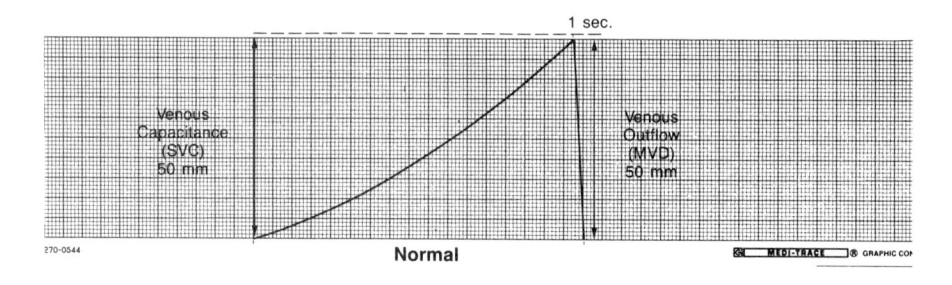

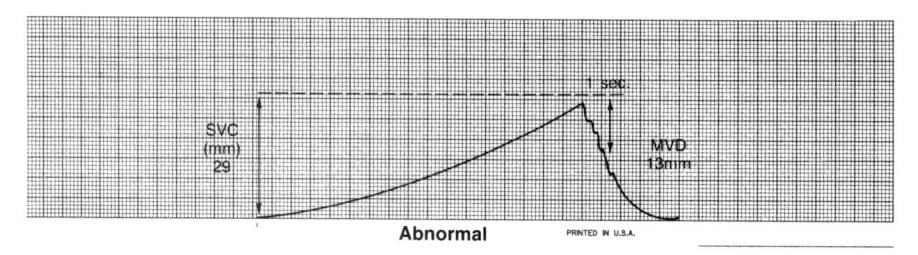

Figure 12-38 Schematic representation of normal and abnormal venous PVR.

the PRG in acute DVT and an increase in volume in a proximal area after foot cuff inflation is present in acute DVT.[23]

As in Doppler studies, plethysmography is highly accurate in diagnosing proximal thrombi, but remains insensitive to minor calf and non-hemodynamically significant thrombi.

Venous Reflux Plethysmography (Chronic)

Venous insufficiency may be relatively quantified and diagnosed by PPG, SPG, or other calf volume techniques.*

Technique. The patient is positioned sitting on the edge of an examining table or stretcher. A PPG transducer and/or strain gauge, and/or calf cuff, and/or calf electrodes are applied to the calf (PPG close to medial malleolus). The patient then dorsiflexes five times and venous refilling time may be determined. If the study is abnormal the test is repeated with a proximal tourniquet.

*Wexler SH, Oliver MA, Castronuovo JJ: Personal communication, 1985

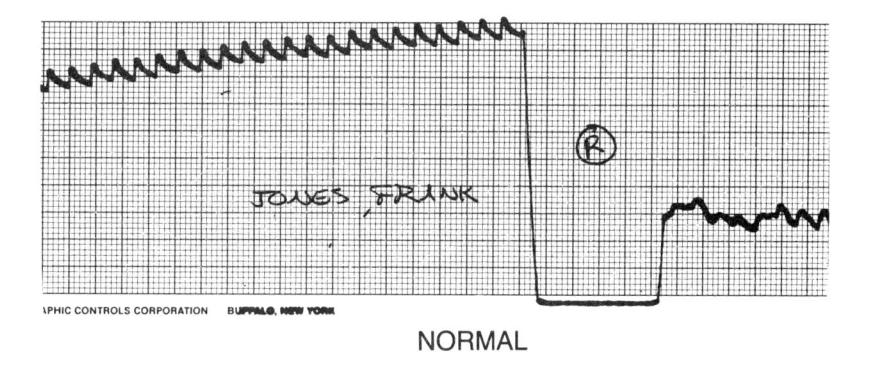

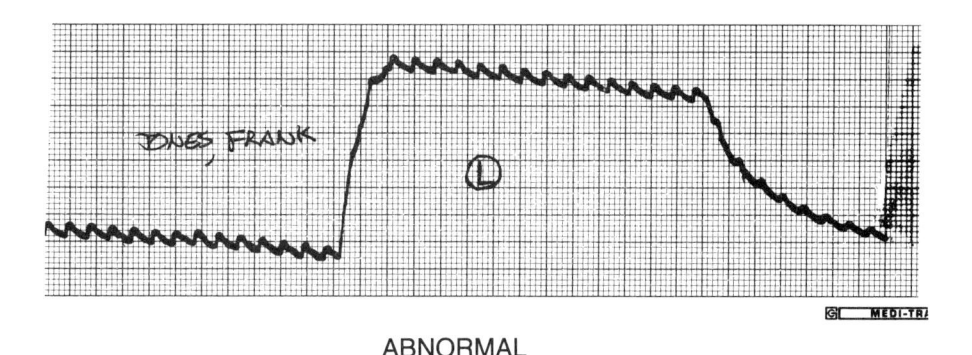

Figure 12-39 (A) Normal and abnormal PVR (patient with leg swelling).

(Continued)

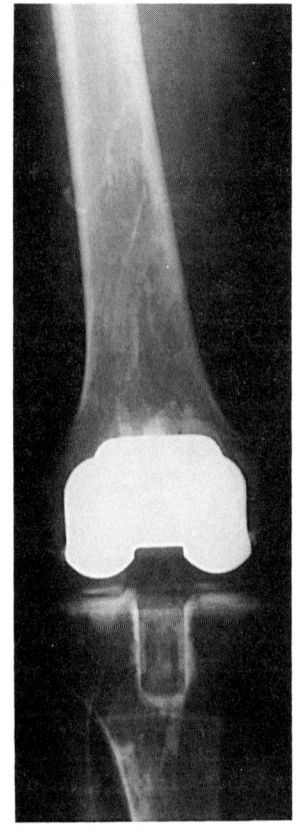

Figure 12-39 (B) Venogram showing popliteal occlusion (absence of dye visualized).

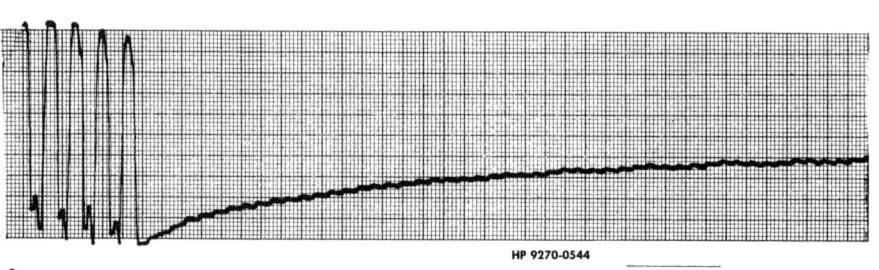

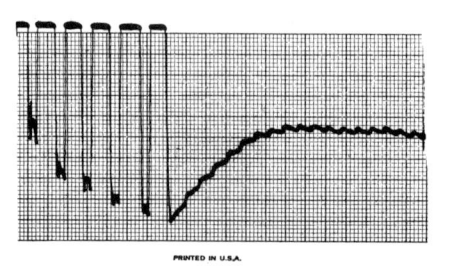

Figure 12-40 (A) Normal venous refilling time (VRT). (B) Abnormal VRT.

Interpretation. A normal venous refilling time (VRT) for PPG is generally >20 seconds and for SPG, IPG, or PVR >10 seconds (Figure 12-40).

The PPG generally reflects the perforating and superficial veins whereas the SPG, IPG, PVR (calf volume methods) generally reflect deep veins, although there is some overlap. If an abnormal VRT corrects after application of tourniquet, the abnormality is considered involving the superficial venous system.[24]

Duplex Scanning

Duplex scanning (real-time B-mode images with Doppler) has become an excellent technique for the evaluation of extracranial carotid disease. In a preliminary report in 1981, Talbot introduced the clinical application of real-time B-mode imaging in venous disease evaluation.[25]

Technique. The veins of the upper leg are best examined in a supine position with reversed Trendelenburg, if possible. The popliteal, peroneal, posterior, and anterior tibial veins can then be evaluated with the patient in the sitting position with the leg resting on the examiner's chair. Transverse views and the sagittal views are obtained. Veins of the upper extremity may best be examined with the patient in the flat supine position.

Interpretation. *Normal* veins will compress with probe pressure, have no thrombosis present, have normal Doppler signals, and may have blood flow with a normal valve motion that may be visualized.

Abnormal veins do not compress with probe pressure, have visualized thrombosis and, in occlusive disease, have no Doppler signal present (Figure 12-41).[26]

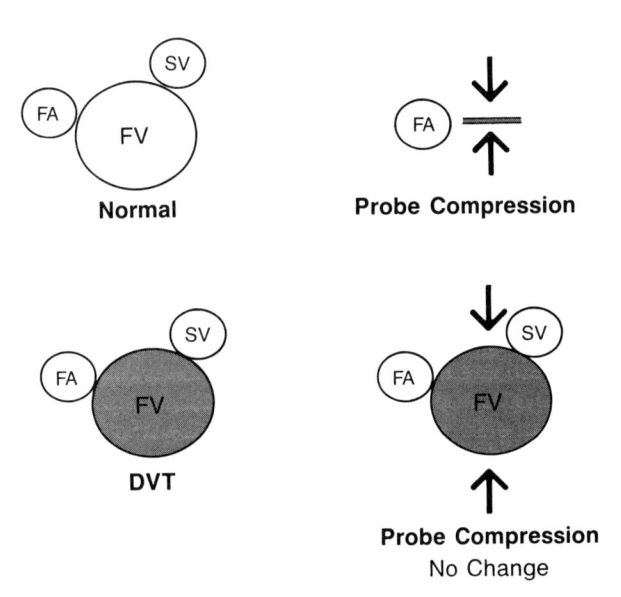

Figure 12-41 Normal and abnormal ultrasonic imaging of femoral veins.

374 Peripheral Vascular Testing

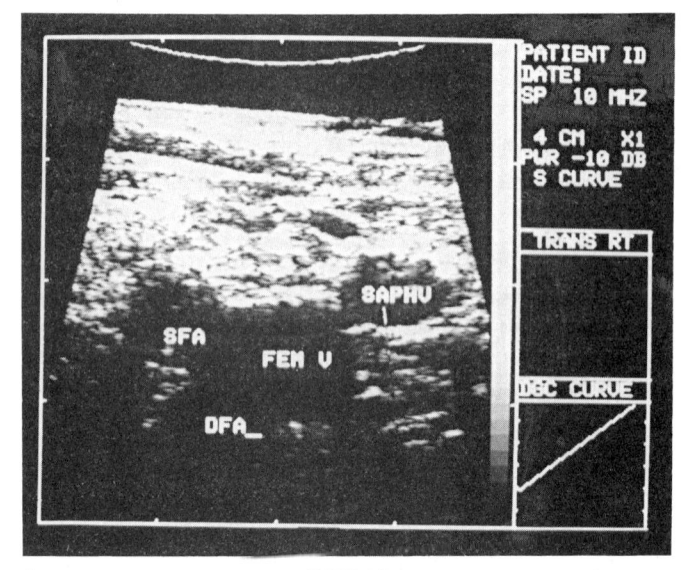

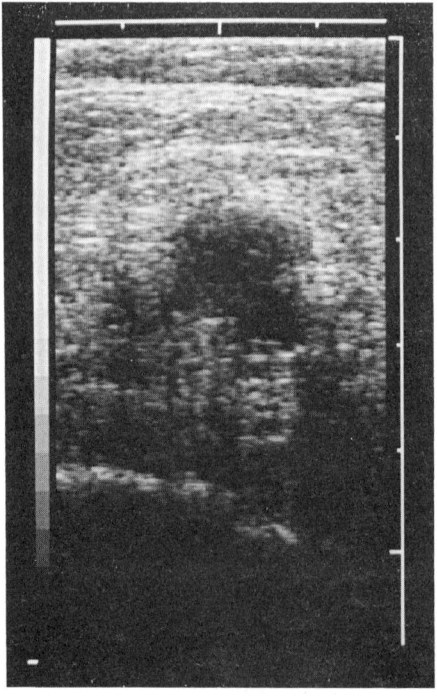

A. POP V

B. POP A

Figure 12-42 (*A*) Normal ultrasound image in femoral area. (*B*) Abnormal ultrasound image (transverse view) of popliteal vein shown in Figure 12-39. (POP V = Popliteal vein with occlusive thrombus. POP A = Popliteal artery.)

Table 12-3

Venous	Normal	Abnormal
Doppler ultrasound	Phasicity Augmentation Competency Spontaneity ō Pulsatility	Mainly loss of phasicity and/or augmentation and/or competency
Plethysmography	ACUTE IPG Normogram PVR-Raines point system (in general MVO > 30 mm Hg)	IPG Normogram PVR-Raines point system (MVO < 30 mm Hg)
	CHRONIC PPG-VRT > 20 secs PVR SPG ⟩ VRT > 10 secs IPG	VRT < 20 secs VRT < 10 secs
Duplex scanning	Compressible No clot Normal blood, valve motion Normal signal	Noncompressible Dilated with clot Clot, loss of valve motion Occluded—no signal

Acute thrombosis may have a tail present, may tend to be smooth with a homogeneous texture and the vein is generally very dilated (Figure 12-42).

With *chronic thrombi*, the clot becomes more irregular and heterogeneous and the vein may be the same size or smaller.[27]

In summary, duplex scanning has been found to be an excellent adjunctive tool in venous testing and with the advancements in technology, can produce both pertinent anatomic and physiologic information. This information can thus be utilized in the diagnosis and management of venous disease (Table 12-3).

References

1. Barber FE, Baker DW, Nation AWC, Standness DE et al: Ultrasonic duplex echo-Doppler scanner. IEEE Trans. Biomed. Eng (21):109, 1974
2. Barnes RW: Noninvasive Diagnostic Technique in Peripheral Vascular Disease (5). Richmond, Medical College of Virginia of Virginia Commonwealth University, 1980
3. Satomura S: Study of flow patterns in peripheral arteries by ultrasonic. J Acoust Soc Jpn (15):151, 1959

4. Mozersky DJ, Hokanson DE, Baker DW et al: Ultrasonic arteriography. Arch Surg (103):663, 1971
5. Brodie TG, Russell AE: On the determination of rate of blood flow through an organ. J Physiol (32):47, 105
6. Cremer H: Uber die Resistrierung mechanischer Vorlange auf electrischem Wege, Spziell mit Hilfe des Saitengavonometers and Saiterelektrometers. Munch. Med. Wochenschr (54):1629, 1907
7. Nyboer J: Electrical Impedance Plethysmography, 2nd ed. Springfield, IL, Charles C Thomas, 1970
8. Darling CR, Raines JK, Brener JB et al: Quantitative segmental pulse volume recorder: A clinical tool. Surgery (72):873–877, 1973
9. Strandness DE, Jr: Peripheral Arterial Disease: A Physiologic Approach, p 112. Boston, Little, Brown & Co, 1969
10. Raines JK, Darling RC, Buth J et al: Vascular laboratory criteria for the management of peripheral vascular disease of the lower extremities. Surgery (79):12–29, 1976
11. Winsor T: Influence of arterial disease on the systolic blood pressure gradients of the extremity. Am J Med Sci (220):117, 1950
12. Yao JST, Holbs JT, Irvine WT: Ankle systolic pressure measurements in arterial disease affecting the lower extremities. Br J Surg (56): 176, 1969
13. Kempczinski RF: Role of the vascular diagnostic laboratory in the evaluation of male impotence. Am J Surg (138):278–282, 1979
14. Sumner DS, Strandness DE, Jr: The relationship between calf blood flow and ankle blood pressure in patients with intermittent claudication. Surgery (65):763, 1969
15. Barnes RW, Russell HE, Bone GE, Slaymaker EE: Doppler cerebrovascular examination: Improved results with refinements in technique. Stroke (8): 468–471, 1977
16. Gee W: Physiologic principles of ocular pneumoplethysmography. In Bernstein EF (ed): Noninvasive Diagnostic Techniques in Vascular Disease, pp 57–66. St. Louis, CV Mosby, 1982
17. Kartchner MM, McRae LP: Auscultation for carotid bruits in cerebrovascular insufficiency. JAMA (210):494–497, 1969
18. Kartchner MM, McRae LP, Morrison FD: Noninvasive detection and evaluation of carotid occlusive disease. Arch Surg (106):528–535, 1973
19. Hayes AC. Calculation and implication of accuracy measurements. Bruit (IX):178–182, 1985
20. Fells G, Phillips DJ, Chikos DP, Hailey JD, Thiele BL, Strandness DE, Jr: Ultrasound duplex scanning for disease of the carotid artery. Circulation (64):191–195, 1981
21. Barnes RW, Russell HE, Wilson MR: Doppler Ultrasound Evaluation of Venous Disease: A Programmed Audiovisual Instruction, 2nd ed. Iowa City, University of Iowa Press, 1975
22. Wheeler HB, Patwardhan NA, Anderson FA, Jr et al: Occlusive impedance plethysmography in the diagnosis of venous thrombosis. In Bergan JJ, Yao JST (eds): Venous Problems, pp 145–158. Chicago, Year Book Medical Pub 1978
23. Cranley JJ, Canos AJ, Sull WJ et al: Phleborrheographic technique for diagnosing deep venous thrombosis of the lower extremities. Surg Gynecol Obstet (141):331, 1975

24. Miles C, Nicolaides AN: Photoplethysmography: Principles and development. In Nicolaides AN, Yao JST (eds): Investigation of Vascular Disorders, pp 501–515. New York, Churchill Livingstone, 1981
25. Talbot S: Use of real-time imaging in identifying deep venous obstruction: A preliminary report. Bruit (6):41–42, 1982
26. Oliver MA: Duplex Scanning in venous disease. Bruit (IX):206–209, 1985
27. Sullivan ED, Peter DJ, Cranley JJ: Real-time B-mode venous ultrasound. J Vasc Surg (1):465–471, 1984

Suggested Reading

Barnes RW, Wilson MR: Doppler Ultrasonic Evaluation of Cerebrovascular disease: A programmed Audiovisual Instruction. Iowa City, University of Iowa Press, 1975

Barnes RW, Russell HE, Wilson MR: Doppler Ultrasonic Evaluation of Venous Disease: A Programmed Audiovisual Instruction. Iowa City, University of Iowa Press, 1975

Bernstein EF: Noninvasive Diagnostic Techniques in Vascular Disease. St Louis, CV Mosby, 1982

Hershey FB, Barnes RW, Sumner DS: Noninvasive Diagnosis of Vascular Disease. Pasadena. Appleton Davis, 1984

Kempczinski RF, Yao JS: Practical Noninvasive Vascular Diagnosis. Chicago, Year Book Medical Pub 1982

Kremkau FW: Diagnostic Ultrasound. New York, Grune and Stratton, 1984

Moore WS: Vascular Surgery A comprehensive review. New York: Grune & Stratton, 1983

Nix ML, Barnes RW: Noninvasive Peripheral Vascular Laboratory Diagnostic Technique. Richmond, Medical College of Virginia of Virginia Commonwealth University, 1980

Pirisky et al: Imaging of the Peripheral Vascular System. New York, Grune & Stratton, 1984

Zwiebel WJ: Introduction to Vascular Ultrasonography. New York, Grune & Stratton, 1982

Index

Abbokinase, 36
aberration, 138–139
absorption, 27
accidents
  cardiovascular, 45
  electrical, 57–61
accuracy, in ultrasonic arteriography, 361
acoustic gel, 357
acquired mitral stenosis, 230–232
acrocyanosis, 41
actin filaments, 71
actin/myosin protein filaments, 84
action potential, 77–84
acute arterial occlusion, 334
acute, defined, 41
Adalat (nifedipine), 33
adrenalin, 41
Adrenalin (epinephrine), 35, 47
adrenergic pharmacology, 34–37
afterload, 29
air plethysmography, 330
akiasing, 278
akinetic area, 225
Aldomet, 37
Allen Test, 41
alpha-adrenergic blockers, 34
alpha-adrenergic receptor stimulators, 35
amaurosis fugax, 41
Amicar, 36
amiodarone, stress test, effects on, 156
amplitude
  defined, 41
  echocardiographic, 174
analogue recording, 329
anatomy
  in catheterization, 283–287
  cellular, 69–84

  functional, 8–11
  geographic, 12–14
  internal, 8–11
aneurysm
  coronary, 22
  defined, 41
  dissecting, 153
  testing for
    peripheral vascular, 334
    stress, 153
  ventricular, 154
angina pectoris
  defined, 24, 41
  stress testing for, 150
  in terminating stress testing, 154
Anginyl (diltiazem), 33
angiocardiography, 41
angioplasty
  catheterization and, 320–321
  coronary artery, 281–282
ankle/arm index, 41
ankle/brachial index, 343
anomalous left coronary artery, 307
anorexia, 41
anoxia, 41
antagonists, calcium, 36, 155
antegrade flow, 41
anterior fascicle, 69
anterior infarction, 117–120
anterior interventricular sulcus, 13
anterior/ventral, defined, 38
antianginal agents, 35–36
antiarrhythmic agents, 32, 156
anticoagulants
  defined, 42
  listed, 33, 36
antifibrinolytic agents, 36
antihypertensive agents

  defined, 42
  listed, 36–37
  stress test, effects on, 155
anulus fibrosus, 10, 69, 76
aorta
  arch of, 42
  blood flow in, 248–251
  coarctation of
    angioplasty for, 282
    catheterization in, 314–315
    defined, 45
  defined, 5, 8, 42
  insufficiency of, 42
  stenosis of, 42
  valve of, 42
aortic sclerosis, 210
aortic stenosis. *See* stenosis, aortic
aortography, 42
apex
  defined, 42
  views of
    five-chamber, 197–198
    four-chamber, 192–197
    long axis, 197, 199
    two-chamber, 197, 199
apoplexy, 42
Apresoline (hydralazine), 32, 37
Arfonad, 37
arm, right, segmented voltage of, 87
array
  linear, 175
  phased, 175
arrhythmia
  from catheterization, 283
  defined, 42
  on ECG pattern, 127–149
  exercise-induced, 168–169
  in myocardial infarction, 21
  stress testing for, 150, 154
  supraventricular, 154

379

Index

arterial blood, 42
arterial compliance, 42
arteries. *See also* coronary artery disease
  anatomy of, 5, 14–17
  auscultation of, 338
  axillary, 16
  basilar, 43
  brachial
    anatomy of, 16
    defined, 44
  carotid, 16, 17, 44
  common iliac, 5, 16
  coronary
    anatomy of, 15–16
    angioplasty of, 281–282
    defined, 46, 114
    left, anomalous, 307
    spasm of, 21
  defined, 42
  dorsalis pedal, 16
  evaluation of, 334–349
  femoral, 16, 48
  great, 318–319
  hardening of, 42
  iliac, 49
  inferior mesenteric, 5
  innominate, 16, 49
  internal iliac, 16
  internal mammary, 16
  laboratory studies of, 339–349
  left circumflex, 16
  occlusion of, 24, 42, 334
  ophthalmic, 50
  palpation of, 338
  physical examination of, 337–338
  pulmonary, 8, 51
  radial, 16
  renal, 5
  vertebral, 16
Arteriograph, Hokanson's Ultrasonic, 329
arteriography, 358–361
arterioles, 5, 42
arteriosclerosis, 42
arteritis, temporal, 336
artifact, 278
ASD. *See* atrium, septal defect of
Ashman phenomenon, 139
asthenia, 159–160, 163–164
atenolol (Tenormin), 34, 36
atheroma, 43
atherosclerosis, 22–24, 43, 46
atria, 8, 13–14
atrial fibrillation, 135
atrial flutter, 134
atrial hypertrophy, 98–100
atrial premature contraction, 43, 127, 129
atrial pressure, 296
atrial septostomy, Rashkind balloon, 322–323

atrioventricular block, 139–141, 154
atrioventricular bundle, 43
atrioventricular dissociation, 138
atrioventricular fistulas, 334
atrioventricular node, 11, 68
atrioventricular valves, 10, 43
atrium
  defined, 43
  ectopic rhythms of, 133
  right, 13
  septal defects of, 19
    catheterization in, 282, 309–312
    Doppler evaluation of, 276–277
audio processing, 329
augmentation, 43
augmented leads, 86–87
auriculoventricular bundle, 43
auscultation, 43, 338
automaticity, cellular, 76–77
autonomic nervous system, 43
AVR, 87
axillary artery, 16
axis
  celiac, 5
  QRS, 94–95

Bachmann's bundle, 68
back pressure, 43
bacterial endocarditis, 43, 224–225
barbituate, 43
Barlow's syndrome, 210–214
basilar artery, 43
basilic veins, 16
beats, escape, 130–132
benzothiadiazine, 43
beta-adrenergic blockers, 34, 35
beta-adrenergic receptor stimulators, 35
beta blockers, 155
beta-lipoproteins, 23
bicuspid valve. *See* valve, mitral
bidirectional Doppler, 327
bifurcation, 43
bilateral, defined, 43
biopsy, 281
bipolar leads, 86
Blocadren (timolol), 34, 36
block
  atrioventruicular, 139–141, 154
  defined, 48
  left anterior fascicular, 110–111
  left bundle branch
    on ECG, 106–109
    on echocardiography, 229
    on stress test, 158
  left posterior fascicular, 110–113
    ST abnormalities of, 168
  right bundle branch
    on ECG, 103–106, 113, 118, 121

    ST abnormalities of, 165, 167
    stress testing and, 154
  sinoatrial, 142
blockers
  beta-adrenergic, 33–34
  calcium channel, 33
blood
  arterial, 42
  flow of
    aortic, 248–251
    mitral, 246–247
    pulmonic, 252–253
    tricuspid, 254–258
  venous, 52
blood pressure. *See also* hypertension; hypotension
  defined, 43
  in terminating stress testing, 154
blue babies, 43–44
B-mode imaging, 332–333
body systems, 40–41
brachial artery, 16, 44
brachiocephalic branches, 5
bradycardia
  defined, 44
  sinus, 128, 130
  in terminating stress testing, 154
branches
  brachiocephalic, 5
  bundle, 69
bretylium (Bretylol), 32, 36
Bruce protocol, 151–153
bruit, 44
Buerger's disease, 336
bundle
  atrioventricular, 43
  auriculoventricular, 43
  Bachmann's, 68
  of His
    anatomy of, 11, 69
    defined, 43
    electrical impulses of, 91
  Kent's, 69
bundle branches, 69
bypass grafting, 150

CAD. *See* coronary artery disease
Calan (verapamil), 33, 36
Calciparine, 36
calcium antagonists, 36, 155
calcium channel blockers, 33
calculations, catheterization, 298–299
calibration markers, 278
capillaries
  anatomy of, 5, 14–17
  defined, 44
Capoten, 37
cardiac afterload reducers, 37

Index

cardiac arrhythmia. *See* arrhythmia
cardiac biopsy, 281
cardiac catheterization. *See* catheterization
cardiac cycle, 44
cardiac enlargement, 154
cardiac glycosides, 37
cardiac index, 301
cardiac muscle, 10
cardiac output
   defined, 29, 44
   measurement of, 300–304
   stroke volume and, 146
cardiac preload reducers, 37
cardiac rehabilitation, 150
Cardilate, 36
cardiomyopathy
   congestive, 26, 233–235
   constrictive, 27
cardiovascular, defined, 44
cardiovascular accidents, 45
cardiovascular-renal disease, 44
carditis, 44
Cardizem (diltiazem), 33, 36
carotid arteries, 16, 17, 44
carotid body, 44
carotid phonoangiography, 357
carotid sinus, 44
Catapres, 37
catheterization
   anatomy in, 283–287
   calculations in, 298–299
   defined, 44
   diseases confirmed by, 305–319
   laboratory instrumentation in, 292–296
   placement in, 287–288
   Swan-Ganz, 281, 321–322
   technical aspects of, 287–304
   uses of
      diagnostic, 281
      invasive, 282–283
      therapeutic, 281–282, 319–322
catheters
   defined, 44
   flow-directed, 288
   placement of, 287–288
   uses of, 288–292
cauterization, 44
Cedilanid-D, 37
celiac axis, 5
cells
   anatomy of, 69–84
   contractile, 69–74
   electrophysiologic properties of, 76–84
   P, 74, 82–83
   Purkinje's
      action potential of, 83–84
      anatomy of, 75
central, defined, 38

central alpha$_2$-adrenergic agonists, 37
central venous pressure, 45
cephalic veins, 16
cerebral "drains," 17
cerebral vascular accident, 45
cerebrovascular evaluation
   documentation in, 349–352
   laboratory studies in, 354–361
   physical examination in, 353–354
chemicals, 75–76
chemotherapy, 45
cholesterol, 45
chordae tendineae
   anatomy of, 10
   defined, 45
   ruptured, 235–236
chronic arterial occlusive disease, 334
chronotopic reserve, 146
circle of Willis
   anatomy of, 17
   arterial flow in, 355
   defined, 45
circulation
   collateral, 45
   extracorporeal, 47–48
   pulmonary, 51, 283–285
   renal, 51
   systemic, 52, 283
circulatory, defined, 45
claudication, 45, 334
clots, 233
coagulation, 45
coarctation, aortic. *See* aorta, coarctation of
collagen, 21
collateral circulation, 45
commissurotomy, 45
common iliac artery, 5, 16
compensation, 45
complete atrioventricular block, 140–141
complex, QRS, 91–92
compliance, arterial, 42
conduction
   cellular, 75
   heart, 67–69
   intraventricular, 103–113
congenitally corrected transposition, 319
congestive cardiomyopathy, 26, 233–235
congestive heart failure. *See* heart, congestive failure of
constriction, 45
constrictive cardiomyopathy, 27
constrictive pericarditis, 46
continuous wave Doppler, 243, 326
contractile cells, 69–74
contractile proteins, 46
contractility, 29

contractions, premature, 127–130
contralateral, defined, 46
controls, echoscape, 173–174
conus branch, 15
Corgard, 35–36, 155
coronary artery disease
   catheterization in, 305–307
   risk factors in, 149
   stress testing for, 150
coronary atherosclerosis, 46
coronary care units, 64
coronary occlusion, 46
coronary sinus, 8, 10
coronary sulcus, 13
coronary thrombosis, 46
cor pulmonale, 46
Coumadin, 33, 36
coumarin, 46
coupling gel, 174
CPA. *See* carotid phonoangiography
cross-bridges, 84
cross-sectional echocardiography. *See* echocardiography, two-dimensional
Crystodigin, 37
cuffs, pneumatic, 343
cusps, 10

death from catheterization, 283
decompensation, 46
deep venous thrombosis, 364
defibrillator, 46, 296
depolarization, 89
depression
   J-point, 160
   ST, 160–162
detectors, signal, 329
dextrocardia, 46, 125–126
diabetes mellitus, 149, 154
diagnosis
   arterial, 334–349
   catheterization in, 281
   cerebrovascular, 349–361
diastole, 46
dibenzyline, 34
diffuse hypokinesia, 235
diffusion, 4
digestive system, 40
digitalis
   cardiac glycoside, 37
   defined, 46
   on ECG pattern, 121
   stress testing and, 153, 155–156, 158
Dilantin (phenytoin), 32
dilatation, 309
dilation, 46
Dilatrate ST, 36
diltiazem (Herebessor), 33, 156
diphasic waves, 92

382 Index

direct cerebrovascular testing, 357–361
directional Doppler, 327
disease
  Buerger's, 336
  Takayasu's, 336
disks, intercalated, 70
disopyramide (Norpace), 32, 36
display, spectral, 239
dissecting aneurysm, 153
dissociation, atrioventricular, 138
distal, defined, 38, 47
diuresis, 46
diuretics, 46, 155
documentation
  arterial, 334–337
  cerebrovascular, 349–352
  venous, 362–364
Doppler echocardiography. *See* echocardiography, Doppler
Doppler frequency shift, 239
Doppler probe, 296
Doppler ultrasound
  noninvasive, 325–329
  venous, 364–370
Doppler wave forms, 345–346
dorsal pedal artery, 16
dorsum, 47
downsloping ST depression, 160–161
"drains," cerebral, 17
drugs
  antianginal, 35–36, 155
  antiarrhythmic, 32, 156
  anticoagulant, 33, 36, 42
  antihypertensive, 36–37, 42, 155
  for stress testing, 154–155
D-TGA. *See* transposition of the great arteries
D-to-E slope, 208
ductless glands, 41
ductus arteriosus
  anatomy of, 19–20
  defined, 47
  patent, 315–316
ductus venosus, 17
duplex scanning
  arterial, 349
  in plethysmography, 332–333
  venous, 373–375
DVT. *See* deep venous thrombosis
dynes, 299
dysfunction, 47
dyskinetic area, 225
dyspnea, 47, 154

echocardiography
  cross-sectional, 171–172
  disease states on, 209–238
  Doppler
    examination by, 244–273
    gradients in, 271–272
    other uses of, 278
    terminology of, 278–279
    velocities in, 278
  machine control in, 172–174
  m-mode, 171, 175–187
    derivation of, from two-dimensional, 201–206
    left ventricular, 205–208
    measurement in, 207–209
    tricuspid valve, 205
  real-time, 171–175
  two-dimensional, 171–172, 188–201
Echoflow Doppler signal detector, 329
echoscape controls, 173–174
ectropy, 154
edema, 47
effusions, pericardial, 227–228
electrical accidents, 57–61
electric cardiac pacemaker, 47
electricity
  basic, 54–56
  in myocardial stimulation, 76
  precautions in, 62–64
  shock from, 56–61
electrocardiograms, resting, 148
electrocardiography
  configuration, 12-lead in, 95
  defined, 47, 86
  electrical conduction in, 89–92
  graph paper in, 92–113
  heart rate determination in, 93–94
  infarctions on, 116–121
  injury on, 114
  ischemia on, 114
  leads for, 86–87
  measurements in, 92–113
  miscellaneous patterns on, 121–126
  sinus rhythms on, 127–143
electrodes, 147
electrolyte, 47
electronic real-time echocardiography, 174–175
electrophysiology, 69–84
embolism, 47, 153
endoarterium, 47
endocarditis
  bacterial, 43, 224–225
  defined, 47
endocardium, 10, 47
endocrine system, 41
endothelium, 47
end systolic volume, 29
enlargement, cardiac, 154
enzyme, 47
epicardium, 10, 47

epidemiology, 47
epinephrine (Adrenalin), 35, 47
equipment, stress testing, 146–147
erythrocyte, 47
escape beats, 130–132
escape rhythms, 130–132
essential hypertension, 47
etiology, 47
E-to-F slope, 208
eustachian valve, 10
examination, physical. *See* physical examination
excessive medications, 153
excitability, myocardial, 75–79
excitation-contraction coupling, 84–85
exercise-induced arrhythmias, 168–169
exercise physiology, 145–146
exercise testing. *See* testing, stress
external, defined, 38
external iliac artery, 16
external saphenous vein, 16
extracorporeal circulation, 47–48
extrasystole, 48, 127, 129

failure
  monitoring, 154
  myocardial, 27–30
false-negative rate, 48
false-positive patients, 151
false-positive rate, 48
family history, 149
fascicles, 11, 69
fatigue, 154
femoral artery, 16, 48
fever
  rheumatic, 25–26, 51
  stress testing in, 153
fibers, Purkinje's, 11, 51
fibrillation
  atrial, 135
  defined, 48
  ventricular, 138
fibrin, 48
fibrinogen, 48
fibrinolysin, 48
fibrinolytic, 48
fibrosis, valvular, 25
fibrotic ring, 10
fibrous ligamentus arteriosus, 20
fibrous tissue, 10
Fick principle, 301
filaments
  actin, 71
  myosin, 71
first-degree atrioventricular block, 139–140
fistula, 48, 334

five-chamber apical view, 197-198
flail mitral valve leaflet, 235-236
flecainide, 156
flow
  antegrade, 41
  pulmonary, 298-299
  systemic, 298-299
flow-directed catheters, 288
fluid transport, 4-5
fluoroscopy, 48
flutter
  atrial, 134
  ventricular, 136-137
foramen ovale
  anatomy of, 8, 17
  defined, 48
  patent, 19
force, shear, 23
four-chamber view
  apical, 192-197
  subcostal, 197, 200
frequency shift, 239, 326
functional anatomy, 8-11

gain, overall, 174
gallop rhythm, 48
gangrene, 48
gel
  acoustic, 357
  coupling, 174
genetics, 48
geographic anatomy, 12-14
glands, ductless, 41
glycosides, cardiac, 37
gradients, 271-272
graft, 48
grafting, bypass, 150
grating, range, 243
great arteries, transposition of, 318-319
great vessels, 8

HDL. See high-density lipoproteins
heart
  anatomy of, 8-14
  congestive failure of, 27-30, 45, 153
  electrical conduction in, 67-69, 89-92
  rates of, 93-94
  regional vascularization, 14-17
heart attack, 20-21
hemangioma, 48
hemiblock, left anterior, 110-111. See also block
hemiparesis, 48
hemodynamics, 48
hemoglobin, 48

hemorrhage
  agents in, 36
  from catheterization, 282
  defined, 48
heparin, 33, 49
Herebessor, 33, 156
hertz, 278
hexaxial reference system, 94-96
high blood pressure. See hypertension
high-density lipoproteins (HDL), 23-24
high-grade atrioventricular block, 140-141
His, bundle of. See bundle of His
history, for stress testing, 148-149
Hokanson's Ultrasonic Arteriograph, 329
horizontal, defined, 39
horizontal ST depression, 160
hospital, electric shock in, 57-61
hydralazine (Apresoline), 32, 37
Hylorel, 37
hypercalcemia, 125-126
hyperemia testing, reactive, 347-349
hyperkalemia, 121, 124
hyperkinetic area, 225
hyperlipoproteinemia, as risk factor, 149
hyperplasia, muscular, 23
Hyperstat I.V., 37
hypertension
  in coronary artery disease, 23
  essential, 47
  malignant, 49
  as risk factor, 149
  secondary, 51
  stress testing in, 154
hypertrophic subaortic stenosis, idiopathic. See idiopathic-hypertrophic subaortic stenosis
hypertrophy
  atrial, 98-100
  in cardiomyopathy, 26
  defined, 49
  ventricular, 101-103, 158
hyperventilation, 159-160
hypocalcemia, 125, 158
hypokalemia, 121, 124
hypokinesis, diffuse, 235
hypokinetic area, 225
hypotension, 49
hypothermia, 49
hypovolemia, 49
hypoxia, 49

idiopathic hypertrophic subaortic stenosis. See stenosis, idiopathic hypertrophic subaortic

iliac artery, 49
imaging, 329, 332-333
impedance plethysmography, 49, 330-331
incompetent valve, 49
Inderal (propranolol), 34, 35, 36
  stress test, effects on, 155
Inderal-LA, 36
index
  ankle/arm, 41
  ankle/brachial, 343
  cardiac, 301
  pulmonic, 298
indirect cerebrovascular testing, 354-357
infarct, 49
infarction
  from catheterization, 282
  defined, 114
  myocardial, 20-21, 49
  stress testing for, 150, 153
  varieties of
    anterior, 117-120
    inferior, 116-121
    lateral, 116, 118
    posterior, 119
infection from catheterization, 282
infectious disease, stress testing in, 153
infective endocarditis, 43, 224-225
inferior, defined, 38
inferior infarction, 116-121
inferior mesenteric artery, 5
inferior vena cava, 5, 8
injectors, pressure, 292
injury
  acute myocardial, 154
  defined, 114
innominate artery, 16, 49
inotropic reserve, 146
instrumentation, catheterization, 292-296
insufficiency
  aortic
    Doppler view of, 259-266
    on echocardiography, 220-221
  mitral, 49, 307
  myocardial, 50
  pulmonic, 259-266
  valvular, 307
intensive care units, 64
intercalated disks, 70
internal, defined, 38
internal iliac artery, 16
internal mammary artery, 16
internal saphenous vein, 16
internodal pathways, 11, 68
intervals
  PR, 93
  QRS, 93
interventricular septum, 49

interview, patient, 147–148
intima, 49
intracardiac pressures, 285–286
intraventricular conduction, 103–113
intraventricular septum, 229–230
involuntary nervous system, 43
ions, 79–82
Iponeratril (verapamil), 33
ipsilateral, defined, 49
ischemia, 49, 114
ischemic neurologic deficit, reversible, 350
Ismelin, 37
isoelectric line, 92
isoproterenol (Isuprel), 35
Isoptin (verapamil), 33, 36
Isordil (isosorbide dinitrate), 31, 36
isosorbide dinitrate (Isordil), 31, 36
Isuprel (isoproterenol), 35

jet effect dilatation, 309
J-point depression, 160
jugular veins, 17, 49
junctional premature contraction, 130
junctional rhythms, 135–136

Kabinase, 36
Kawasaki's syndrome, 22
Kent's bundle, 69

laboratory studies
  arterial, 339–349
  venous, 364–375
Lanoxicaps, 37
Lanoxin, 37
lateral, defined, 38
lateral infarction, 116, 118
LDL. See low-density lipoproteins
leads
  augmented, 86–87
  bipolar, 86
  precordial, 87–89
  standard, 86
  stress test, 146–147
  unipolar, 86–87
left anterior fascicular block, 110–111
left bundle branch block. See block, left bundle branch
left circumflex artery, 16
left coronary artery, 15–16
left main disease, 154
left posterior fascicular block, 110–113

left-to-right shunting, 287
left ventricle. See ventricle, left
leukocytes, polymorphonuclear, 21
Levarterenol (norepinephrine), 35
Levophed (norepinephrine), 35
lidocaine, 32
line, isoelectric, 92
lipid, 49
lipoproteins
  defined, 49
  high density, 23–24
  low density, 23
long-axis view
  apical, 197, 199
  parasternal, 188
Loniten, 37
Lopressor (metoprolol), 34, 36, 155
low blood pressure, 49
low-density lipoproteins (LDL), 23
L-TGA. See congenitally corrected transposition
lumen, 49

macroshock, 56, 57–58
malignant hypertension, 49
markers, calibration, 278
maximal stress testing, 151–153
measurement
  m-mode echocardiographic, 207–209
  ST segment, 93
mechanical excitability, myocardial, 76
mechanical real-time echocardiography, 174–175
medial, defined, 38
medications, excessive, 153
MET, 145
metabolic disease, 154
metabolism, 49
methoxamine (Vasoxyl), 35
metoprolol (Lopressor), 34, 36
mexiletine (Mexitil), 32
microshock, 56–57
midsagittal, defined, 39
Minipress (prazosin), 32, 34, 37
  stress test, effects on, 155
mitochondria, 72
mitral blood flow, 246–247
mitral insufficiency. See insufficiency, mitral
mitral regurgitation. See regurgitation, mitral
mitral stenosis, 49, 230–232
mitral valve. See valve, mitral
mitral valvulotomy, 50
m-mode echocardiography. See echocardiography, m-mode
Mobitz block, 140–142

monitoring
  failure of, 154
  oxygen consumption, 295–296
motion, paradoxical septal, 229–230
multifocal atrial tachycardia, 133–134
multifocal extrasystoles, 127
murmur, 50
muscles
  cardiac, 10
  papillary, 8, 10
muscular hyperplasia, 23
muscular system, 40
myocardial failure, 27–30
myocardial infarction. See infarction, myocardial
myocardial injury, 154
myocardial insufficiency. See insufficiency, myocardial
myocardial perfusion, 169–170
myocarditis, 50, 153
myocardium, 10, 50
myofibrils, 70–71
myosin filaments, 71

Naughton protocol, 152
neargain, 174
negative predictive value, 361
Neosynephrine (phenylephrine), 35
nervous system
  autonomic, 43
  defined, 41
  involuntary, 43
  parasympathetic, 50
  sympathetic, 51
neurologic deficit, reversible ischemic, 350
nifedipine (Procardia), 33, 36
Nipride (sodium nitroprusside), 31, 37
nitrates, 36
nitrites, 50
Nitro-Bid, 36, 37
Nitrodisc, 36
Nitro-Dur, 36
nitroglycerin, 31, 155
Nitrol Ointment, 36
Nitrostat, 36, 37
nodes
  atrioventricular, 11, 68
  sinoatrial, 11, 67–68
nonconducted atrial premature contraction, 127, 129
nondirectional Doppler, 327
noninvasive peripheral vascular testing, 325–333
norepinephrine (Levarterenol), 35
Norpace (disopyramide), 32, 36, 156

obesity, 149
occlusion
  arterial, 24
  coronary, 46
  defined, 50
ocular plesthymography, 356–357
Ointment, Nitrol, 36
operating room, 63–64
OPG. *See* ocular plesthymography
ophthalmic artery, 50
organic heart disease, 50
ostium primum, 310
ostium secundum, 310
output, cardiac, 29, 44
ovale, foramen. *See* foramen ovale
overall gain, 174
oximeter, 295
oxygen capacity, 300
oxygen consumption, 295–296, 300
oxygen saturation, 286–287, 301
oxygen step-up, 287
oxyhemoglobin, 48

pacemaker
  defined, 50
  electrical, 89
palpation
  arterial, 338
  defined, 50
palpitation, 50
pancarditis, 50
Panwarfin, 36
paper speed, in echocardiography, 174
papillary muscles
  anatomy of, 8
  defined, 50
paradoxical septal motion, 229–230
parasternal views
  long-axis, 188
  short-axis, 188–192
parasternal short-axis view, 188–192
parasympathetic nervous system, defined, 50
parietal, defined, 38
parietal pericardium, 50
paroxysmal tachycardia
  atrial, 133
  defined, 50
patency, 50
patent *ductus arteriosus*, 315–316
patent foramen ovale, 19
pathways, internodal, 11, 68
patients
  in stress testing
    interviewing, 147–148
    selection of, 153–154
P cells
  action potential of, 82–83

anatomy of, 74
PDA. *See* patent *ductus arteriosus*
pectoris, angina. *See* angina pectoris
percutaneous Seldinger catheterization, 287–288
perfusion, 27–28, 169–170
pericardial effusions, 227–228
pericarditis
  constrictive, 46
  defined, 50
  on ECG pattern, 121, 123
pericardium
  anatomy of, 13
  parietal, 50
periorbital Doppler, 354–356
peripheral, defined, 38
peripheral resistance, 50
peripheral vascular testing. *See* testing, peripheral vascular
peripheral vasodilators, 37
Peritrate, 36
Persantine, 36
pharmacology, adrenergic, 34–37
phased array, 175
phenomenon, Ashmann, 139
phenylephrine (Neosynephrine), 35
phenytoin (Dilantin), 32
phlebitis, 50
phonoangiography, carotid, 357
photoelectric plethysmography, 331–332
physical examination
  arterial, 337–338
  cerebrovascular, 353–354
physiologic pressure recorder, 294
physiology
  in catheterization, 283–287
  exercise, 145–146
plasma, 50
plethysmography
  air, 330
  impedance, 49, 330–331
  ocular, 356–357
  photoelectric, 331–332
  strain gauge, 330
  venous, 370–371
  venous reflux, 371–373
  water, 331
pneumatic cuffs, 343
polyarteritis *nodosa*, 336
polymorphonuclear leukocytes. 21
popliteal artery, 16
position, echocardiographic, 174
positive predictive value, 360–361
posterior/dorsal, defined, 38
posterior fascicle, 69
poststenotic dilatation, 309
postural changes, 159–160
potential, action, 77–84
prazosin. *See* Minipress

precordial leads, 87–89
predictive values, 360–361
prefixes, 39–40
preload, 29
premature contractions, 127–130
pressor, 51
pressure
  atrial, 296
  back, 43
  blood, 43
  central venous, 45
  intracardiac, 285–286
  physiologic recording of, 294
  segmental limb, 340–345
  venous, 296
  wedge, 296
pressure injectors, 292
pressure wave forms, 296–297
primary hypertension. *See* hypertension
principle, Fick, 301
PR interval, 93
probe, Doppler, 296
procainamide, 32, 156
Procan SR, 36
Procardia (nifedipine), 33, 36
processing, audio, 329
prolapse, mitral valve, 210–214
Pronestyl, 36
propranolol (Inderal), 34, 35, 36
proteins, contractile, 46
protocols, stress testing, 151–153
proximal, defined, 38
pseudoclaudication, 334
psychotropic drugs, 153
pulmonary artery, 8, 51
pulmonary circulation, 51
pulmonary flow, 298–299
pulmonary hypertension, 154
pulmonary resistance, 299
pulmonary to systemic flow ratio, 298–299
pulmonary valve, 51
pulmonary veins, 8, 51
pulmonic flow, 252–253
pulmonic index, 298
pulmonic stenosis, 269–271, 282
pulmonic valve, 205
pulsatility, 369–370
pulse, 51
pulsed Doppler, 326
pulsed repetition frequency Doppler, 243
pulsed repetition rate, 278
pulse pressure, 51
Pulse Volume Recorder, 330, 340
pulse wave Doppler. 243
Purkinje's cells, 75, 83–84
Purkinje's fibers, 11, 51
Purodigin, 37

QRS axis, 94–95
QRS complex, 91–92
QRS interval, 93
Quinaglute, 36
Quinidex, 36
quinidine
  on ECG pattern, 121, 122
  stress test, effects on, 156
  uses of, 32

radial artery, 16
radionuclide ventriculography, 170
range grating, 243
Rashkind balloon atrial septostomy, 281, 322–323
ratio, pulmonic to systemic flow, 298–299
Raynaud's syndrome, 336–337
reactive hyperemia testing, 347–349
real-time B-mode imaging, 332–333
real-time echocardiography, 172–175
receptor-stimulating drugs, 35
recorder, physiologic pressure, 294
recording, analogue, 329
reference system, hexaxial, 94–96
refractory period, 77, 79
regional vascularization, 14–17
regitine, 34
regurgitation
  defined, 51
  mitral
    Doppler view of, 259–266
    on echocardiography, 233
  tricuspid, 259–266
rehabilitation, cardiac, 150
reject, 174
renal arteries, 5
renal circulation, 51
repolarization, 89
reproductive system, 40
reserve
  chronotropic, 146
  inotropic, 146
resistance
  defined, 302
  peripheral, 50
  systemic, 299
respiration, ST depression with, 165
respiratory system, 40
resting electrocardiograms, 148
resting ST abnormalities, 158
reticulum, sarcoplasmic, 72–74
reversible ischemic neurologic deficit, 350
Reynold's syndrome, 164
rheumatic fever, 25–26, 51
rheumatic mitral stenosis, 230–232

rhythms
  atrial, 133–135
  bradycardias, sinus, 128, 130
  escape, 130–132
  extrasystoles, 127, 129
  gallop, 48
  junctional, 135–136
  premature contractions, 127–130
  tachycardias
    multifocal atrial, 133–134
    paroxysmal, 133
    sinus, 128
  ventricular, 136–139
  WPW syndrome, 143
right atrium, 13
right bundle branch block. See block, right bundle branch
right coronary artery. See arteries, coronary
right ventricle. See ventricle, right
RIND. See reversible ischemic neurologic deficit
ring, fibrotic, 10
risk factors, for coronary artery disease, 149
roots, 39

SA node, 11
sacromere, 70, 71–72
saphenous vein, external, 16
sarcolemma, 70
sarcoplasmic reticulum, 72–74
sarcosomes, 72
saturation, oxygen, 286–287, 301
scanning, duplex. See duplex scanning
sclerosis
  aortic, 210
  defined, 51
secondary hypertension, 51
second degree block, 139–142
segment, ST. See ST segment
segmental limb pressures, 340–345
Seldinger catheterization, percutaneous, 287–288
selection, patient, in stress testing, 153–154
semilunar valves, 10
sensitivity
  in stress testing, 151
  in ultrasonic arteriography, 3360
sensory system, 41
septal motion, paradoxical, 229–230
septostomy, Rashkind balloon atrial, 281, 322–323
Serpasil, 37
shear force, 23
shift, frequency, 239, 326
shock, electrical, 57–61

short-axis view, parasternal, 188–192
shunt
  defined, 51
  left-to-right, 287
signal detectors, 329
sinoatrial node, 11, 67–68
sinus bradycardia, 128, 130
sinuses
  carotid, 44
  coronary, 8, 10
  Valsalva, 10, 51
sinus node, 67–68
sinus tachycardia, 128
skeletal system, 40
slope, echocardiographic, 208
slow channel blockers, 33
smoking, 149
sodium nitroprusside (Nipride), 31, 37
Sone's catheterization, 288
Sorbitrate, 36
specialized conductive tissue, 10–11
specificity, 151, 360
spectral analysis, 329, 357–358
  carotid Doppler with, 357–358
  in Doppler ultrasound, 329
spectral display, 239
speed, paper, in echocardiography, 174
spontaneity, venous flow, 369
ST abnormalities, resting, 158
standard leads, 86
stenosis
  aortic
    defined, 42
    on echocardiography, 216–219
    stress testing in, 153, 154, 158
    Doppler evaluation of, 269–271
    idiopathic hypertrophic subaortic, 221–224
  mitral, 49, 230–232
  pulmonic, 269–271, 282
  subaortic, 26–27
  tricuspid, 269–271
  valvular, 25, 307–309
step-up, oxygen, 287
stethoscope, 51
Stokes-Adams Syndrome, 51
strain gauge plethysmography, 330
Streptase, 36
streptokinase, 33, 320
stress testing. See testing, stress
stroke, 42, 45, 283
stroke volume
  cardiac output and, 146
  defined, 51
  in heart failure, 29
ST segment
  abnormalities of, 165–166

defined, 91
depression of
　downsloping, 160–161
　horizontal, 160
　measurement of, 93
　with respiration, 165
　upsloping, 160
　in women, 162
elevation of, 165–166
measurement of, 93
subaortic stenosis, 26–27
subcostal four-chamber view, 197, 200
subclavian artery, 16
submaximal stress testing, 151–153
subxiphoid view, 197, 200
suffixes, 40
sulcus, anterior interventricular, 13
superior, defined, 38
superior mesenteric artery, 5
superior venae cavae, 5, 8
supersternal view, 197–201
supraventricular arrhythmia, 154
Swan-Ganz catheterization, 281, 321–322
sympathetic nervous system, 51
sympatholytics, 37
syncope, 52
syndrome(s)
　Barlow's, 210–214
　Raynaud's, 336–337
　Reynold's, 164
　thoracic outlet, 336
　WPW, 143, 158
　X, 165
systemic circulation, 52
systemic flow, 298–299
systemic hypertension, 154
systemic resistance, 299
systems
　endocrine, 41
　muscular, 40
　reproductive, 40
　respiratory, 40
　sensory, 51
　urinary, 40
systole, 52
systolic volume, end, 29

tachyarrhythmias, 21
tachycardia
　defined, 52
　junctional, 135–136
　paroxysmal, 50, 133, 168
　sinus, 128
　ventricular
　　exercise-induced, 169
　　in sinus rhythm, 136–137
　　stress testing in, 153, 154

Takayasu's disease, 336
technetium 99m, 169
temporal arteritis, 336
Tenormin (atenolol), 34, 36, 155
terminology, 39–40
testing
　peripheral vascular
　　arterial, 334–349
　　cerebrovascular, 349–351
　　noninvasive, 325–333
　　reactive hyperemia, 347–349
　stress
　　contraindications to, 153–154
　　goals of, 144–145
　　indications for, 148–151
　　interpretation of, 156–159
　　maximal, 151–153
　　medications for, 154–155
　　patient interview in, 147–148
　　patient selection in, 153–154
　　protocols for, 151–153
　　submaximal, 151–153
　　termination of, 154
　　thallium, 158, 169–170
　　treadmill, 346–347
tests, Allen, 41
tetralogy of Fallot, 52, 316–318
thallium stress testing, 158, 169–170
thebesian valve, 10
thermodilution, 301–302
thoracic outlet syndrome, 336
thrombogenesis, 24
thrombolytic agents, 33, 36
thrombophlebitis, 153
thrombosis
　coronary, 46
　deep venous, 364
thrombus, 52
time gain-compensation, 174
timolol (Blocadren), 34, 36
tissue
　fibrous, 10
　specialized conductive, 10–11
tocainide, 32
Tonocard, 36
trabeculae, 8
transcutaneous, defined, 52
transcutaneous pO_2 monitor, 296
Transderm-Nitro, 36
transducer, 52, 172–174
transient ischemic attack, 52
transitional cells, 75, 83–84
transport, fluid, 4–5
transposition of the great arteries, 318–319
transverse, 39
treadmill testing, 346–347
Trental, 36
tricuspid flow, 254–258
tricuspid stenosis, 269–271

tricuspid valve. See valve, tricuspid
Tridil, 36, 37
troponin-tropomyosin, 84–85
true claudication, 334
true-positive patients, 151
T wave, 93, 168
twelve-lead ECG configurations, 95
two-chamber apical view, 197, 198
two-dimensional echocardiography, 171–172, 188–201

ulnar artery, 16
Ultrasonic Arteriograph, Hokanson's, 329
ultrasonic arteriography, 358–361
ultrasound, Doppler. See Doppler ultrasound
unidirectional Doppler, 327
unifocal extrasystoles, 127
unipolar leads, 86–87
upsloping ST segments, 160
urinary system, 40
U waves, 168

Valsalva, sinuses of, 10, 51
valves
　anatomy of, 10
　atrioventricular
　　anatomy of, 10
　　defined, 43
　bicuspid aortic, 214–215
　disorders of, 25–26
　eustachian, 10
　insufficiency of, 49
　mitral
　　anatomy of, 10
　　defined, 49
　　flail leaflet of, 235–236
　　m-mode views of, 201–205
　　prolapse of, 25
　　on echocardiography, 210–214
　pulmonic, 205
　stenosis of, 25, 307–309
　surgery on, 229
　thesbian, 10
　tricuspid
　　anatomy of, 10
　　defined, 52
　　m-mode view of, 205
valvuloplasty, 282, 321
vascularization, regional, 14–17
vasculitis, 336
vasoconstrictor, 41, 52
vasodilators, 31, 37, 52
　stress test, effects on, 155
vasoinhibitor, 52

vasopressor substance, 41, 47
vasoregulatory asthenia, 159–160, 163–164
Vasoxyl (methoxamine), 35
vectorcardiography, 52
vegetations, 26
  bacterial, 43, 224–225
veins
  anatomy of, 5, 14–17
  basilic, 16
  cephalic, 16
  deep thrombosis of, 364
  defined, 52
  evaluation of, 362–375
  flow characteristics of, 369–370
  jugular, 17, 49
  laboratory testing of, 364–375
  physical examination of, 362–364
  saphenous, external, 16
velocity, Doppler, 278
vena cava, 52
venous blood, 52
venous pressure, 296
venous valves, 10
ventricles
  anatomy of, 8, 13
  left
    anatomy of, 13
    clots of, 233
    dysfunction of, 225–226
  m-mode view of, 205–208
  right, volume overload in, 229
  septal defects of
    catheterization in, 312–314
    Doppler evaluation of, 272–275
ventricular aneurysm, 154
ventricular arrhythmia, exercise-induced, 168
ventricular ectopy, 154
ventricular hypertrophy, 101–103
ventricular premature contraction, 130
ventricular rhythms, 136–139
ventricular septum, 19, 49
ventricular tachycardia. *See* tachycardia, ventricular
ventriculography, radionuclide, 170
venule, 52
verapamil (Isoptin), 33, 36, 156
vertebral artery, 16
very low-density lipoproteins (VLDL), 24
vessels
  damage to, from catheterization, 282
  great, 8
visceral, defined, 39
Visken, 36
VLDL. *See* very low-density lipoproteins

volume plethysmography, 370–371
VSD. *See* ventricles, septal defects of

water plethysmography, 331
wave forms
  Doppler, 345–346
  pressure, 296–297
waves
  diphasic, 92
  T, inversion of, 168
  U, 168
wedge pressure, 296
Wenckebach block, 139–142
Willis, circle of. *See* circle of Willis
Wolff-Parkinson-White syndrome
  rhythm of, 143
  ST abnormalities of, 168
  on stress test, 158
WPW syndrome. *See* Wolff-Parkinson-White syndrome
Wytensin, 37

X, syndrome, 165
xylocaine, 36

zero-shifting, 279